LifeSpan-Plus

LifeSpan-Plus

900 NATURAL TECHNIQUES TO LIVE LONGER

By the Editors of

PREVENTION

Magazine

Rodale Press, Emmaus, Pennsylvania

If you have any questions or comments concerning this book, please write:

Rodale Press
Book Reader Service
33 East Minor Street
Emmaus, PA 18098

Library of Congress Cataloging-in-Publication Data

LifeSpan-plus : 900 natural techniques to live longer / by the editors of Prevention magazine.
    p.   cm.
  ISBN 0–87857–908–7 hardcover
  1. Health. 2. Longevity. I. Tkac, Debora. II. Faelten, Sharon.
III. Michaud, Ellen. IV. Prevention (Emmaus, Pa.) V. Title: LifeSpan-plus.
RA776.L732   1990
613—dc20   90–35849
                                         CIP

Distributed in the book trade by St. Martin's Press

2 4 6 8 10 9 7 5 3 1   hardcover

Notice

This book is intended as a reference volume only, not as a medical guide or manual for self-treatment. If you suspect that you have a medical problem, please seek competent medical care. The information here is designed to help you make informed decisions about your health. It is not intended as a substitute for any treatment prescribed by your doctor.

Editor: Debora Tkac

Compiled and written by: Don Barone and Sharon Faelten

Project research assistant: Dawn Horvath

Research and fact-checking staff: *Research Chief,* Ann Gossy; *Senior Research Associates,* Staci Hadeed, Karen Lombardi; *Research Associates,* Anna Crawford, Christine Dreisbach

Production editor: Jane Sherman

Copy editor: Sally Roth

Cover and interior design: Jerry O'Brien

Office staff: *Office Manager,* Roberta Mulliner; Karen Earl-Braymer, Eve Buchay

Publisher: Pat Corpora

Editor in chief: William Gottlieb

Executive editor, *Prevention* Magazine Health Books: Carol Keough

CONTENTS

THE
GIFT
OF MORE
LIFE

Nine out of ten deaths in America are caused by people killing themselves. The other cause of death is suicide.

Yes, I'm exaggerating—but only a little. Fact is, many people in the United States *do* kill themselves. They don't use six-guns, they use six-packs. They don't drown in rivers, they drown in fat. They don't take a sleeping pill, they take a puff. Here's how the scientists put it:

"Nine of the ten leading causes of [early death] in the United States are linked to one or more of six behaviors: cigarette smoking, misuse of alcohol, lack of exercise, not wearing seat belts, overeating, and failure to control high blood pressure."

That quote is from a report in the *New York State Journal of Medicine.* It's one of the many medical reports we used in writing *Life-Span-Plus*—reports that started appearing a few years back and gave us the idea for this book. They show—remarkably—that *you* have the power to extend your life. All you have to do is emphasize specific healthy actions and reduce or eliminate unhealthy ones.

And *LifeSpan-Plus* is perhaps the best tool ever produced to help you do just that.

We've compiled 900 specific, practical, how-to tips to live a healthier, happier, longer life. Tips to keep every part of you strong and vital—your heart, your immune system, your bones, your brain. As you browse through the book and choose the best tips for you, think of each one of them as a postcard of positivity and encouragement from your friends at *Prevention* magazine and Rodale Books. We write these books so it will be easier for you to change your life for the better. And we hope this book fulfills that purpose—to give yourself the greatest change for the better: better health, and the years to enjoy it.

Yours for personal empowerment,

Bill Gottlieb

Bill Gottlieb
Editor in Chief, Rodale Books

C H A P T E R · 1

101 FOODS TO HELP YOU LIVE LONGER

The human body was built to last roughly 120 years—but it never seems to make it. It never seems to make it because, to a large extent, we lose a little time every time we sit down to eat.

How? By what we put in our mouths. We eat too many calories, too much cholesterol, too much fat, and too little fiber. We eat too many additives, too much salt, too much junk, and too few vitamins and minerals. The result is that three out of every four of us—that's 75 percent—will die of heart disease, high blood pressure, stroke, cancer, diabetes, kidney failure, or complications arising from osteoporosis. Rather than living to 120, many of us will be lucky if we make it halfway.

Study after study reveals that what we do or do not eat condemns us to an early grave. Too much cholesterol and saturated fat? Congratulations—that deadly duo can cause atherosclerosis, the artery-clogging disease that sets the stage for heart attacks and strokes. Too many calories? Step right up—overweight is the single biggest risk factor for diabetes. Too little fiber, not enough calcium? You qualify—that just about doubles your risk of colon cancer.

The list goes on and on. Yet the truth is that we can help prevent almost *one-third* of the premature deaths caused by these diseases simply by changing the way we eat.

The Right Stuff

We can load up on fruits that are rich in potassium, the potent nutrient that can help prevent strokes and reduce blood pressure. We can load up on vegetables that are bursting with carotene, the plant form of vitamin A that can help prevent cancer. We can load up on grains that contain a bushel of fiber, the substance that reduces the likelihood of colon cancer and obesity. We can load up on fish that are high in omega–3's, the fatty acids that have been linked to a reduced risk of heart disease. And we can load up on low-fat dairy products that are rich in calcium, the mineral that keeps bones strong and can help bring blood pressure down.

All told, we can take a great step toward preventing many of the major diseases that kill us before our time by eating the right foods. So here are 101 foods that have the "right stuff"—the stuff that will help us live long, productive, and vibrant lives.

Foods for a Longer Life

1. Apples

Apples are one of the best sources of pectin, a soluble fiber. It's the kind of fiber that helps prevent heart disease and stroke by keeping cholesterol levels low and also prevents wide swings in blood sugar levels, which can help keep diabetes under control. Apple pectin is also the kind of fiber that slows digestion and fills you up quickly, making it an ally in weight control. At 81 calories per apple, this fruit is definitely a shining symbol of good health.

2. Apricots

Apricots are a rich source of carotene and fiber, a cancer-busting duo. They also contain plenty of potassium, which fights high blood pressure and stroke. A handful of dried apricots—about ten halves—contains only 83 calories, making them a sweet treat for the weight watcher.

3. Artichokes

One medium artichoke contains more fiber than a bowl of oat bran—and *three times* as much as an oat muffin! That plus a pinch of calcium and good amounts of potassium and magnesium makes artichokes a valuable ally in the fight against cancer, diabetes, high blood pressure, stroke, and heart disease.

4. Asparagus

A cup of these stately spears packs a solid punch of carotene and potassium to help fight cancer and high blood pressure. And with no fat, no cholesterol, and a decent amount of fiber, asparagus also helps prevent heart disease, stroke, diabetes, and obesity, at only 44 calories a cup.

5. Avocados

A single avocado is quite possibly the most potent source of potassium you can find, making it the champion in the battle against high blood pressure. Unfortunately, its high calorie content (324 per fruit) can work against you, so consider it an occasional treat. Avocados often take a bad rap because of their high fat content. Actually, a majority of the fat is unsaturated, the type that has been found to be good for your health, mainly because of its ability to lower cholesterol.

6. Bananas

Two small bananas provide as much fiber as a slice of whole wheat bread—plus a hefty dose of blood pressure–lowering potassium. Low in fat and sodium, with a dash of vitamins A and C, bananas belong in every diet that purports to fight cancer, stroke, heart disease, diabetes, and obesity. A single banana has about 100 nutritious calories.

7. Barley

Barley comes in two forms: pearled, which has had its entire outer husk removed, and pot—also known as Scotch—which has had only a single layer of its outer husk removed. Weighing in at 170 calories per cup of cooked grain, barley is low in fat and sodium and is a good source of protein and fiber. Added to soups and stews, it can be a hearty substitute for meat at a meal.

8. Beans

It would be hard to find a bean that isn't good for you. Whether they're pink, red, white, or brown, these legumes are so packed full of soluble fiber that a diet that includes a single, daily, 4-ounce serving has the ability to drop high cholesterol levels significantly. They're also a terrific source of potassium and a good source of calcium. Beans are also high in protein and contain very little fat, making them a perfect replacement for high-fat meats at meals.

9. Beets

Next time your salads start to get boring, slice up a half cup of these purple beauties and tuck them around the edge of your greens. Not only will you perk up both color and taste, but the added shot of potassium and fiber will stoke your antistroke program. And with barely any calories to speak of, they'll fill you up without filling you out.

10. Blackberries

Tipping the scales at just 74 calories per cup, these sweet treats from the berry patch have a hefty amount of fiber, a healthy amount of potassium, almost no salt, and only a smidgen of fat, making them a class act against high blood pressure and obesity.

11. Broccoli

Broccoli is called the number one anticancer vegetable because a single cup is brimming with carotene, vitamin C, calcium, and potassium. All those nutrients, plus its low fat, low sodium content, put broccoli on duty against a squadron of diseases: high blood pressure, stroke, heart disease, and osteoporosis. And at 24 calories per cup, this deep green beauty can help keep obesity at bay. With all these attributes, broccoli could quite possibly be the number one good-for-you food.

12. Brown Rice

Think of each small grain of brown rice as ammunition against heart disease, diabetes, high blood pressure, stroke, and cancer. But the explosive compound inside a grain of brown rice is not gunpowder—it's fiber. You won't find fiber, or many nutrients, in its stripped-down "white" form, however, so when it comes to rice, make it brown.

13. Brussels Sprouts

These little garden gems provide a good shot of vitamins A and C. They have little sodium, little fat, and moderately high levels of potassium and fiber. At 55 calories a cup, they make the weight-control patrol.

14. Buckwheat

Like all good grains, nutty-flavored buckwheat is low in fat and sodium and high in fiber, qualities that put grains in league against heart disease and cancer. But buckwheat may have a benefit that other grains may not. One study found that a buckwheat diet had a beneficial effect on sugar tolerance, which can be beneficial to those with diabetes. Cook the buckwheat and toss it with shredded spinach in a salad, or buy it ground into flour and use it as a substitute for all-purpose flour in cooking and baking. It makes super-tasting pancakes and crepes.

15. Bulgur

Bulgur is wheat that has been parboiled, dried, and cracked. It's frequently sprinkled over salads or used as a major ingredient in Middle Eastern dishes such as *tabouli*. A single cup of bulgur made from club wheat or hard red winter wheat will yield a hefty shot of potassium to help you prevent stroke and lower your blood pressure.

16. Cabbage

Green leaf cabbage is one of those premier vegetables that seem to inspire good health on every level. A single cup of shredded raw leaves has a nice amount of calcium, potassium, and vitamin A. It has virtually no sodium or fat, only 16 calories, and ample fiber, and it contains various compounds that fight the effects of cancer-causing agents. In fact, studies indicate that people who don't eat cabbage are three times more likely to develop colon cancer than those who munch on it at least once a week. All this goodness also puts cabbage in the prevention plan against high blood pressure, stroke, heart disease, diabetes, and obesity.

17. Canola Oil

Also known as rapeseed oil, this mostly monounsaturated oil lowers cholesterol so well that it helps fight stroke and heart disease. It *is* high in calories—120 per tablespoon—so use it in place of, not in addition to, other fats in your diet.

18. Cantaloupes

This sunny apricot-colored melon is so packed with nutrition that just half of one provides you with a hefty supply of cancer-fighting vitamins A and C. It's also super-rich in potassium and low in salt and fat, making it an ideal food for someone trying to control high blood pressure. And at 94 calories a half, obesity is out the door.

19. Carrots

Carrots are champion disease fighters on every level. They're the most widely available source of cancer-preventing carotene. Significantly, the risk of lung cancer is three times higher among smokers who don't eat carrots than among those who do. They are rich enough in potassium and fiber to effectively help fight stroke and high blood pressure. They contain a nice amount of soluble fiber, the kind so important in controlling diabetes. And with virtually no fat and a paltry 31 calories each, they're the ideal weight-control snack.

20. Casaba Melons

Even a single slice of the casaba melon is a plentiful source of potassium and vitamin C, a combination that helps prevent stroke and keep blood pressure down. And at 43 calories a slice—45 for a whole cup of cubed fruit—casaba is a weapon in the war on obesity.

21. Cauliflower

Cauliflower is low enough in fat and sodium and punched with enough potassium and fiber to make it a good choice for those trying to control blood pressure and prevent a stroke. But everyone should eat it because of its cancer-fighting potential. Cauliflower is a member of the cruciferous (cabbage) family of vegetables, which, studies have shown, contain cancer-preventive qualities.

22. Celery

Those crunchy green stalks are the mainstay of dieters everywhere. When you consider it's only 6 calories a stalk, celery is a good source of cancer-fighting vitamin A and blood pressure–controlling potassium. It also contains a modest amount of bone-building calcium. What it doesn't contain is any fat. When you think of it, that's a lot of first-rate action for such a second-class food.

23. Cheese

Cheese is the catch–22 of foods. It's chock-full of nutrients: plenty of bone-protecting calcium, lots of stress-fighting B vitamins and cancer-protecting vitamin A. But it's also full of fat, and mostly the saturated variety. The way around it, however, is to eat only the low-fat, low-salt varieties. And eat it sparingly—a 1-ounce helping is plenty. The lighter in color and softer in texture, the less fat. Your best bet: dry curd cottage cheese.

24. Cherries

Sweet cherries are nature's gift to those with a sweet tooth— and they contain virtually no sugar and fat! But they do contain as much vitamin A as many vegetables, putting them up front in the fight against cancer. They're a good source of potassium, which helps prevent stroke and control blood pressure.

25. Chestnuts

Chestnuts are not just for roasting over a Christmas Eve fire. Start enjoying them the minute they drop off the trees every autumn. At 846 milligrams per cup of rich, shelled nuts, they're one of the best sources of potassium you can find to help prevent high blood pressure and stroke. But if you're watching your weight, beware—that cup will cost you 310 calories.

26. Chicken Breast

Chicken breast is low in calories, low in fat, and low in sodium—a perfect source of protein for anyone trying to fend off heart disease, high blood pressure, stroke, or obesity. Half a roasted chicken breast without skin has 142 calories.

27. Chick-Peas

Often used as a substitute for meat because they're loaded with protein, a cup of boiled chick-peas also has a fair amount of calcium, super fiber content, and an incredible amount of potassium—making chick-peas one of the best foods available to lower blood pressure and prevent stroke. Studies also indicate that chick-peas lower cholesterol to the extent that they may help reduce heart disease. A half cup comes in at 134 calories.

28. Collard Greens

Collards are a many-splendored green. A single cup of boiled collards is a great source of calcium, which fights osteoporosis. It's a good source of potassium, which protects against stroke and high blood pressure. It contains almost a full day's supply of the Recommended Dietary Allowance (RDA) for vitamin A, which pits it against cancer. And it's so low in fat, it's a natural promoter of health and slim living. Not bad for a green that measures only 27 calories per cup, cooked.

29. Corn

Corn has enough vitamin A and fiber—plus only 66 calories per half cup—to play an important role in any diet designed to defeat cancer, stroke, heart disease, diabetes, and obesity.

30. Cowpeas

These tiny little gifts from the South, also known as black-eyed peas, are also a gift of health-promoting nutrients. They are high in stress-fighting B vitamins and blood-building iron. They are also high in fiber and potassium and low in fat and salt, pitting them against stroke and high blood pressure.

31. Dandelion Greens

Dandelion greens are a good low-fat, low-sodium source of calcium and potassium. A single cup of raw dandelion greens, at only 35 calories, provides a two-day supply of the RDA for vitamin A. And that makes dandelions a true ally in the war against cancer.

32. Eggplant

This deep purple vegetable has a good amount of potassium to help prevent high blood pressure and stroke. At 27 calories a cup, it belongs on any weight watcher's menu.

33. Figs

Figs are such a good low-fat source of fiber that experts feel they can fight obesity by helping you feel full for a longer time. And three canned figs, which have only 42 calories, provide as much fiber as a whole bowl of 40% bran flakes.

34. Flank Steak

Surprised? You don't need to banish red meat from your diet, as long as you exercise restraint. Just stick to the lowest-fat cuts and eat them in moderation. A well-trimmed flank steak, which has 276 calories for an 8-ounce portion, is a good source of stroke-preventing potassium and blood-building iron.

35. Flounder

This flaky, white-fleshed flatfish contains almost no saturated fat, little sodium, and only 100 calories per 3-ounce serving. Put it high on your list of protein-rich, heart-healthy, low-calorie entrees. And it's got enough B vitamins to help you fight stress.

36. Garlic

Garlic's big taste is matched by its cholesterol-busting ability to fight heart disease and its potential to enhance the process by which our bodies break up stroke-causing blood clots. At 4 calories a clove, it's one of the least expensive insurance policies around.

37. Grapefruits

One of the most popular diet foods of all time—second only to celery—grapefruit helps fight obesity by virtue of its feeling-full fiber and low-calorie profile—only 38 calories per half. Moreover, it has enough potassium to help keep stroke and high blood pressure at bay. One grapefruit provides more than a day's supply of the RDA for vitamin C.

38. Halibut

A member of the same flatfish family as flounder, halibut offers the same healing qualities: virtually no saturated fat, plenty of protein, a nice amount of B vitamins, and few calories—only 120 per 3-ounce serving.

39. Hearts of Palm

Out in the backcountry, this little vegetable is better known as swamp cabbage. And for those who learn to love it, the hearts provide an entire day's supply of the RDA for cancer-fighting vitamin A, at only 21 calories a cup.

40. Honeydew Melons

This pale, lime-colored melon is such a rich source of potassium that it belongs on the menu of anyone concerned about stroke and high blood pressure. And at 46 calories a slice, it'll help keep you thin, too.

41. Kale

A single cup of boiled kale is a great source of calcium, potassium, and vitamin A. At 43 calories, that cup of kale becomes a major weapon in the fight against obesity.

42. Kiwifruit

Also known as Chinese gooseberry, kiwifruit is an excellent source of vitamin C and a good source of potassium. Its exotic, luxuriant color is also a super antidote to dieter's boredom. Each fruit contains approximately 55 low-fat calories.

43. Kohlrabi

Kohlrabi literally translates as "cabbage turnip" in German. And indeed, it is a member of the cancer-fighting cabbage family. It's also a good source of potassium and vitamin C. It has almost no fat, little salt, and only 48 calories per cup. All in all, it's a good way to fight stroke, obesity, and high blood pressure.

44., 45. Lemons and Limes

These citrus fruits are healthy because of what they *don't* have: no fat, no salt, and no calories to speak of. And that makes them a key player in the war on obesity because they can frequently serve as a flavorful substitute for fats: Use lemon or lime juice instead of butter on fish, for example, or as a zesty alternative to high-fat dressings on salads.

46. Mackerel

This is the fish of choice for those who are looking for the best source of heart-protecting omega–3 fatty acids. It's also a good source of potassium, making it good for your blood pressure as well. A 3-ounce serving is 223 calories.

47. Mangoes

Deep green mangoes are a gift from the tropics. They're packed with vitamin A, stuffed with potassium, and finished with a dash of fiber. All at only 135 calories per tropical delight. They belong in a diet aimed at preventing cancer and holding down blood pressure.

48. Milk

A single glass of low-fat milk packs a hefty shot of both calcium and potassium to help keep osteoporosis, stroke, and high blood pressure at bay. It may also help reduce your risk of intestinal cancer. At least one study indicates that men who ate foods containing both calcium and vitamin D—vitamin D helps your body absorb calcium and is routinely added to milk—had about one-third the cancer risk of those who didn't. Just remember to stick to the low-fat kind. Whole milk is so high in saturated fat that it just about cancels out any nutritional benefits.

49. Mushrooms

Mushrooms are a source of potassium that has virtually no fat, no sodium, few calories, and a modest amount of magnesium. Add them raw to your salad.

50. Nectarines

A single glowing nectarine packs a wallop of vitamin A and potassium with a modest amount of magnesium. At 67 calories for a single fruit, they'll also help keep you slim.

51. Nuts

That is, almonds, hazelnuts, macadamia nuts, pecans, and pistachios. Although high in calories (about 170 per ounce) and fat, the fat they contain is mostly monounsaturated, the kind that has been found to be beneficial to the heart. They should be used sparingly—sprinkled over stir-fries, for example—with other heart-healthy foods. These nuts have another benefit: They contain modest amounts of potassium and magnesium, which can help blood pressure.

52. Oat Bran

Studies show that those with high cholesterol can lower it significantly by eating a cup of oat bran a day. Studies also show it can also help reduce or eliminate the need for insulin in diabetics. The secret, of course, is fiber—oat bran is packed with soluble fiber that is credited with helping to lower harmful LDL (low-density lipoprotein) cholesterol and raise beneficial HDL (high-density lipoprotein) cholesterol.

53. Oatmeal Cereal

Not quite as healthful as oat bran, oatmeal still packs a hefty amount of cholesterol-lowering fiber. It's a good alternative at breakfast for those seeking a better-tasting way to get the benefits of oat bran.

54. Olive Oil

The ability of this golden liquid to prevent heart disease is nothing short of amazing. It's been found to help lower LDL cholesterol without altering HDL cholesterol. But don't forget that it's still a fat and loaded with calories—120 a tablespoon. Use it only as a substitute for other fats in your diet.

55. Onions

Studies indicate that the chemical components of onions can help prevent heart disease by helping to raise levels of beneficial HDL cholesterol. And its oils are believed to inhibit cancer-producing activity. It may even have anti-asthmatic properties.

56. Oranges

Most people associate oranges with vitamin C and its ability to fight a cold. But you should also think of oranges and vitamin C for their potential to help fight cancer. Opt for the whole fruit—at only 65 calories—instead of juice, for its fiber benefits.

57. Oysters

The pearl in most oysters is not a luminous jewel but the disease-fighting zinc that keeps your immune system on its toes. Steam a dozen—never eat them raw—and for only 117 calories, you'll receive a nice shot of reinforcements to your body's defensive forces.

58. Papaya

This popular tropical fruit has more health-giving nutrients packed into its flesh than almost any other food. It contains a hefty dose of potassium and fiber, one-quarter of the calcium found in a glass of milk, more than an entire day's supply of vitamin A, and a *three-day* supply of vitamin C.

59. Parsley

Its deep green color should give you the clue that this flavor enhancer is much more than a garnish. It's a good source of vitamins A and C, making it a major player in the war against cancer. It's the main attraction in *tabouli,* a popular Middle Eastern salad.

60. Parsnips

A single parsnip contains enough fiber to give bran cereals a run for their money. And although a little high in calories—130 each— the lowly parsnip contains a good amount of calcium and a hefty shot of potassium, making it good for your bones and blood pressure.

61. Pasta

With just a trace of fat and only 200 calories per serving, why shouldn't pasta be considered a healthy food! Pasta has finally shed its image as a fattening food and gained a notable place in the healthy foods lineup. It's high in B vitamins and contains respectable amounts of iron and zinc. Just make sure you don't spoil all its healthfulness by topping it with a heavy creamy sauce. A simple tomato sauce is your best bet.

62. Peaches

A peach is—well, a peach of a treat for your body. This fuzzy fruit yields a fair share of vitamin A and potassium. It has a modest amount of fiber, provided you eat it fresh: A peach loses much of its fiber during processing. At 37 calories for a medium peach, it's a perfect low-calorie snack.

63. Pears

A single 98-calorie pear has as much fiber as most whole-grain cereals. Pears are also naturally low in sodium and contain modest amounts of potassium and calcium, making them a perfect fruit for those watching their blood pressure.

64. Peas

The green pea is just about perfect when it comes to healthfulness. The vitamin A, potassium, and fiber in peas are helpful against cancer, stroke, heart disease, high blood pressure, and diabetes. Plus, peas contain little or no fat, sodium, or cholesterol. One half cup serving of cooked peas contains only 67 calories.

65. Peppers

Green or red, sweet or hot, peppers have more cancer-fighting vitamin C than an entire glass of orange juice. The jalapeño, although high in sodium, contains more vitamin A and fiber than other varieties. Use any of the peppers to spice up your appetizers, salads, or entrees.

66. Persimmons

Fresh Japanese persimmons rank with papayas and parsnips right at the top of our fiber-foods list. They're also loaded with vitamin A, putting them in the anticancer league.

67. Plantain

What could be better than a banana for blood pressure-protecting potassium? Try the plantain, a first cousin to the banana in looks. But its similarities end there. Plantains are not sweet, and they cannot be eaten raw. They are also high in calories—one fresh plantain has 218 calories. A Caribbean vegetable, plantains are often combined with rice and beans for a fiber-packed main dish.

68. Plums

A single cup of canned purple plums delivers half the necessary supply of daily vitamin A—along with a shot of potassium and a great deal of sweet, tongue-tingling pleasure. Fresh from the tree or stewed in a compote, plums can help prevent cancer, high blood pressure, and stroke.

69. Pomegranates

A good low-fat, low-sodium way to get the stroke-busting potassium your body needs. At only 104 calories each, they may also deter obesity.

70. Popcorn

Pop a movie in the VCR and enjoy this high-fiber snack, which has only 25 calories per popped cup. Add a low-calorie seasoning such as Mrs. Dash, then spray lightly with butter-flavored Pam to help the seasoning stick. It's the perfect heart-healthy, weight-watching snack.

71. Potatoes

Potatoes are one of the best sources of potassium there is, putting them up front in the battle against stroke and high blood pressure. The lowly potato is also low in sodium and low in fat. Add it all up, and potatoes rank high in your eat-to-live program. Here's a tip: To keep potassium in potatoes, don't boil them. Bake or steam instead. And don't forget to eat the skin.

72. Prunes

These dark, wrinkled pendants of the fruit world can take the place of bran when it comes to disease-fighting fiber. But unlike bran, they are loaded with all-important vitamin A, iron, and potassium.

73. Pumpkin

Carotene-rich pumpkin is probably the best cancer-fighting vegetable on your produce stand. One half cup of even the canned variety is so overflowing with health that it will give you nearly a *five-day* supply of the RDA for vitamin A. It's also a good source of fiber and contains moderate amounts of potassium and calcium. It's also low in calories, fat, and sodium, making it a perfect diet food.

74. Rainbow Trout

Low in fat and containing modest amounts of the omega–3 fatty acids, rainbow trout can help you fight heart disease and stroke. To avoid fish that are contaminated by toxic chemicals as a result of polluted lakes, shop for trout raised on a fish farm.

75. Raspberries

Beat the birds to your backyard raspberry bush next summer and pick yourself a bushel of health. Red or black, these berries are a super source of disease-fighting fiber. The best thing about them is that they're so low in calories, you can eat them to your heart's content.

76. Rhubarb

A single cup of diced, bright pink stalks from the rhubarb plant can help you prevent stroke and high blood pressure. Whether it's thrown into a pot and simmered or chucked into a pie and baked, rhubarb will give you a good shot of potassium and fiber. And it has almost as much calcium and half the calories you'd find in half a glass of milk.

77. Romaine Lettuce

When it comes to salad greens, pass on pale iceberg and go for deep-colored varieties such as romaine. The dark green color is the clue that they are loaded with carotene, the form of vitamin A that's believed to help prevent cancer. And calories, sodium, and fat are virtually nonexistent.

78. Safflower Oil

Safflower oil is another of the healthy monounsaturated oils that can help lower your cholesterol level. Like any other oil, it is high in calories—120 per tablespoon—so be sure to use it judiciously.

79. Salmon

Fresh or canned, salmon is one of the richest sources of heart-healthy, cholesterol-lowering omega–3 fatty acids. When eating the canned variety, eat the bones along with the flesh: You'll get just about as much bone-building calcium as you would in half a glass of milk.

80. Sardines

Sardines can give you a double dose of prevention. Their oil is rich in omega–3 fatty acids, which goes a long way in protecting your heart. And their bones are a rich source of calcium, making sardines the best nondairy food against osteoporosis.

81. Spinach

Popeye knew what he was doing when he reached for this particular vegetable. A good source of vitamin A, spinach also contains a moderate supply of calcium and potassium. With no fat or calories to speak of—12 calories per cup, raw—it's probably best noted for its waist-trimming potential.

82. Sprouts

One cup of raw alfalfa sprouts at 10 calories is a healthful way to dress up your salads without adding calories or fat. Try other varieties of sprouts such as mung bean sprouts, which are high in magnesium and calcium, minerals that can help reduce blood pressure. And don't forget the wheat sprout: Studies indicate that this innocuous little sprout can inhibit the genetic damage to cells caused by some cancer-causing agents.

83. Stone-Ground Wheat Crackers

An ounce of stoned-wheat crackers has more fiber than a slice of whole-wheat bread, and some makers are beginning to substitute heart-healthy canola oil in place of saturated fat. Some brands even contain wheat germ and sesame seeds—adding more good fiber. Served with low-fat cheese, they make a nutritious snack.

84. Strawberries

Besides adding the luscious taste of warm spring to everything with which they're served, strawberries also add a special measure of cancer protection. That's because they contain ellagic acid, a compound that seems to block the effects of some of the carcinogens found in cigarette smoke, bacon, and peanut butter. And at 45 calories a cup, you can eat them forever and not get fat.

85. Sunflower Seeds

A handful of sunflower seeds contains as much fiber as a slice of whole-wheat bread. Sprinkle them over your breakfast cereal or luncheon salad, but don't overdo it. That handful of seeds has 165 calories.

86. Sweet Potatoes

The South shall rise again indeed if its inhabitants keep growing such healthful vegetables as sweet potatoes. A single baked "sweet'un" contains 24,877 milligrams, or five times the RDA of vitamin A, making it a perfect vegetable to power your body's cancer-prevention efforts. With a modest amount of calcium, magnesium, and potassium and as much fiber as two slices of mixed-grain bread, sweet potatoes are also a potent weapon against stroke, heart disease, high blood pressure, obesity, and diabetes.

87. Swiss Chard

A single leaf of Swiss chard packs 20 percent of a day's supply of vitamin A, plus a dusting of fiber, calcium, and potassium. It also has no fat and few calories. Mix it with other vitamin A-rich greens in your salads.

88. Tangerines

Like the orange, a tangerine is known for its vitamin C. But unlike the orange, a single cup of tangerine sections will provide a generous serving of vitamin A, making it an even stronger soldier in the fight against cancer. And at only 86 calories a cup, it can go into combat against obesity as well.

89. Tofu

Use this food in place of high-fat meat and cheese, and you'll take a giant step toward a longer life. Tofu is high in protein, low in fat and sodium, and contains a generous supply of calcium. As a substitute for cheese, it has been shown to help lower cholesterol. Tofu is a perfect food for any program designed to fight heart disease, high blood pressure, and osteoporosis.

90. Tomatoes

Whether they're from California, New Jersey, or your own backyard, freshly picked tomatoes are one of nature's gifts to health. They're loaded with vitamin A, vitamin C, potassium, and fiber, and they're low in fat and sodium. That makes them all-around disease fighters. And at 24 calories per red, shining globe, they're a succulent way to fight obesity as well.

91. Tuna

Albacore tuna is right up there with mackerel and salmon as a rich source of the omega–3 fatty acids that help prevent heart disease and stroke. It also contains a healthy measure of potassium, making it good for your blood pressure as well. If you're buying it canned instead of fresh, make sure you buy it packed in water to save on unnecessary calories and fat.

92. Turnips

One half cup of cooked turnips has almost no fat and no calories, and it's loaded with fiber. Add it to one half cup of cooked turnip greens—which has almost a whole day's supply of vitamin A—and you've got a strong supporter against cancer, stroke, heart disease, diabetes, and obesity.

93. Turkey

When it comes to animal flesh, the white, skinless meat of turkey is as low in fat and calories as it gets. That means it should be *your* meat of choice at the dinner table.

94. Watercress

This popular soup green is noted more for what it doesn't have—no fat, no salt, no calories. But a single one half cup serving will give you modest amounts of calcium, potassium, and vitamins A and C. Mix it with other dark greens in your salads, or use it as an alternative to lettuce on turkey or tuna fish sandwiches.

95. Watermelon

An icy slice of watermelon on a hot summer's day is more than a way to cool your dusty throat. It's also a flavorful way to load up on vitamins A and C, as well as potassium and calcium. And since a nice-size slice has about 150 calories, it's a delicious way to watch your weight.

96. Wheat Bran

Wheat bran should be a part of your live-longer eating program because it is one of the best sources of insoluble fiber, the type that keeps your digestive system running smoothly and can prevent colon trouble, such as diverticular disease and cancer. Although you can eat it pure—stirred in juice or sprinkled on stews, for example—your tastiest choice is cereal. But choose high-bran cereals such as 100% Bran or 40% Bran Flakes to ensure you're getting the health-promoting benefit.

A ¼-cup serving of wheat bran is a fine source of blood-building iron and stress-fighting B vitamins. Its high-potassium, low-sodium ratio means it can help lower blood pressure as well. If you're watching your blood pressure, though, be sure you read the label on the cereal box to check for any added salt.

97. Wheat Germ

A single ounce of wheat germ has as much fiber as six slices of whole-wheat bread or a whole bowl of even the healthiest bran cereal. Sprinkle it on or in just about anything to increase fiber content and help prevent cancer, stroke, heart disease, diabetes, obesity, and high blood pressure.

98. Whole-Grain Cookies

Not just any cookies, mind you, but homemade cookies that are high in fiber and low in saturated fat. You can add one quarter cup of bran, a few tablespoons of psyllium seed, and a handful of sunflower seeds to almost any standard cookie recipe. Just remember to reduce the dry ingredients by as much as you add—excluding any nuts. And substitute monounsaturated oils such as rapeseed oil for any butter or margarine the recipe calls for. It's a tasty way to help you prevent cancer, stroke, heart disease, diabetes, high blood pressure, and (in moderation) obesity.

99. Whole-Wheat Bread

The traditional source of fiber goodness, whole-wheat bread also offers a healthy helping of B vitamins and iron. It's also low in fat. Make it a permanent staple in your home.

100. Winter Squash

The deep orange flesh of acorn and butternut squash is brimming with anticancer nutrients in the form of carotene, vitamin C, and fiber. It also contains a good supply of stroke-preventing potassium and enough calcium to qualify as a bone-building vegetable.

101. Yogurt

Yogurt is a super source of calcium and potassium. Eaten regularly as part of a low-fat diet, it can help you prevent osteoporosis and stroke while it keeps the lid on your blood pressure. But not all yogurts are created equal. Some varieties are so high in fat that their disease-fighting capabilities are almost lost. So make sure the yogurt you choose is marked "low fat."

C H A P T E R · 2

REJUVENATE YOUR HEART

One in three. Those aren't very good odds if what you're up against is something to fear. Like heart disease, or more precisely, *death* from heart disease. But, like it or not, those are *your* odds.

Today in the United States, 1 out of every 3 people dies from heart disease, making it the number one killer of Americans. It is so prevalent that it is responsible for more deaths than all other causes combined.

Startling facts? They shouldn't be. Unless you've been living on an uninhabited island in the South Pacific for the past 30 years, you already know that heart disease is dogging the country like a rampant assassin. It hides in wait around deli counters, living room recliners, smoking lounges—all the places it can find an easy mark. Then it starts to infiltrate, slowly and steadily. A friend becomes a victim. Then someone at work. The neighbor across the street. Maybe a parent. Sooner or later you think, Could I be next? Could this happen to me?

You are about to find out. And if the answer is yes, you're about to find out how to make sure it *doesn't* happen.

The Heart of the Problem

Not too many years ago, most people assumed that heart disease was as normal to aging as gray hair and wrinkles. But recent declines in the number of people over the age of 75 who, despite the odds, *don't* develop heart trouble show that heart disease is not an inevitable consequence of age. Instead, it's an inevitable consequence of the way its victims live their lives.

The main cause of heart disease is atherosclerosis, or "hardening of the arteries," a condition created by the insidious buildup of cholesterol-laden sludge that tends to cling to the inner walls of coronary arteries like dried oatmeal sticks to a cereal bowl.

If allowed to accumulate over a lifetime, this buildup can leave your arteries hard and narrow, pinching down the blood flow to your heart and impeding the smooth-working condition of this most important life-sustaining organ. If the arteries get too hard or too narrow, the blood can't pass through at all. And if blood can't reach your heart, it stops working altogether. Heart disease claims another victim.

Who gets marked for heart disease is actually determined by a number of markers. Genetics, of course, counts big. If two people in your immediate family—parents, brothers, or sisters—have had heart attacks before the age of 55, your risk of developing early heart disease is five to ten times higher than that of people whose families are free of heart attacks, say University of Utah researchers, who conducted one of the largest studies ever of inherited heart disease. But lifestyle factors, say doctors, count even more.

High cholesterol levels, caused chiefly by a diet high in saturated fat, head the list. A study of 356,000 men in 18 cities across the

FACT OF LIFE

Meet Joe Heart Disease

Ever wonder who's been voted most likely to succumb to heart disease? According to the National Center for Health Statistics, the typical heart disease victim is a man over age 65 who doesn't work, suffers from high blood pressure, and lists assets of less than $50,000.

United States revealed that the higher your cholesterol, the higher your risk of dying of heart disease. Also implicated are smoking, high blood pressure, stress, overweight, and being sedentary—yes, hearts *like* to be worked hard.

Deaths Are Down

All the news about heart disease is not bad, however. Since 1950, deaths from heart disease have decreased dramatically—nearly 50 percent. One reason is advanced medical technology: Successful drugs like cholestyramine, lovastatin, and tissue plasminogen activator (TPA) have helped treat the disease, and coronary bypass surgery and an artery-clearing procedure called balloon angioplasty have played a part. And the development of coronary care units—hospital wards specializing in medical care for heart patients—is also credited with saving lives.

Better medical treatment of existing heart problems explains only part of the decline, however. Fewer people are getting heart disease in the first place, or they're slowing its course before drugs or surgery are ever necessary. Over the years, the public has become increasingly aware of the importance of such things as diet, exercise, and a smokeless environment in avoiding heart disease. Each day, new people are making these and other lifestyle improvements. Many experts can't help but feel that these healthy lifestyle practices are also responsible for at least some of the decline in coronary death rates.

Preventing heart disease isn't complicated. Risk factors tend to build upon each other like a house of cards—and, like those cards,

FACT OF LIFE

Male-Female Odds: 6 to 1

In a 26-year follow-up of more than 5,000 people studied in the famous Framingham Heart Study, the incidence of heart disease in men aged 35 to 44 was more than six times greater than in women of the same age. Nevertheless, approximately 250,000 women in the United States die of heart attacks each year.

eliminating one can topple many others. Reducing dietary fat, for example, not only lowers serum cholesterol but also helps the heart further by aiding weight loss. Learning to relax can help lower blood pressure and maybe even reduce the desire to drink and smoke. Quitting smoking not only does arteries a huge favor but also improves your "wind" and can make you feel more like exercising, which in turn lowers your risk.

You get the idea: You *can* escape heart disease. A case in point: Members of a test group were put on a low-fat diet by researchers at the University of California at San Francisco. They also practiced yoga or other relaxation techniques, walked regularly, and stopped smoking. The results are encouraging for all of us: Within a year, their cholesterol levels dropped significantly—by almost 100 points. Best of all, their narrowed arteries *widened.*

Here's what it takes to get on the road to a healthy heart.

Weighing Your Risk

102. Get a Medical Checkup

Periodic medical checkups will protect you from heart disease by detecting it early, as well as revealing the presence of cardiovascular risk factors—something that varies tremendously from one person to the next. Your risk of heart disease will vary, to some degree, with your age or sex. High cholesterol and obesity, for example, seem to be more of a risk factor for men than women, while diabetes seems to be more of a risk factor for women than men.

103. Feeling Fine Is No Protection

You should have a checkup even if you have no symptoms and think you're relatively safe. A long-term study indicates that silent ischemia (a symptomless type of heart disease) is both riskier and more likely to bring on a heart attack than heart disease accompanied by preliminary chest pains.

Ischemia is a blood deficiency in part of the heart muscle. The flow of blood to that area of the heart may be blocked due to spasms or obstruction of the arteries.

Who should be tested for silent ischemia? "Middle-aged men who smoke, who have a family history of high cholesterol and high blood pressure, or who have diabetes," says Peter F. Cohn, M.D., of the Health Sciences Center of the State University of New York, Stony Brook.

104. Have Your Cholesterol Tested

Doctors have found that reducing a high cholesterol level reduces the risk of heart attack. Too much cholesterol in your blood winds up as layers of plaque that can narrow arteries, slow blood flow to a trickle, and possibly end in a fatal heart attack. In many cases, all this occurs without so much as a hint of trouble beforehand. So a cholesterol test is and should be part of any evaluation for heart disease. It's like a sneak preview that gives you a chance to avoid a bad movie.

What your ideal cholesterol level should be is determined by your age and sex, and it varies accordingly. For men and women aged 50 to 54, for example, a desirable cholesterol level would be lower than 200. Women aged 45 to 49, though, should shoot for a level less than 191, while men the same age would be fine with a level still less than 200.

A cholesterol test consists of having a small tube of blood drawn from your arm—about 10 cc, or ⅓ ounce. The sample is then analyzed for lipids, or blood fats, at a laboratory. The test can be done in the doctor's office or a laboratory (usually with a doctor's authorization) and requires an overnight fast.

Instant "pin-prick" testing is becoming readily available in schools, shopping malls, and churches in many communities, but these tests are not always accurate. Ten percent of all finger-prick cholesterol tests give false high readings, says Phillip Greenland, M.D., of the University of Rochester School of Medicine and Dentistry.

105. Ask for a Complete Lipid Profile

Fifteen percent of heart attack deaths occur in people whose total cholesterol levels are below the so-called safe level of 200 milligrams, according to the Framingham Heart Study. So ask your doctor to have your cholesterol test broken down to high-density lipo-

How Does Your Cholesterol Rate?

Once you have your cholesterol tested, the following table can help you size up the results. In particular, you should note your total cholesterol/HDL ratio. (Divide total cholesterol by HDL cholesterol.) This gives you a better picture of your heart disease risk than total cholesterol alone.

For a male over age 40, a healthy ratio should not exceed 4.5. An optimal ratio is 3.5. (By comparison, vegetarians often have ratios in the 2.9 range, and Boston marathoners, 3.5. On the other hand, men with coronary heart disease customarily show up with ratios around 5.8.)

By the way, one study found that people under age 50 whose total serum cholesterol levels were below 180 had a much greater chance of still being alive 30 years later than others whose cholesterol levels were above 180.

Component	Age	Optimal Level	High-Risk Level
Total cholesterol	20–29	Below 152	above 220
	30–39	below 166	above 240
	over 40	below 190	above 260
HDL cholesterol	20 and over	above 50	below 35
Total cholesterol/HDL ratio	20–29	below 3.0	above 6.0
	30–39	below 3.3	above 6.5
	over 40	below 3.5	above 7.0
Triglycerides	20 and over	below 100	above 250

SOURCE: Adapted from *The Aerobics News,* an official publication of the Institute for Aerobics Research, Dallas, Texas.

protein (HDL) cholesterol and low-density lipoprotein (LDL) cholesterol, not just total cholesterol. A detailed breakdown is more meaningful for assessing your true risk, which is actually the ratio between the two. (For more details, see "How Does Your Cholesterol Rate?" above.)

Evidence suggests that low amounts of HDL may put you at risk for heart disease *even if your total cholesterol is fine.* Robert D. Abbott, Ph.D., a coauthor of the Framingham Heart Study, believes that everyone over age 50 should have HDL screenings. Some scientists go so far as to say that *everyone* should find out his or her HDL level.

A complete lipid profile will also include a measure of your level of triglycerides, another blood fat that has been implicated in heart disease. If you're being tested for triglycerides, you'll be asked not to eat anything after 6:00 P.M. the night before the test.

106. Aim for High HDL Cholesterol

Is there such a thing as a good type of cholesterol? Researchers believe there is.

HDL works sort of like a vacuum cleaner in your arteries by removing harmful cholesterol particles and keeping them from attaching to your arterial walls. The less harmful cholesterol that attaches, the less buildup there will be in your veins.

High levels of HDL decrease your risk of atherosclerosis and stroke, and the higher the level, the safer you'll be. Men should shoot for HDL in the 45-milligram range; women should try to keep their level around 55 milligrams.

107. Keep Your LDL Cholesterol Low

Here's the bad guy of cholesterol. LDL is not the type of cholesterol you want floating around in your veins. High levels of LDL increase your risk of atherosclerosis and stroke, so you want to keep LDL levels low.

What level of LDL is good for you is determined again by your sex and age. For men age 50 to 54, look to keep LDL in the less-than–135 range. Women in the same age category should try to keep their LDL level below 127.

108. Be Honest about Yourself

For the best results, schedule your lipids test during a time you're eating your usual diet, not when you're gaining or losing weight.

"People say, 'Oh, I'm gonna get my cholesterol measured,' and start changing their diet to the way they think they should eat," says John W. Farquhar, M.D., director of the Stanford Center for Research in Disease Prevention at Stanford University. "It's better to see what it is on your usual diet. Then if you want to experiment, you can change and see what happens."

Also, make sure to tell your doctor about any medications you may be taking. Heart drugs and androgenic steroids, especially, can change HDL levels dramatically.

109. Don't Take Your Cholesterol Lying Down

Doctors have found that the patient's body position affects the concentration of lipids and lipoproteins in the blood. Lying down can produce falsely high readings.

A prone position dilutes blood, while standing concentrates it, according to researchers at the Bowman Gray School of Medicine in Winston-Salem, North Carolina, the Institute for Aerobic Research, and the University of Texas Health Science Center, both in Dallas. This is true for both men and women.

The researchers say that a physician should consider your body position during the test—and the length of time you spent in that position—when interpreting test results for serum cholesterol and lipids.

110. Once Is Not Enough

Have your cholesterol test repeated once or twice over the subsequent two weeks after the first test, then average the results. Just as your body weight and blood pressure can vary from day to day, so can your cholesterol. Also, test results can vary from lab to lab or within a single lab. Dr. Farquhar recommends having the test done three times and taking the average.

Thereafter, have your cholesterol retested in five years (if the results are acceptable) or once a year (if they aren't). If your cholesterol is too high, you will also want to recheck it after a major change in weight, diet, or exercise patterns, to monitor your progress.

111. Be Aware That Cholesterol Changes Seasonally

Your blood cholesterol level tends to be higher in winter months and lower in the summer, according to the results of a decade-long study. The seasonal difference is small but distinct—an average of 7.4 points, reports David J. Gordon, M.D., of the National Heart, Lung, and Blood Institute.

You and your physician should know that the slight difference can affect not only your test results but also your dietary attempts to control cholesterol.

Dr. Gordon points out that a patient whose level was 240 in the summer could reduce that level to 190 through a low-fat diet—only to find that, in winter, the level would rise to 200, even if he stuck to his diet.

112. Keep Your Blood Pressure under Control

Blood pressure is the force your blood exerts against artery walls as it courses through the arteries. High blood pressure means that your heart is working harder than normal to pump blood, putting your arteries under considerable strain.

Unrelenting high blood pressure—140/90 or above—can leave the artery walls scarred, hardened, and less elastic, accelerating atherosclerosis. It also makes it harder and harder for your heart to pump enough blood and oxygen to organs and tissues. When forced to work harder than normal for months or years, the heart tends to enlarge. There's also the dangerous possibility that a blood clot can become lodged in a narrowed coronary artery, triggering a heart attack.

High blood pressure is insidious because you can have it and feel fine. So have your blood pressure checked frequently. (If you have high blood presssure, the tips in chapter 6 will help you get it under control.)

113. Control Your Weight

Scientists now believe that being overweight is harder on your heart than once expected. And dropping weight (even a little!) does more good than anyone realized.

"Being overweight is a more important risk factor in heart disease than we thought at first," says Joseph Stokes, M.D., of the Boston University Medical Center and the Framingham Heart Study. "It's a causative factor, partly because it raises blood pressure and cholesterol, which are risk factors in themselves."

Morning Is Heart Attack Time

Most fatal heart attacks occur between 7:00 A.M. and 11:00 A.M., according to a study done by Harvard Medical School researchers. Doctors speculate that this is due to the fact that the morning is the most physiologically stressful time of the day because the body is gearing up for the day's demands. Blood pressure goes up, heart rate increases, and blood platelets are more likely to clot.

114. If You Snore, See a Doctor

Here's a risk factor you may not have heard about: Heavy snorers are at 1.7 times greater risk of heart disease than silent sleepers and at 2.08 times greater risk of heart disease and stroke combined, say Finnish researchers who studied more than 4,000 men.

One reason behind these statistics is that superloud snoring reduces the amount of circulating oxygen in the blood. Lack of oxygen not only boosts blood pressure temporarily but also alters cholesterol and metabolism, leading to heavier concentrations of harmful LDL cholesterol.

The Finnish researchers speculate that the squeeze snoring puts on the cardiovascular system could be one reason why heart attacks are three times more likely to occur first thing in the morning than at any other time of day.

115. Stop Smoking Now

If you smoke cigarettes, you're significantly lowering your body's level of HDL. But if you quit, the levels of HDL cholesterol in your blood may increase, reports Stephen P. Fortmann, M.D., in the *American Journal of Epidemiology*.

Components of cigarette smoke injure artery walls and then encourage blood platelets to stick to these sites of injury, thus increasing the risk of potentially fatal clots.

A study of more than 2,500 people between the ages of 65 and 74 showed current cigarette smokers were more likely to die of heart

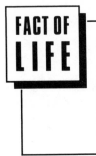

FACT OF LIFE

Smokers: Now Hear This

It doesn't matter how long or how much you've been smoking. If you quit smoking now, you'll reduce your risk of heart disease by 70 percent in a year or two, says Daniel Levy, M.D., director of the cardiology laboratory for the Framingham Heart Study.

disease than nonsmokers, even after taking into consideration other risk factors like age, sex, weight, presence of diabetes, and family history of heart disease.

116. If You Drink, Read This

Moderate drinking—two or fewer drinks a day—may actually be good for the heart as a reducer of both stress and cholesterol levels. But heavy drinking—defined as anything more than two beers, two glasses of wine, or two cocktails a day—can begin to sabotage the heart in several ways. It can raise blood pressure, it can adversely affect the heart muscle, and it can damage the nerves responsible for making the heart beat in the first place.

The end result is that heavy drinkers—whether they drink beer, wine, or liquor—have more heart attacks than light drinkers and nondrinkers.

117. Men, Check Your Testosterone

Older men, especially those with a history of alcohol consumption, should be checked for serum-testosterone levels. Why? Heavy drinking can lower testosterone, and a low testosterone level adds to the risk of having a heart attack—a risk similar to smoking or high blood pressure, according to a report in the *Journal of the American Geriatric Society*.

What's a low testosterone level? Well, an average reading for older men is about 500. The prevalence of heart attacks was higher in all men with testosterone of 438 and less.

118. Listen to Your Doctor

This advice seems obvious, but it bears emphasis. Following your doctor's advice can save your life.

A study done by the World Health Organization split 60,000 middle-aged men into two groups. The first group was advised to lower their cholesterol intake, control smoking, reduce weight, monitor their blood pressure, and get regular exercise; the second group was not. Six years later, the men who'd received heart-protective advice had 10.2 percent less heart disease than the others. Also, 6.9 percent fewer had died of heart disease, and 14.8 fewer had suffered nonfatal heart attacks.

Conquering Fat and Cholesterol

119. Adopt a New Way of Eating

If you put your mind to it, you can change your cholesterol level for the good—and lower your risk of heart disease. With the right dietary changes, it's possible to drop your blood cholesterol significantly in a relatively short period of time, such as a month.

Your likelihood of dropping, say, 30 points in 30 days depends on many individual factors, including your current cholesterol levels. If your blood cholesterol is under the generally considered safe level of 200, it probably won't drop much further. The higher your cholesterol, however, the more it's likely to drop in response to dietary change.

In other words, people who have the most to lose—those with the highest cholesterol readings—have the most to gain by following a diet designed to lower cholesterol in the blood.

Of course, to keep your cholesterol at its new level (or to get it even lower), you should consider your dietary changes your new way of eating—permanently.

120. Shun Saturated Fat

Dietary strategies often center around cutting out foods high in cholesterol, like sour cream and eggs. And that's important. But it's even more important to cut down on all sources of saturated fat. The

How to Recognize a Heart Attack

More than 300,000 heart attack victims die each year before they reach the hospital. Don't make the same fatal mistake. Know the warning signs.

While symptoms of heart attack can vary, here are the most common. If you experience any of the following for 2 minutes or more, call your local emergency medical service immediately, or get to the nearest hospital or cardiac-care unit as soon as possible.

- A pain in the center of the chest that can range from a mild feeling of tightness to an agonizing, crushing sensation
- Pain that comes on suddenly *or* appears gradually, and which may be continuous or intermittent, fading then returning every few minutes
- Pain that spreads to the shoulders, arms, jaw, neck, or stomach
- Possible dizziness, sweating, fainting, nausea, shortness of breath, chills, or a feeling of severe indigestion, with or without the pains mentioned above

fact is, saturated fat can drive up your blood cholesterol levels faster and higher than consuming cholesterol itself.

"Studies have shown that watching your saturated fat intake is definitely more important than even cutting your cholesterol intake," says Thomas Pickering, M.D., of the Helmsley Cardiovascular Center at New York Hospital.

One study sponsored by the National Heart, Lung, and Blood Institute gave researchers a chance to actually peek into living human arteries and see the damage being done. Pictures of the arteries of a group of men suffering from severe atherosclerosis were taken, and then the men were divided into two separate groups. One group was put on a low-fat diet and was also given a cholesterol-lowering drug. The other group was also put on a low-fat diet but was given a placebo (an inactive drug look-alike) instead.

After two years, pictures were taken again, and the researchers found that not only had the atherosclerosis slowed in the diet-only group, but in some cases their arteries were less clogged than before.

Men in the diet-plus-drug group also enjoyed a benefit, but fully 37 percent of the diet-only men saw their atherosclerosis stop. Low fat got the fat out.

121. How Low Should You Go?

We're not talking cold turkey here when it comes to giving up fat. Most nutrition experts recommend that only a little less than a third, or 30 percent of your daily calories, come from fat.

Right now, if you're a typical American, you probably have a diet that contains about 40 percent fat. That extra 10 percent could be all that's standing between you and heart disease.

What does this mean when you're about to sit down at the kitchen table? Margo Denke, M.D., a cholesterol researcher at the University of Texas Southwestern Medical School, uses the following formula: The average adult American man eats 2,400 calories a day. Thirty percent of total calories is 720 calories. Since 1 gram of fat is equal to 9 calories, you should be getting no more than 80 grams of fat per day. That's approximately the amount of fat you'd find in 1½ pounds of french fries.

122. Avoid High-Cholesterol Foods

The American Heart Association recommends that you limit the amount of cholesterol you eat a day to 300 milligrams. The quickest way you can do that is to avoid eating the foods highest in cholesterol, like liver (410 milligrams a serving) or eggs (274 milligrams each).

Basically, you can cut down on cholesterol by decreasing your intake of animal products (the major source of cholesterol) and increasing your intake of fruits and vegetables (which contain no cholesterol).

123. Defat Dairy Products

Choose low-fat and nonfat milk and yogurt over whole milk products. And use evaporated skim milk instead of heavy cream or half-and-half. Avoid high-fat cheddar and cream cheeses. Instead, try low-fat ricotta, skim-milk mozzarella, and low-fat cottage cheese.

When you shop for cheese, read the labels. Buy cheese that contains 6 grams or less of fat per ounce. True low-fat cheeses will have 3 grams or less of fat per ounce.

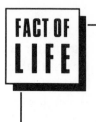

FACT OF LIFE

The Older, the Wiser

A Gallup survey found that 85 percent of those 50 and older have their cholesterol checked regularly, compared to 50 percent of those between 35 to 49. Among *all* ages, only 1 in 3 adults of the 900 polled knew their cholesterol level.

124. Skim Milk Is Special

By the way, if your cholesterol is over 230, you may benefit from drinking skim milk. In a study of 67 people, drinking a quart of skim milk every day for 12 weeks reduced serum cholesterol by an average of 8 percent.

125. Low-Fat Milk May Do It, Too

In another study, 15 healthy men at the Chicago Medical School who drank 1 quart of 2 percent milk a day increased the proportion of good to bad cholesterol in their blood by 19.5 percent after three months. The ratio increased by 31 percent after six months. Fifteen other men who ate the same number of calories a day but skipped the milk were unaffected. Total cholesterol, by the way, did not change in this study.

Researchers, however, say that studies on larger numbers of people are needed before these results can be put to practical use.

126. Don't Bother with Butter

To help cut back on your intake of saturated fat, choose tub or squeeze margarine as an alternative to butter, advises Dr. Denke. The softer the margarine, the less hydrogenation it has undergone. Hydrogenation increases the saturated fat content of margarine. Margarines with liquid corn or soybean oil listed as the first ingredient are the best choices.

If you must have stick margarine, look for products made of pure corn or soybean oil, or choose one of the "light" whipped brands. Stay away from sticks that are part butter.

127. Replace Fat with Flavor

Contrary to what your taste buds may be telling you, you don't need butter and other fats to get flavor out of your food. Heart-healthy food doesn't have to be bland. Learn to experiment with herbs, spices, and other flavorings, such as juices and mustards. To get you started, here are a few ideas.

- Brush a smidgen of mustard on broiled fish or chicken. Add a little paprika, red pepper, or parsley.
- Add pineapple, mandarin oranges, or other fruits to chicken dishes. Brush orange juice concentrate on broiled fish or chicken. Instead of piling on the mayo, add mango, papaya, a few pine nuts, and a little honey to chicken salad. A fruit salad dressing of pureed bananas, yogurt, poppyseeds, and orange juice contains only 30 calories per tablespoon.
- Use pureed cooked potatoes, carrots, or beans instead of cream, butter, and flour to thicken soups.
- Add flavor extracts of almond, vanilla, or rum to boost flavor in pies, cakes, cookies, and pudding to make up for cutbacks in salt, fat, and sugar.
- Instead of moistening hot cereal with butter and milk, use cinnamon and fruit butters, or Butter Buds.
- Add texture and taste to foods with sesame seeds, sunflower seeds, or water chestnuts.

128. Beware of Misleading Labels

The fact that a food product is labeled as cholesterol-free doesn't always mean that it is a heart-healthy food. Cholesterol can be found in animal fats only, but foods like coconut and palm kernel oil, although cholesterol-free, are extremely high in saturated fat. Hydrogenated oil also means saturated fat. So watch out for hidden fats.

129. Using Jelly Will Keep You out of a Jam

If you can't eat bread without butter on it, and you haven't quite developed a taste for margarine just yet, use jelly. Jams and jellies are good substitutes for butter in that they are tasty, have fewer calories, and have no fat.

130. Put Your Recipes on a Diet

The next time you make a dish, try cutting the fat in it by 25 percent. The trick to *successfully* cutting fat from your diet is not to merely remove it, but to replace it with a substitute that's equally satisfying.

Here are some pointers.

- Use ground turkey (without skin) in meat loaf or spaghetti sauce. Use less meat and more vegetables and grains in casseroles. Remember that for the same 5 grams of fat, you can eat either 3 ounces of skinless chicken breast, 10 ounces of haddock, or 6 cups of kidney beans.
- Substitute the same amount of low-fat yogurt or buttermilk for sour cream, milk, or butter. Help retain moisture in muffins and pancakes by adding moistened oatmeal or bran.
- Use egg whites with a little added vegetable oil and nonfat dry milk powder in place of whole eggs.
- For flavor, use a few walnuts or a small amount of sesame oil or Butter Buds, a commercial butter substitute.
- Use pine nuts in pesto sauce, pasta dishes, stir-fries, and other dishes that can benefit from their nutlike flavor. Low in saturated fat and with no cholesterol, pine nuts are an ideal food source for people modifying their fat intake. They're also high in omega–5 fatty acids, compounds that may turn out to benefit the heart.

131. Splash on the Olive Oil

Olive oil, along with avocados and nuts, is high in monounsaturated fat—a special fat that actually lowers cholesterol. Even more surprising is that foods high in this kind of oil selectively lower the bad cholesterol, leaving the good kind intact.

As with all oils, olive oil tends to be calorie-dense. So how do you reap the benefits? Start by maintaining a low-fat diet, the less-than-30-percent-fat variety. Once you've trimmed your diet, "supplement" it with about 2 to 3 tablespoons of olive oil a day—or an equivalent amount of mono-rich foods: 3½ tablespoons of almonds, half an avocado, 4 teaspoons of canola (rapeseed) oil, 2½ tablespoons of peanut butter, or 1½ tablespoons of peanut oil.

That doesn't mean dump on the oil. Instead, use monos to replace some of the other fats remaining in your diet.

132. Choose Oils Carefully

Ten-to-40-weight oil is good for a car; humans, on the other hand, need to buy oil that is a little lighter. If you're reaching for some salad oil or adding oil to a recipe, choose the one that is the least saturated. The following is a list of oils that range from least saturated to most, or best to worst.

- Canola (rapeseed) oil
- Safflower oil
- Sunflower oil
- Corn oil
- Olive oil
- Hydrogenated sunflower oil
- Sesame oil
- Soybean oil
- Peanut oil
- Cottonseed oil
- Palm oil
- Palm kernel oil
- Coconut oil

133. Avoid Those Tropical Oils

Thought you'd cut down on calories by having a couple of snack crackers instead of a bowl of potato chips, did you? You might be surprised to learn that snack crackers made with palm or coconut oil have twice the saturated fat of beef.

Many commercially prepared crackers and baked goods are made with palm or coconut oil, which contains no cholesterol. But they have nearly double the amount of saturated fat that meat has.

Look for foods that contain polyunsaturated fat. It's found mainly in vegetable oils and has been shown to lower blood cholesterol levels.

134. Give Your Cracker the Fat Test

Here's an easy way to gauge the fat content of your favorite cracker: Rub it with a paper napkin. If it leaves a grease stain, it's high in fat.

135. Pass Up the Prime

Fancier cuts of meat are your worst choices when it comes to heart health, because the more fat in a meat, the better "grade" it gets. This system discriminates against lean beef by giving the best-sounding, highest grades, such as "prime" and "choice," to the fattiest cuts, not the healthiest.

For lean beef cuts, buy flank steak, round steak, or sirloin steak, round roast (top, bottom, or eye of round), rump roast, or sirloin tip. Another good choice is extra-lean ground round.

In pork, pick loin chops (also called center-cut pork chops), or fresh ham (pork leg), Canadian bacon, or lean boiled center-slice ham. (Rinse Canadian bacon and ham in water to remove some salt.)

136. Cut Off the Fat

Eaten in moderation, meat can be part of a cholesterol-lowering diet, concludes a study in the *British Medical Journal.* The secret is to trim all fat off before cooking. The result will be a dietary-fat content of 27 percent—well below the 40 percent most people consume.

Another way to eat less meat is to cut down on the portions that you eat. Slice it, chop it, or sliver it into other dishes so that it becomes just a part of the meal, not the star.

Then serve it less. The American Heart Association recommends that you eat 6 ounces of meat or less a day. A good way to do that is to cut it out of your breakfast menu. When you're used to that, cut it slowly out of your lunch menu. Instead of a corned beef or salami sandwich, have turkey or tuna fish on rye.

137. Consider Becoming a Vegetarian

Meat eaters seem to have higher cholesterol levels than people who don't eat meat, according to a British study.

Researchers in England measured the blood cholesterol levels in more than 3,000 people. They found that meat eaters had the highest cholesterol levels of all the participants. Vegetarians and people who ate fish but no meat had lower levels. Vegans, those who eat no meat, dairy products, or eggs, had the lowest levels.

"The differences in total cholesterol concentration suggest that the incidence of coronary heart disease may be 24 percent lower in lifelong British vegetarians and 57 percent lower in lifelong vegans than in meat eaters," say the researchers.

Here's another argument for eating less meat: By substituting soybean protein (with added lecithin) for protein-providing meat sources, members of a Swedish study were able to reduce their cholesterol levels by an additional 22 percent below the level they achieved by following a typical cholesterol-reduction diet.

Not only did this diet lower the LDL level, it tended to increase the level of beneficial HDL. For some people this diet may be an effective substitute for cholesterol-lowering drugs. Please check with your doctor to consider the health benefits this type of diet may offer.

138. Vegetarian Diets Offer Double Protection

Vegetarians tend to have lower blood pressure and cholesterol levels—two well-known risk factors for heart disease. It's been assumed that both these benefits were simply the result of abstaining from meat. But Frank M. Sacks, M.D., at Harvard Medical School, says his experiments show that low-fat, low-meat diets account only for the lower levels of blood cholesterol seen in vegetarians. He suspects that it's the higher levels of minerals—magnesium, calcium, and potassium—in the fruits and vegetables vegetarians eat that protect them from high blood pressure.

139. Develop a Taste for Fish

Fish is good for your heart, for two reasons. First, fish is lower in saturated fat than beef, pork, or lamb, so it's a good substitute for meat. Second, many fish contain significant amounts of omega–3 fatty acids—a special heart-protecting substance.

In the 1970s, population studies of Greenland Eskimos, who eat a high-fat diet consisting mainly of fatty fish, suggested that eating marine fish—and the omega–3 fatty acids contained in fish oils—was associated with a lower-than-average incidence of coronary artery disease. The theory that fish oils protect against heart disease gained strength when scientists noted that Greenland Eskimos who migrated to Denmark and ate a Danish diet lost their edge against heart disease.

Subsequent experiments found that in some people, omega–3 fatty acids lower blood levels of triglycerides, a blood fat linked to heart disease. Omega–3's can lower elevated triglycerides by approximately 30 to 40 percent within as little as two weeks, according to Carlos A. Dujovne, M.D., director of the Lipid and Atherosclerosis Prevention Clinic, University of Kansas Medical Center, Kansas City.

Other studies suggest that introducing omega–3's to the diet widens arteries, lowers blood pressure, decreases blood-clotting tendencies, and exerts other beneficial effects on the heart and arteries.

The biochemistry behind the omega–3 fatty acid link is very complex, and the evidence isn't entirely conclusive. Nevertheless, many doctors say they have good reason to believe that consuming omega–3 fatty acids in the form of fish can reduce an individual's risk of coronary artery disease, especially when done as part of an overall heart-disease-prevention strategy.

"There's no question that eating fish instead of meat will lead to less coronary disease," says Stuart Rich, M.D., a cardiologist at the University of Illinois.

So the prescription from the experts is to dine on fish at least twice a week. Salmon, tuna, mackerel, herring, anchovies, sardines, shad, and trout are rich in omega–3 fatty acids.

140. Go for the Albacore

Tuna ranks right up there with salmon and sardines in heart-healthy omega–3 fatty acids, according to scientists from MIT's Sea Grant Program.

Solid white albacore was found to be the best omega–3 source, containing approximately twice as much as other tuna varieties. And tuna packed in water proved a better source than tuna packed in oil, due to fewer omega–3's being lost to drainage. Water-packed tuna lost only about 3 percent of its beneficial fatty acids when drained, while oil-packed tuna lost 25 percent.

141. Say Yes to Soy

One of the fatty acids in soybean oil may be converted by the body into the same kind of heart-healthy fatty acids found in fish, report researchers at the U.S. Department of Agriculture's Northern

Regional Research Center in Peoria, Illinois. The key ingredient is linoleic acid, which is converted into the same omega–3 oils found in fish, depending upon the body's need for this element.

Good sources of linoleic acid are liquid (nonhydrogenated) soybean oil and canola oil.

142. Try Nuts, Beans, and Seeds

For those who don't care for the taste of fish, there are alternatives. Walnuts, walnut oil, soybeans, tofu, beans, butternuts, canola (rapeseed) oil, and purslane (a creeping, flowering, little succulent plant), are all good sources of omega–3's.

143. Check Out Chicken

Another way to improve your overall diet is to eat less beef and more chicken. Next to fish, chicken is the best option as a substitute for beef. Although it doesn't contain omega–3's, it has a lot less saturated fat than red meat.

When cooking chicken, it's better to use it in a casserole or stew than it is to roast or bake it with the skin on. The skin of the chicken contains most of the fat, so cook it without the skin, or at least remove the skin before you eat the bird.

144. Pass the Lemongrass

Lemongrass oil, used as a flavoring in oriental cooking, reduced serum cholesterol by more than 10 percent in one-third of those who participated in a study at the University of Wisconsin-Madison. A compound in the oil apparently decreases synthesis of cholesterol from fats just as some fruits and vegetables do, says Charles Elson, M.D., who conducted the study.

145. Fill Up on Fiber

People who eat the most dietary fiber have the lowest death rates due to heart disease.

Eating 16 grams of fiber or more a day may reduce risk from heart disease-related death, researchers report in the *American Jour-*

nal of Epidemiology. Even upping daily dietary fiber intake from 12 grams to 18 grams reduced heart-disease death risk by 25 percent in a study of 859 elderly people. (Fiber has also been credited with preventing colon cancer and other diseases.)

Scientists are still searching for a reason behind this phenomenon. "We know that certain kinds of fiber, such as oat bran, are more effective in lowering cholesterol than other kinds," says Elizabeth Barrett-Conner, M.D., from the School of Medicine at the University of California, San Diego. "But we think that fiber does more for the heart than just lower cholesterol. It's been suggested, for example, that fiber might hinder the formation of blood clots that can lodge in the arteries causing heart attacks and strokes."

146. Eat More Oats, the Top Cholesterol Fighter

An amazing ability to help lower cholesterol levels has garnered newfound fame for oats and oat bran. Oats have the ability to lower cholesterol because they are a concentrated source of soluble fiber (soluble means it dissolves in water).

Scientists know soluble fiber increases the output of bile, a digestive fluid made with cholesterol, in the stool. They theorize that the liver then has to make more bile, using more cholesterol. That leaves less cholesterol to circulate in the blood and gum up your arteries. Other theories hold that soluble fiber helps reduce the liver's cholesterol production.

Research shows that eating 2 ounces of oats a day along with a diet low in saturated fat can lower blood cholesterol levels in people with high levels of blood fats.

FACT OF LIFE

It's Cheap and Effective

Oat bran has been found to be just as effective at lowering cholesterol as drugs—and plenty cheaper. The amount of oat bran needed to lower cholesterol by 13 percent in a year (1½ cups daily) would cost $249. A year's supply of the cholesterol-lowering drug cholestyramine needed to achieve that same reduction would cost $1,442; colestipol would cost $879.

Oat bran, however, does not stop its work with cholesterol. It also has potential to lower triglycerides.

Medical students participating in a study showed an 8.3 percent reduction in their triglyceride levels after eating two oat bran muffins a day for four weeks. Muffins made of wheat bran or a wheat and oat bran mix had no effect.

147. Advice for New Converts to Oat Fiber

To introduce oat fiber to your diet, James Anderson, M.D., a noted fiber researcher from the University of Kentucky, offers this advice.

- The first week, add about ⅓ cup of dry oat bran to your daily diet. You can get that amount in two oat bran muffins.
- Drink lots of fluids—at least eight glasses a day. Fiber normally draws water into the intestine. Without enough water, fiber can block the intestines.
- To round out the diet, consider taking a multivitamin and mineral supplement. "Since we don't know the long-term effects of fiber on vitamin and mineral absorption, we prescribe a supplement as a precaution," says Dr. Anderson.
- At week two, if your body has adjusted to the increase in fiber so far, double your intake of soluble fiber. If you like oat bran, aim for ⅔ cup of oat bran a day. That's about four oat bran muffins or two muffins and ⅓ cup of oat bran cereal per day.

148. Add Beans to Your Menu

Beans also contain considerable amounts of soluble fiber and can be as potent as oats when it comes to fighting cholesterol.

In one study, a team of researchers led by Dr. Anderson studied 20 men, aged 34 to 66, with an average cholesterol level of 260. The men split into two groups. For three weeks, one group added 1½ cups of pinto and navy beans (cooked or in soup) to their daily diets. The other group added a cup of dry oat bran—served as hot cereal and in five muffins—each day.

The men's total cholesterol fell, on an average, 60 points for both groups. LDL dropped 46 points.

In another study, Dr. Anderson evaluated ten men with cholesterol levels averaging 309 to find out how oat bran and beans work in the long run. Six months into the study, the men's cholesterol had dropped an average of 76 points. Their LDL averaged 52 points lower.

In men who were monitored for two years, cholesterol and LDL had fallen slightly more. And HDL had gained 3 points, another indicator of improved protection from heart disease.

Don't worry about getting bored with beans. Legumes are among the most versatile of all foods. You can eat them in purees, dips, casseroles, soups, stews, salads, sauces, curries, croquettes, burritos, stir-fries, sandwich spreads—whatever you like.

149. Scout Out Corn Bran

If you get bored with oatmeal, eat corn flakes instead. In a report in the *Journal of the American Dietetic Association*, researchers at Georgetown University Hospital say people who added corn bran— like that found in some breakfast cereals—to their low-cholesterol diets experienced a 20 percent drop in serum cholesterol levels and a 31 percent dip in triglycerides within 12 weeks. (Popcorn counts, too.)

150. Make Barley Soup

Preliminary research suggests that barley may have cholesterol-lowering qualities similar to oats. Barley contains one of the same components present in oat bran but absent in wheat bran.

In one study of men aged 35 and older, one group was assigned to a barley diet and the other a wheat-bran diet for four weeks. Cholesterol levels dropped in the barley group. Cholesterol levels rose, however, in the wheat-bran group.

151. Seek Out Soy Fiber

Add soy fiber to the list of dietary fibers that lower cholesterol. Cholesterol levels dipped 5 percent in people who added 25 milligrams of soy fiber to a low-fat, low-cholesterol diet, say researchers at Washington University School of Medicine in St. Louis.

152. Mix and Match Your Top Fibers

One cup of cooked beans contains the same amount of soluble fiber as ⅔ cup of oat bran. So, if you like beans, you can substitute beans for some of the oat bran in your diet. Two oat bran muffins for breakfast and a bowl of chili containing ½ cup of cooked beans for lunch, for example, will easily fill the bill.

153. Two Carrots a Day Keep Cholesterol Away

Carrots are yet another excellent way of lowering cholesterol levels, say researchers for the Department of Agriculture. Two carrots eaten daily can reduce cholesterol by as much as 20 percent. The reason behind this lies in the calcium pectate found in carrot fiber, which helps speed up the body's metabolism of cholesterol.

Other good cholesterol fighters are onions, broccoli, and cabbage.

154. Go for the Grapefruit, Not the Juice

Research at the University of Florida in Gainesville suggests that grapefruit pectin—a type of soluble fiber found in the rind and fleshy parts of the fruit—may be a cholesterol fighter.

In a study there, 27 participants took either placebos or capsules (equivalent to 3 tablespoons) of concentrated grapefruit pectin each day. After two months, cholesterol levels that started at about 275 dropped an average of 7.6 percent in the group taking pectin. And for some, cholesterol dropped more than 10 percent. Total cholesterol in the placebo group stayed the same.

155. Brewed Coffee Is Preferred

A study in the professional journal *Modern Medicine* reported that cholesterol and LDL rose significantly in people who drank coffee that was boiled (percolated).

The researchers found no significant changes in cholesterol or LDL when people consumed coffee that was drip-brewed. Their theory is that the filtering process of brewing may remove the detrimental compounds.

156. Treat Your Blood to Garlic and Onions

"Clinical studies seem to be pretty much in agreement that there's something in garlic that helps prevent blood from clotting," says Eric Block, Ph.D., chairman and professor of the Department of Chemistry at the State University of New York at Albany. Components of garlic have been found to change the surface membrane of platelet cells so that they're less likely to stick together and form the kinds of blockages that can spell disaster for people with heart and circulatory disease.

Right now the best way to take advantage of garlic's blood-thinning effects is to eat whole bulbs, Dr. Block says. Ready-made garlic preparations are less likely to have anticlotting action.

You might also want to load up on onions, which seem to have similar, although less potent, chemical properties, Dr. Block says.

157. Exercise Fat Away

When you eat a high-fat meal, you can lower its damaging effect by exercising afterward, suggest researchers at Rockefeller University. Exercising after a high-fat meal reduces triglyceride levels by 32 percent. These dietary fat particles normally remain high for up to 8 hours after eating.

158. Make Hard Water Your Drink of Choice

There may be a relationship between the hardness of the water you drink and your risk of getting heart disease, according to the World Health Organization and the National Academy of Sciences. Specifically, harder water has been linked to decreased mortality from heart disease.

Some studies have shown that the high-calcium content of hard water might influence the rate of heart disease. Calcium might be protective against high-blood cholesterol levels and high blood pressure. Another possible explanation is that while hard water may not be protective, soft water is detrimental. Because of its low-calcium and magnesium content, soft water is more acidic. Toxic metals are more likely to dissolve in it, and water softeners place an overdose of sodium in the water.

If your house does have a water softener, you can avoid the problem. Have a hard-water line connected to your cold-water kitchen faucet and use that as your source of drinking water. If you live in a soft-water area and are concerned about heavy metals, you can install a water filter that removes them, or you can use bottled water.

Exercise to Your Heart's Content

159. Exercise Is as Good as Diet

Exercise can reap the same results as dietary restrictions when it comes to lowering your risk for heart disease, according to the results of one study.

Researchers at Stanford University and Washington University set out to examine the effects of exercise without dieting as well as dieting without exercise on 155 overweight men. They found that both dieting alone and and exercising alone are equally effective in boosting beneficial HDL cholesterol, lowering harmful triglycerides, and reducing body weight and body fat—all of which are risk factors in heart disease.

Men in both groups experienced increases in HDL levels, but no significant increase on LDL levels. Both groups also experienced weight loss and significant reduction of body fat, but the dieting group also experienced loss of muscle tissues, whereas the exercising group did not.

A combination of dieting and exercise is still the best, notes Peter Wood, D.Sc., Ph.D., principal author of the study and *The California Diet and Exercise Program.* In an either-or situation, however, exercise is the more effective because people are more likely to become hooked on exercise than dieting.

160. Exercise Plus Diet Is Best

Just because you exercise doesn't mean that you can follow a bad diet without suffering some consequences, especially if your cholesterol level is already too high.

A University of Rochester study revealed that exercisers following a high-cholesterol diet for four weeks showed an average increase of 7 percent in serum cholesterol levels—despite their regular workouts.

The bottom line: Regular exercise *combined* with a low-fat diet is still your best bet.

161. Moderate Exercise Will Do

You don't have to be an exercise fanatic to reduce your heart risk. Moderate activity will suffice. One study of 5,930 men and women showed that those who regularly did exercises like walking and stair climbing had more heart-healthy factors going for them than sedentary people. In general, moderate exercisers were less overweight, had lower blood pressure, lower cholesterol, and lower triglyceride levels than their less active peers.

162. Don't Use Age as an Excuse

All ages benefit from regular exercise, but it appears that fitness benefits older people even more—at least in preventing heart disease. A 12-year study from the Honolulu Heart Program found that men age 65 or older who exercised regularly cut their incidence of heart disease by half compared with the sedentary counterparts. Middle-aged men saw a 30-percent improvement when they practiced regular workouts.

163. Disease Doesn't Count You Out, Either

If you've been told you have heart disease, ask your doctor about an exercise prescription.

"We know that patients with coronary artery disease benefit considerably from a prescribed exercise training regimen," says Terence Kavanagh, M.D., medical director of the Toronto Rehabilitation Centre and associate professor in the department of rehabilitation medicine, University of Toronto.

A study done at Duke University Medical Center backs up his assertion. Researchers studied the effects of exercise on 49 people over the age of 64 who had heart disease, high blood pressure, or

Exercise a Big Benefit for Heart Attack Victims

Before 1950, doctors prescribed bed rest—and lots of it—for anyone who'd suffered a heart attack. Now they recommend a progressive, medically supervised program of exercise, along with dietary changes, smoking cessation, relaxation training, and stress reduction.

In fact, studies have found that heart attack victims who are put on a rehabilitation program that includes exercise are less likely to die from a second heart attack. Researchers came to this conclusion after following more than 4,500 heart attack victims over three years.

If you have a heart attack, you can expect an exercise test as early as two weeks afterward to test your tolerance for exertion. Then you'll be prescribed a regimen designed to gradually build up your heart to working at 85 percent of maximum capacity. And you'll be expected to follow this strategy for the rest of your (hopefully long) life.

Doctors now say that a combination of early detection, immediate treatment, follow-up drug therapy, diet modification, and exercise can improve the quality—and perhaps the quantity—of life for people who've had heart attacks.

other chronic health problems. The participants exercised for 90 minutes, three days per week. Activities included walking, stationary cycling, stretching, and weight training. After four months, heart function and other measures of health improved significantly.

"This study demonstrates that elderly individuals, including those with chronic diseases, who participate in an exercise program will experience improvements in cardiovascular fitness, strength, and flexibility," conclude the researchers.

164. Walk Away from Heart Disease

Evidence continues to mount that walking is just about the best thing you can do for your heart. For example, researchers at the University of Minnesota found that HDL levels rose significantly in obese young men who walked briskly for 90 minutes, five days a week, for 16 weeks.

At the University of North Carolina at Chapel Hill, research on

2,802 women found that those who exercise are only one-third as likely to die of a heart attack than those who are sedentary. The study, conducted by Lars Ekelund, M.D., Ph.D., also found that active women had lower blood pressure than nonexercisers. His advice is to walk 3 miles a day three to five days a week.

165. Swimming Is Swell for the Heart

For exercise that's as heart-healthy as jogging but spares your joints undue wear and tear, try swimming.

Researchers at the University of Texas Health Science Center, Dallas, put a group of previously inactive middle-aged adults through 12 weeks of intense swim training. They swam six days a week and trained with weights three days. At study's end their cardiovascular fitness had improved considerably. Maximal oxygen uptake (an important measure of their cardiovascular fitness) increased by an average of about 20 percent. Plus, each contraction of the heart muscle pumped a greater volume of blood through the arteries without elevating blood pressure.

166. The Key Is Calorie-Burning Activity

Aerobic exercises such as jogging, swimming, and walking aren't the only ways you can exercise yourself to a healthier heart. Leisure activities can help the heart, too, says Stanford University's William Haskell, M.D., but only when they burn between 200 and 300 calories a day—about what you would use in an hour of vigorous gardening.

FACT OF LIFE

Death Rate Highest in New York

New York State leads the nation in deaths from heart disease—with 320 of every 100,000 men dying of artery-blocked heart disease. New Mexico has the lowest death rate, with 151 deaths per 100,000, says the Centers for Disease Control. Geographically, the Northeast and Midwest have the highest incidences of heart-disease deaths, while the West has the lowest.

Calorie-burning activities you can do around the home include chopping wood, cleaning windows, scrubbing floors, gardening, washing and polishing the car, or shoveling snow. The trick is to maintain a daily minimum of 30 minutes.

In fact, researchers in the Netherlands found that people who lovingly tend their plants have significantly fewer heart attacks than those who never stop to smell—or grow—the roses.

167. Tally Your Exercise Calories

You can keep track of your exercise quota by tallying the calories you burn via exercise over the course of a week.

A study of 146 men 30 to 55 years old concluded that the "threshold dose of exercise effective for prevention of coronary heart disease" was a total weekly output of 1,000 to 1,499 calories.

168. Lift Your HDL

Heart-healthy HDL cholesterol may get a lift from weights. Researchers at West Virginia University Medical Center found that after eight weeks of pumping iron, participants' HDL had increased 14 percent. Harmful LDL cholesterol levels had dropped 8 percent.

169. Don't Be a Type-A Exerciser

If you're the type of exerciser who feels you always have to finish first, or at least beat your best time, you may be getting less than optimum healthy heart benefits from your workout, says psychologist Walter Buckalew, Ph.D., of Cumberland University in Lebanon, Texas.

Dr. Buckalew compared blood fat levels in relaxed Type-B exercisers with revved-up Type-A exercisers. He found the Type B's had higher levels of HDLs and lower LDL levels than the Type A's had. Normal Type A's who could adopt Type-B behavior while they were exercising had healthier blood fat levels.

If you want to cut down on the internal competition, run on an unmarked course or stop counting swim laps. Instead, set out to exercise for a certain amount of time, or until you come to a natural halt.

170. You Can't Bypass Exercise

If you're a veteran of coronary bypass surgery, don't assume you can retire to the hammock for the rest of your life. You still have to follow your marching orders.

"Post-bypass surgery patients can effectively and safely perform highly intensive upper and lower body aerobic exercise within four to six weeks after surgery," conclude researchers at the Boone Hospital Center in Columbia, Missouri.

They studied 31 coronary bypass patients who progressed from 25 minutes up to 60 minutes of vigorous (about 85 percent of maximum capacity) aerobic exercise, three times a week. Their workouts combined treadmill walking, jogging, rowing, stair climbing, and stationary bicycling. All emerged with substantially lower resting heart rates, an increase in work capacity of over 60 percent, and less flab.

Tips for a Heart-Smart Attitude

171. Find Your Source of Stress

Evidence shows that stress may actually boost your cholesterol levels and throw your blood fats out of balance. Consequently, stress has been linked to heart attacks and "sudden cardiac death."

Before you become stressed out over your stress level, here are some helpful suggestions.

- Don't assume that life in the fast lane is necessarily stressful. Doctors from Harvard Medical School say that calling a hectic pace stressful may actually cause stress where there is none. For some, the best pace may be a fast pace.
- Stop worrying about things that don't matter. Pinpoint what's really important and let the rest take care of itself.
- Rearrange your routine or environment. Sometimes simple changes in your schedule, workload, or surroundings can eliminate big sources of stress.
- Set realistic goals. Aiming too high can lead to a sense of helplessness and hopelessness.
- Don't try to be perfect. You'll only set yourself up for failure—and, in the process, set yourself on a course of higher stress, even burnout.

172. Don't Let Your Marital Status Ruin Your Health

"Separated and divorced persons report the highest rates of hospitalization for heart attack and stroke," says Maurine Venters, Ph.D., of the University of Minnesota. "The loss of a spouse means a loss of social support," she notes. "Ex-marrieds and widowed persons have to create a new network of friends and neighbors—something that the marrieds and never-marrieds never lost. And the loss of stability is one of the things that make this transition a more stressful and less healthy time of life."

Her study also found that a higher proportion of separated and divorced men and women smoked cigarettes and drank more alcohol than people who were widowed, never married, or married. Although they exercised more than any other marital status group, Dr. Venters thinks that these three activities are just attempts to relax and avoid emotional stress.

She recommends that separated and divorced people should concentrate on modifying smoking and drinking habits and on increasing their exercise routines. They should also make an effort to put some social stability back into their lives.

If you fall into one of these categories, don't feel that all the cards are stacked against you, however. The study also found that married men have higher than average levels of blood cholesterol and lower levels of HDL cholesterol than those who have separated or are breaking up.

173. Don't Hang On to a Hostile Heart

At one time, many doctors thought that people with so-called Type-A personalities—always in a hurry, highly competitive, keenly ambitious, and easily annoyed—ran a much greater risk of suffering a heart attack or dying from heart disease than their patient, noncompetitive, and easygoing Type-B counterparts.

But subsequent research at Duke University has revealed that Type A's just may be taking a bum rap. It's not Type A's per se that are setting themselves up for heart failure—it's those who possess a characteristic often associated with the Type-A personality: namely, hostility.

People who are merely ambitious or driven aren't the ones at risk for heart disease, says Redford Williams, M.D., director of Duke's

Cultural Behavioral Medicine Research Center. But people who are hostile—not just irritable, but rude, abrasive, cynical, vengeful, manipulative, or condescending—*are*.

So if hostility is the real heartbreaker, can people change in time to prevent a heart attack? Apparently, they can. Meyer Friedman, M.D., the "grandfather" of Type-A research, offers these tips for rooting out hostility.

- Dump personal myths about hostility—myths that you need hostility to get ahead in the world, that you can't change your hostile ways, that giving and receiving love is a sign of weakness.
- Go out of your way to express your affection and admiration for family members and make a point of accepting any tenderness they show you.
- Make a conscious effort to employ understanding and forgiveness when you encounter people you don't like.
- Take time out every day to examine and appreciate something beautiful.

174. Lower Your Cholesterol with Relaxation Tapes

Relaxation can lower cholesterol, according to one study. In the experiment, heart disease patients were divided into groups that either read for leisure or listened to relaxation tapes twice daily; both groups were also given low-cholesterol diets. By the end of the experiment, the blood pressure and cholesterol levels of the tape group had dropped significantly compared with those of the reading group. Getting the most cardiac benefit were those who initially scored highest on anxiety tests.

175. Take This Crash Course in Patience

With a little practice, people with impatient, hard-driving personalities can cultivate heart-healthy habits. The following drills are divided into two groups. General drills are to be done as often as possible, on no particular timetable. Specific drills are to be done according to schedule—a different drill once a day for seven days, then the sequence repeated week by week throughout the month. Try a different set of seven drills for each month.

For best results, select specific drills from the list below and schedule them throughout a full year. If you're a diehard Type A, these drills will drive you crazy at first, but they're far better than a heart attack.

General Drills

- Announce to your spouse and friends that you intend to turn over a new leaf to whip your Type-A habits (namely, aggravation, irritation, anger, and impatience).
- Start smiling at other people and laughing at yourself.
- Stop trying to think or do more than one thing at a time.
- Play to lose, at least some of the time.
- When something angers you, immediately make a note of it. Review the list at the end of the week and decide objectively which items truly merited your level of anger.
- Listen. Really listen to the conversations of others.

Specific Drills

- For 15 minutes, recall pleasant memories.
- Don't wear a watch.
- At the supermarket, get in the longest checkout line.
- Do absolutely nothing but listen to music for 15 minutes.
- Buy a small gift for a member of your family.
- Cheerfully say "Good morning" to each member of your family and to people you see at work.
- Carefully, slowly scrutinize a tree, a flower, sunset, or dawn.
- Walk, talk, and eat more slowly.
- On two different occasions, say to someone, "Maybe I'm wrong."
- Tape-record your dinnertime conversation, then play back the tape to see whether you interrupt or talk too fast.

176. Take Responsibility for Your Heart Health

Researchers from the University of Connecticut School of Medicine report that heart attack victims who viewed their first attack as their own fault and who thought there might be positive lessons to

Nappers Have Healthier Hearts

A University of Athens Medical School study found that Greek men who napped at least 30 minutes a day were 30 percent less likely to have heart problems than those who didn't nap.

be learned from their ordeal suffered fewer second attacks than people who tended to pass the blame.

People who accept blame for their condition are more likely to take charge of what caused it, the researchers say. The people who blame stress or being victimized by others, conversely, seem less likely to take charge, leaving open the likelihood of a second attack.

The moral? No one is in a better position to protect your heart than you are.

177. Put on a Happy Face

Being happy and having a positive outlook may help people with heart disease avoid heart attacks and other health problems, says Washington University psychologist Robert Carney, Ph.D.

About 1 in 5 coronary heart disease patients is seriously depressed, says Dr. Carney. So patients (and their friends and relatives) should be on guard for depression symptoms that last more than two weeks. These include being listless, being unable to concentrate, eat, or sleep, and losing interest in hobbies.

Nutritional Therapy to Help the Heart

178. Ask Your Doctor about Niacin

More and more doctors are prescribing the B vitamin niacin to their patients with heart disease. Studies have consistently confirmed niacin's ability to lower blood cholesterol and triglycerides. In fact, it's now standard therapy for people with genetically caused superhigh cholesterol.

But be careful. Experts point out that you should never take niacin in doses above the U.S. Recommended Daily Allowance (20 milligrams) without medical supervision. In high doses, niacin is considered a drug and may have many druglike side effects—flushing, stomach upset, elevated glucose levels, and others. Your doctor may be able to minimize these.

By the way, niacinamide, a popular form of niacin, doesn't cause flushing, but neither does it affect blood fats.

179. Look to Vitamin C for Further Protection

In larger-than-life doses, vitamin C packs a one-two punch that may help older people hit cholesterol hard. Researchers at the USDA Human Nutrition Research Center on Aging at Tufts University studied almost 700 people over age 60 and found that a higher level of vitamin C in the blood correlated with a higher level of HDL cholesterol. But the level of total cholesterol was not higher, an indication that harmful LDL was reduced by vitamin C. Studies of other age groups have shown similar results.

The researchers estimate that an intake of about 1 gram (1,000 milligrams) of vitamin C per day could increase HDL levels by 8 percent. Since this is far higher than the Recommended Dietary Allowance (RDA) of 60 milligrams and also much higher than the level of vitamin C found in even the richest food sources, medical guidance is recommended.

180. Get Adequate E

"The amount of vitamin E in blood and blood vessels may be a factor in determining how rapidly you develop atherosclerosis," says Lawrence Machlin, Ph.D., director of Hoffmann-LaRoche's clinical nutrition department.

Preliminary studies show that when subjects (in this case, monkeys) were given supplemental vitamin E, plaque formation slowed, compared with monkeys on the same diet without vitamin E.

Another study from Scotland offers evidence that vitamin E shields red blood cells from oxidation damage brought on by cigarette smoke, a contributing factor in heart disease.

And a study at Brown University adds to previous evidence that vitamin E makes platelets less likely to form blood clots. In a six-week laboratory study by Manfred Steiner, M.D., Ph.D., platelets from ten volunteers given 400 to 1,200 international units of vitamin E were found to be less sticky than normal. Whether vitamin E will have similar effect in people with clotting abnormalities that can lead to heart attacks isn't known, he says.

Taken in large amounts, vitamin E can have a potentially dangerous blood-thinning effect in some people, such as those on anticoagulant drugs and those with a vitamin K deficiency. Check with your doctor before taking vitamin E supplements.

181. Vitamin E May Make Surgery Safer

Bypass surgery is meant to circumvent years of arterial damage caused by heart disease. But this extensive operation also causes some damage. It creates an excess of destructive particles called free radicals, which cause microscopic damage to cells of the lungs and heart.

Researchers at the Mayo Clinic, Rochester, Minnesota, found that patients given 2,000 international units of vitamin E 12 hours before bypass surgery had much lower blood levels of free radicals than patients who did not get vitamin E. They also found that in unsupplemented patients, vitamin E levels plummeted after surgery. In patients who'd received the vitamin E dose before surgery, levels remained normal.

"I'd recommend that patients receive a dose of vitamin E before heart surgery," says the study's main researcher, Nicholas Cavarocchi, M.D., now at Temple University. "An adequate amount of this vitamin could help make this a safer procedure."

182. Make Sure You're Getting Ample Magnesium

People with life-threatening arrhythmias have recovered their natural rhythm with no treatment other than magnesium supplementation. A magnesium-dependent enzyme helps generate the energy that gives each heartbeat its power. In magnesium-deficient people, the enzyme cannot function effectively.

The National Academy of Sciences recommends 300 to 350 milligrams of magnesium daily. If you suspect that you are not getting adequate magnesium (good sources include rice bran, pumpkin seeds, all-bran cereal, tofu, spinach, oysters, and broccoli), discuss it with your doctor.

183. Copper and Zinc Can Help

Trace metals in your diet, especially copper and zinc, seem to help prevent two kinds of dangerous diseases of the heart (cardiomyopathy and angiopathy), suggests a decade of studies conducted at the University of Cincinnati Medical Center. This is especially worrisome because dietary deficiencies of one or both of these essential trace metals are common in the United States.

Good sources of copper include crab, sunflower seeds, almonds, and prunes. Look to oysters, lean ground beef, pumpkin seeds, and Swiss cheese for zinc.

184. Fish Oil Shows Added Protection

Several studies have demonstrated significant benefits for heart patients when they increase their intake of supplemental omega–3 fatty acids.

In one study at the Dallas Veterans Administration Hospital, researchers were curious about the effects of fish oil on men scheduled to undergo angioplasty, a procedure in which plaque-clogged arteries are opened by passing a tube through them. One problem with angioplasty is that, in the months after the procedure, the vessels can accumulate more plaque and close up again, a process called restenosis.

The researchers took a group of 82 men who were scheduled for angioplasty. Half the men were given conventional therapy, which included aspirin and an anticlotting drug. The other half received the aspirin and drug plus 18 fish-oil capsules (3.2 grams) daily. The treatment began seven days before angioplasty and continued for six months afterward.

After three to four months, the researchers found that restenosis of the blood vessels occurred in 36 percent of men in the control groups, but in only 16 percent of the men who received the fish oil supplementation.

The researchers concluded that dietary omega–3 supplementation "is safe and reduces the occurrence of early restenosis" after angioplasty.

Note, however, that the effect of high doses of fish oil supplements is still not known, and they are not recommended without a doctor's prescription.

Life Extension through Drugs

185. It's as Easy as an Aspirin Every Other Day

If you're a man age 50 or older, you may want to talk to your doctor about the possibility of taking an aspirin every other day. Researchers from Harvard Medical School and Brigham and Women's Hospital in Boston, found that taking the drug may cut the risk of heart attack by 44 percent.

They studied the effect of low-dose aspirin (325 milligrams) on 11,037 men over the course of five years. Another 11,034 men received nonactive white tablets that looked like aspirin. None of the 22,071 men had symptoms of heart disease at the beginning of the study. Nevertheless, 239 people taking the placebo suffered a heart attack, while considerably fewer—139—of the people taking aspirin had a heart attack.

The researchers also noticed that the aspirin seemed to benefit only those age 50 and older. Although the experiment was done only on men, the researchers said women probably can get the same benefit.

Presumably, aspirin prevents heart attacks by inhibiting the tendency of blood platelets to form blood clots or artery plaque.

186. Opt for the Laxative with Extra Strength

A common over-the-counter bowel regulator may also help regulate cholesterol levels in people who take it. In a study conducted by Dr. Anderson of the University of Kentucky College of Medicine, men with elevated cholesterol who took a standard dose of Metamucil three times a day dropped cholesterol levels by an average of 15 percent.

Research suggests that the active ingredient in Metamucil, a plant fiber derived from the husks of psyllium seed, is responsible for the reduction. Metamucil and other seed products could be used as an auxiliary treatment when diet alone is not effective, suggests the study. Their advantage is that they don't produce side effects commonly experienced with potent cholesterol-lowering drugs.

187. Drugs Can Lower Cholesterol

If your cholesterol is so high that it becomes a serious, life-threatening problem, there are a number of prescription medications that can bring it down, each in a different way.

"Lovastatin [marketed as Mevacor] is the newest one," says Donald A. Smith, M.D., director of the lipid unit at New York's Mount Sinai Medical Center. Derived from a kind of fungus, lovastatin works by inhibiting an enzyme that plays a part in making cholesterol. The body's cells, which need cholesterol, are then forced to take it from the bloodstream. In tests, lovastatin lowered harmful LDL by 20 to 40 percent.

In one study, adding lovastatin to the usual diet treatment for people with superhigh cholesterol levels provided a dramatic additional drop in cholesterol. At the conclusion of the testing, total cholesterol had been reduced 58 percent from the original levels.

Another drug in the cholesterol-lowering arsenal is gemfibrozil (Lopid). This drug attacks triglycerides. In tests, it lowered triglycerides 40 to 45 percent and raised levels of HDL cholesterol by 8 percent. The combination resulted in a 30 percent decrease in heart disease over five years.

In the Helsinki Heart Study, a five-year trial that followed more than 4,000 men with high cholesterol, half the men took gemfibrozil, half a placebo. Those who took the drug had 34 percent less coronary heart disease than those on the placebo. Their LDL levels dropped 11 percent while HDLs rose by 11 percent compared to the men on the placebos.

Other drugs to ask your doctor about include cholestyramine (Questran) and colestipol (Colestid). Both help the body use up more cholesterol, so there's less in the bloodstream.

Life-Extension Tools

Lifepak 100

The Food and Drug Administration has approved, for at-home use, an automatic defibrillator similar to those routinely used by paramedics and emergency room physicians to revive heart attack victims. (By delivering a precisely measured amount of electricity, these machines can restore normal rhythm to a heart that's gone into ventricular fibrillation—fluttery, disorganized beats that fail to fill the heart with blood and can result in death.)

Called the Lifepak 100, the at-home defibrillator must be prescribed by a physician and is recommended for people who've already had a heart attack or who are at risk of sudden cardiac arrest. A microcomputer within the unit reads the victim's heart rhythm from pads attached to the patient's chest. It instructs the rescuer to "shock" or "don't shock" the patient. Up to three shocks can be given. With this device and the use of cardiopulmonary resuscitation (CPR), a home rescuer may be able to sustain life until help arrives.

The Lifepak 100 costs close to $4,000, and, according to the manufacturer, the cost is covered by many insurance companies. For more information, contact the Physio-Control Corporation, 11811 Willow Road, N.E., P.O. Box 97006, Redmond, WA 98073.

EKG by Phone

It's sometimes tough for doctors to diagnose irregular heartbeat. A patient's heart may flutter and sputter at home but behave normally in the doctor's office. Now it's possible to capture the heart's idiosyncracies within minutes, on paper, with a device called an Event Transmitter and a phone call.

You put the transmitter—a box the size of a small radio—on your chest and call your medical center. Identify yourself and place the telephone mouthpiece on the unit. A machine at the other end monitors your heartbeat, creating an instant electrocardiogram.

Before undergoing drug therapy for cholesterol, however, be sure to thoroughly discuss the treatment with your physician. Cholesterol-lowering drugs do cause side effects, and their long-term effects still are not fully known.

188. Aspirin Plus Drug Can Save a Life

The combination of two standard heart treatments, streptokinase (a clot-dissolving drug given intravenously at the hospital) and aspirin (one-half tablet, or 160 milligrams, daily for a month after a heart attack) can significantly reduce heart attack deaths.

The key to success is to work quickly. Using the therapy within 4 hours of the first heart attack symptom decreased chances of death to 53 percent of the odds for patients who didn't get the treatment.

Even delayed by 24 hours, the therapy reduced the death rate by an impressive 38 percent—better than any other available treatment. Samuel Z. Goldhaber, one of the study's U.S. coordinators, expects an aspirin-plus-clot-dissolver therapy to eventually become standard.

189. TPA: Another Lifesaver

Hundreds of people, including talk show host Larry King, credit the clot-dissolving drug known as TPA (tissue plasminogen activator) for saving their life following a heart attack.

In a one-year study at North Shore University Hospital in Manhasset, New York, TPA reduced the number of heart attack deaths by 60 percent. (Most heart attacks are the result of a blood clot that forms in a coronary artery.) TPA is a genetically engineered protein that can dissolve blood clots in 10 minutes if injected within 6 hours of a heart attack.

190. Hydralazine Helps Delay Surgery

Long-term treatment with hydralazine, an antihypertension drug, partially reverses heart enlargement caused by leaky aortic valves. According to Barry Massie, M.D., at the University of California, San Francisco, treatment with hydralazine may help these patients delay or avoid surgery.

Dr. Massie and Barry Greenbery, M.D., of Oregon Health Sciences University, studied 80 patients over two years. There was an average 18 percent reduction in heart size after 24 months of treatment.

Leaky aortic valves afflict 2 million Americans, and thousands undergo surgery each year to replace faulty valves. Other related drugs continue to be researched to provide patients with the same benefits without some of the side effects.

191. Don't Let Your Nitroglycerin Pill Bomb

When you're faced with a life-threatening cardiac situation, and you reach for your nitroglycerin pill, you need to be sure it'll work. If it's old, or you haven't stored it right, your pill could end up being a dud.

Researchers analyzed nitro pills from more than 150 heart patients and found that 25 percent of the people were carrying around medication that had lost its punch.

For best results, store your pill in the small, amber glass container that it came in. Don't keep cotton or other drugs in the same container. Nitroglycerin can vaporize and be absorbed into these materials.

Keep the container tightly closed and away from heat. Renew your prescription at least every six months.

How do you know if your nitro pill has gone bad? Full-potency nitroglycerin dissolves rapidly, with a distinct tingle, in your mouth. If your pill doesn't do this, it's time to get new pills.

192. Estrogen, a Heart Protector

Estrogen replacement therapy can reduce the risk of heart disease in postmenopausal women, according to the results of a study on 2,188 women. Researchers found that estrogen treatment protected against coronary artery disease independent of other cardiovascular risk factors.

A later study of 1,057 women aged 50 to 79 confirmed that estrogen replacement therapy may lower the risk of heart disease for women. Women on estrogen therapy had higher HDL levels, lower LDL levels, and other favorable measurements than non-estrogen-users.

Estrogen, however, has also been shown to increase the odds of developing endometrial cancer and gallbladder disease—something you and your doctor need to consider.

FACT OF LIFE

Your Emotions and Your Heart

How closely are emotions tied to your heart? Tests done at UCLA found that 6 out of 10 heart patients had constricted coronary arteries and reduced blood flow to their heart following emotionally trying events. This may explain why some people suffer a heart attack immediately following stressful situations, say researchers.

193. Beta-Blockers Can Protect the Stressed

For people constantly feeling the pressures of stress, heart disease becomes a definite possibility. While it's better to make behavioral changes to combat a hard-driving personality than it is to take drugs, studies show that the drug propranolol may protect the hearts of stressed individuals.

Propranolol belongs to a class of drugs known as beta-blockers, used for years to treat high blood pressure. They block the action of adrenaline and other hormones that normally cause the heart to speed up in response to excitement.

In one two-year study, researchers placed both passive and aggressive monkeys in a stressful social environment—a situation practically guaranteed to give the aggressive animals excessive heart disease. But aggressive monkeys that received the drug propranolol didn't develop the expected heart damage.

"If a doctor is debating which hypertensive drug to give his Type-A patient, he may want to consider that beta-blockers could give additional benefits," says Jay Kaplan, coauthor of the study testing propranolol.

Please note that because beta-blockers do "calm" the heart, people who exercise should monitor their pulse. Rates will be lower than normal for their age and/or intensity group.

194. Theophylline May Ease Angina

People suffering from stable angina, chest pain brought on by a shortage of oxygen to a heart under stress, may be able to benefit from theophylline, a drug conventionally used to treat asthma.

In one study, 20 people given intravenous administration of theophylline delayed the onset of exercise-induced angina pain by 46 percent and increased the length of time they could exercise without pain by 24 percent. Taken orally, theophylline delayed onset of pain by 56 percent and increased exercise duration by 35 percent.

195. Repeat: Diet before Drugs

Don't try to coax your doctor into prescribing cholesterol-lowering drugs until you've made an earnest effort to modify your diet.

"No matter how advanced drug therapy becomes, we won't use drugs to lower cholesterol unless we have to," says Robert DiBianco, M.D., of Washington Adventist Hospital, Takoma Park, Maryland, who expects the use of nutritionists by family doctors to increase. "I foresee more doctors referring their heart patients to dietitians who have the time and training to teach people how to make the necessary dietary changes in their lives."

C H A P T E R · 3

LIVE
LEAN,
LIVE
LONGER

Before you postpone your diet (again) until Monday and order that double chocolate fudge cheesecake, listen to this:

"Obesity is linked to heart disease, high blood pressure, non-insulin-dependent diabetes and certain forms of cancer, including colon, rectum, and prostate cancer in men and gallbladder, biliary passage, breast, cervix, uterus, ovarian, and endometrium cancer in women," notes Mel Bircoll, M.D., author of *Freedom from Fat*. "Phrased more bluntly, and quite simply, obesity kills."

Obese? Not you? Well, don't order that cheesecake just yet. Listen to this:

Even an extra 10 or 15 pounds can subtract years from your life. Results from the Framingham Heart Study—the most extensive, long-range study of heart disease among a population—show that for every pound of excess weight you gain after age 30, you shorten your life by six months, and for every pound of excess weight you gain after age 50, you shorten your life by one year.

And that adds up to a lot of potentially lost years when you consider that up to 31 percent of all men and 38 percent of all women in the United States weigh more than they should.

Why Cancer?

Scientists haven't figured out why so many life-threatening diseases are associated with overweight, and the connection is most mysterious with cancer.

In one study, the American Cancer Society kept tabs on 750,000 people for 12 years to see who would get cancer. They discovered an interesting correlation: Those who were the heaviest—40 percent or more over their ideal weight—were most likely to get cancers of the uterus, gallbladder, kidney, stomach, colon, prostate, and breast. And cancer of the uterus was the most prevalent among overweight women. Women who were as little as 10 percent overweight had a 36 percent greater risk of developing this type of cancer than normal-weight women. But for women who were 40 percent or more overweight, their risk skyrocketed to 542 percent, meaning that being fat made them five to six times more susceptible to uterine cancer.

"It could be that a larger person has more body tissue and thus has more cells that could be at risk for cancer," theorizes Demetrius Albanes, M.D., of the Division of Cancer Prevention and Control of the National Cancer Institute in Bethesda, Maryland.

Another popular theory has to do with hormones. Many older overweight women produce extra levels of the female hormone estrogen. After menopause, most of this hormone is manufactured in the fat cells. And the more fat cells you have, the more hormones you can churn out. Some scientists believe high levels of estrogen may cause cancer of the uterus and breast.

Look and Feel Younger

Fortunately, the risks associated with overweight fade when the weight disappears.

"The good news is that once you lose your excess weight, health-risk factors disappear," says Peter M. Miller, M.D., founder of the Hilton Head Institute and author of *The Hilton Head Over–35 Diet*. "At the Hilton Head Institute, we regularly see significant reductions in blood pressure, blood cholesterol levels, and blood sugar levels as clients lose weight. And most of these improvements occur in as little as four weeks!"

Other weight-loss specialists have found similar positive results. "We know that if one of our patients loses 5 pounds, chances are his blood pressure will be lower," says Joseph Stokes, M.D., of the Boston University Medical Center and the Framingham study. "A 1 percent reduction in body weight usually produces a 2-point reduction in blood pressure, and that's a substantial change."

And a Harvard University study of 1,400 overweight people revealed that those who lost just 10 percent of their body weight (that's 15 pounds if you weigh 150) showed big decreases in symptoms of obesity-related diseases, including high blood pressure and diabetes.

If you maintain your proper weight throughout life, you're likely to sidestep a lot of these health problems altogether. Even better, you'll look and feel younger. Without an extra roll of fat around your waist, a pendulous potbelly, or 15 pounds of baggage bringing up the rear, your body will better maintain the firm, slim look of youth. Without that excess poundage to haul around, you'll have energy to spare, enough to do the things you enjoy.

"I've heard so many of my clients tell me that they feel young again after they lose weight," says Dr. Miller. One client told him, "Since I lost 30 pounds, my friends say I look 38 instead of 48! I finally feel in control of my body, and I'm looking forward to being slim for the rest of my life."

Diet Is a Four-Letter Word

One way to avoid overweight, of course, is to eat less, or at least eat *properly*. And that's a start. Studies on eating only enough to maintain a lean body size have proven three things:

- It extends life span.
- It slows down age-related physical deterioration.
- It retards the progress of age-related diseases such as kidney and heart problems.

Of course, most people already know they should eat less. There are millions walking around who have tried and failed. And most have tried *more* than once—a lot more. For those prone to gaining weight, taking it off—and keeping it off—seems to be an endless battle. A study by San Diego University researchers, for example, found that of 400 people who went on a strict diet for six months,

FACT OF LIFE

Go West, Lose Weight?

Nobody knows why, but people living in midwestern states (such as Indiana) tend to be more overweight than people living in western states (such as New Mexico). Health officials at the Centers for Disease Control speculate that regional differences in residents' ethnic backgrounds, diets, and activity levels may account for the differences.

many lost as much as 84 percent of their excess weight. But 30 months later, many had regained up to 82 percent of what they'd lost.

Why are so many weight-loss programs doomed to fail? In the San Diego study, many blamed hard-to-change social environments, such as easy access to fattening foods. (Translated, that means no willpower.) Other popular excuses included stress and boredom. Others blamed it on heredity—they said they were simply meant to be fat.

Weight-loss specialists and researchers will tell you no one is *meant* to be fat. Everyone has the chance to live a lean, long, and healthy life. The secret is knowing the best way to go about it. It doesn't mean going on a diet this week and getting off of it when all the weight's gone. Why? Because dieting doesn't work. At least not permanently. The secret to being lean and staying lean is to adopt a lifestyle of sensible eating habits with which you can live *all the time.*

So, what works? We scoured the books and talked to the experts to find the best weight-control strategies. Here's what we came up with.

A New Way of Eating

196. Eat Lean, Be Lean

Evidence continues to accumulate linking fat intake with the percentage of body fat. In a study of 155 sedentary men whose diets averaged 41 percent fat (11 percent over dietary requirements), body fat ranged from 18.6 to 40.3 percent. (Normal fat level for men is 15 percent.) Researchers found that the men's fat levels and total body weight were not related to their total calorie intake. Instead, the researchers showed that the men's obesity was linked to the unhealthy ratio of fat to carbohydrates in their diet.

In another study, 28 normal-weight premenopausal women ate a 40-percent-fat diet for four months, after which their percentage of body fat was measured. (Normal fat level for women is 18 percent.) Next, they switched to a low-fat diet (20 percent fat) that contained the same number of calories as the high-fat diet. After another four months their body fat was measured again. Although the women's weight remained the same, they reduced the weight of their body fat by an average of 3 percent on the low-fat diet—a reduction that, if continued long term, would result in significant changes in body fat.

Lowering dietary fat intake helps reduce the body's fat stores, the researchers concluded. Replace fat with more complex carbohydrates, such as fruits, vegetables, and whole grains.

197. Choose Oil over Butter

It seems even the *type* of fat you eat can influence weight gain. In one study published in the *American Journal of Clinical Nutrition,* researchers reported that solid fats (such as butter) enhance weight gain more easily than liquid vegetable oils (such as olive oil).

And that's good news. As you've read on page 40, olive oil is a monounsaturated fat that has been linked to heart health. So when your cooking requires oil, make it olive.

198. Eat Low Fat, Eat More

Scientists at Cornell University's Division of Nutritional Sciences tested low-, medium-, and high-fat diets on 24 women. They found that when the women ate low-fat meals, they naturally consumed 627 fewer calories, even though they were eating as much as they wanted. That led them to lose a pound every two weeks.

"Most diets put restrictions on the *amount* of food people eat," explains David Levitsky, Ph.D., of Cornell. "People lose weight but then gain it back. Low-fat could be the kind of diet people can live with permanently to keep the weight off."

By the way, the women also rated their low-fat meals tops in taste.

Eating low fat means increasing your intake of fruits, vegetables, and grains and decreasing your consumption of meats and dairy products. (For more information on adopting a low-fat lifestyle, see the section "Conquering Fat and Cholesterol" in chapter 2.)

199. Snack without Guilt

One visit from a Girl Scout on a cookie drive can undo days of good deeds. But snacking can be an excellent way for calorie counters to sneak much-needed nutrients (but little fat and calories) into their diet. Here's a list of ten snacks (including cookies!) you can eat without worrying about carrying them around on your hips for weeks.

Popcorn, unbuttered, one handful (6 calories)
Asparagus, raw, four stalks (12 calories)
Seedless grapes, ten (34 calories)
Green pepper, one, sliced (36 calories)
Casaba melon, one wedge (38 calories)
Tangerine, one (46 calories)
Sweet cherries, raw, ten (47 calories)
Gingersnaps, two (58 calories)
Nectarine, one (88 calories)
Pineapple, raw, two slices (88 calories)

FACT OF LIFE

Dieters Switching to Light

Fewer Americans are dieting than ever before, says the Calorie Control Council, an association that keeps tabs on the diet food industry. One in 4 adults are on a diet at any given time. That's down 26 percent since 1986. Another trend, however, seems to be emerging. More people than ever before are incorporating low-calorie foods and beverages into their lifestyle.

200. Crackers: Favor Whole-Wheat Flavor

Love crunching on crackers? So much so that you can't bear to give them up? You don't have to! Just choose whole-wheat matzo crackers or German or Scandinavian crackers to munch on. They have the lowest calories per ounce—90 to 100, compared with 140 calories-plus per ounce for softer, richer crackers. And they're fat-free!

201. Drink Yourself Thin

If you don't take beverage calories into account, you may have trouble with your weight and not know why. Did you know that a glass of whole milk has more calories than a brownie, for example? Yes, 159 versus 97! To start you thinking about the calories you drink—which may account for half the calories you consume all day—here is a representative sampling of some popular beverages, showing how greatly they can vary in caloric content per serving.

Club soda (0 calories)
Herb tea, unsweetened, 4 ounces (4 calories)
Instant tea, unsweetened, 4 ounces (4 calories)
Coffee, with half-and-half, 6 ounces (24 calories)
Tomato juice, 4 ounces (24 calories)
Nonalcoholic white wine, 4 ounces (28 calories)
Vegetable juice cocktail, 4 ounces (28 calories)
Grapefruit juice, fresh, 4 ounces (48 calories)
Cream sherry, 1 ounce (59 calories)
Gin, rum, vodka, whiskey, 80 proof, 1 ounce (70 calories)
Skim milk, 8 ounces (88 calories)
White wine, 4 ounces (92 calories)
Light beer, 12 ounces (98 calories)
Kahlua, 1 ounce (119 calories)
Sundance apple cooler, 10 ounces (119 calories)
Classic Coke, 12 ounces (144 calories)
Beer, 12 ounces (156 calories)
Pepsi-Cola, 12 ounces (160 calories)
Chocolate shake, 8 ounces (352 calories)

Looking at these comparisons, even a "high-calorie" drink like a light beer might find a niche on a weight-control program—*if* you can limit yourself to one or two. Think about it: When was the last time you sat at the bar and drank a six-pack of grapefruit juice, which is about equal to beer in calories? Clearly, putting your beverages on a diet is as much a matter of *how much* you drink as what you select.

202. Fall in Love with Vegetables

No one ever got fat eating broccoli—unless, of course, it was dripping with cheese sauce or dipped in sour cream. So make it a habit to eat vegetables at every meal, but learn to enjoy their natural flavor. Drowning them in fat- and calorie-laden accoutrements will only defeat the purpose.

203. Eat a Little, Often

"Avoid large intakes of food at one time," cautions Peter Vash, M.D., of the UCLA Medical Center and vice president of the American Society of Bariatric Physicians. "Space smaller meals throughout the day. This reduces the hormonal signal that causes fat cells to multiply.

"By increasing the frequency of meals and decreasing the amount of each meal, you reduce the amount of insulin released, and that reduces the stimulus for the body to make new fat cells," he says. "Also, smaller and more frequent meals lower the amount of triglycerides [a blood fat] and insulin released to the blood, so there is less available to be converted into fat cells. In effect, your body handles food more efficiently and has less insulin and triglyceride left over for the storage and generation of new fat cells."

FACT OF LIFE

Ads Say "Buy, Eat, Drink"

A survey of 15,010 consumers, conducted for *Advertising Age*, showed that the ads people most frequently remembered were for potential diet-wreckers: Two were for soft drinks, three were for beer, and two were for fast-food chains.

Count Calories the Easy Way

Sure, counting calories is important. But you don't have to be compulsive about it. You can get a good idea of the amount of calories you take in during a day by following the easy guidelines established by June Roth and Harvey M. Ross, M.D., authors of *The Executive Success Diet*. They've grouped most common foods into three basic calorie categories.

200 to 400 Calories

Meat. Nearly all 4-ounce servings of meat fit into this range, with extremely lean cuts at about 250 calories and fatty ones like short ribs at 400.

Poultry. Count 4 ounces of poultry, prepared without the skin or any added fat, as 200 calories.

Fish. Count 200 calories for 4 ounces of unfried fish, prepared with no added butter.

Pies and cakes. Figure 300 calories for fruit pies, 200 for plain cake, and 400 for frosted cake.

100 to 200 Calories

Cheese, milk, and ice cream. Count 100 calories for 1 ounce of most hard cheeses. One cup of whole milk is 160 calories; skim milk is 90. One half cup of regular ice cream is 150 calories.

Cereals and grains. Count all cereals as 100 calories per 1-ounce serving. Pasta is 210 calories for each 5-ounce cooked serving without sauce. Add 30 calories for plain tomato sauce; 150 for meat sauce.

0 to 100 Calories

Eggs. Count 80 calories for a plain egg.

Cream and yogurt. Count 50 calories for 1 tablespoon of most types of cream, including sweet, whipped, and sour. Low-fat plain yogurt is 10 calories a tablespoon.

Vegetables. One half cup serving of most vegetables is 20 calories. Potatoes are 90 calories each.

Fruits. Apples, pears, and bananas are 100 calories each. Grape-

(continued)

Count Calories the Easy Way—*Continued*

fruits and oranges are 50 calories. Peaches, wedges of melon or pine-apple, and ½ cup of berries are 30 calories each.

Breads. Count 60 calories for one slice of bread. Rolls and muf-fins are 150. Crackers are 25 each.

Beverages. Coffee and tea are 0 (15 calories for each teaspoon of sugar). Count all 8-ounce sodas as 100 calories. Count beer as 125 calories per 8 ounces, and wine as 70 calories per 3 ounces. Hard liquor is 100 calories per ounce.

Fats and oils. Count all butter, margarine, shortening, and oils at 100 calories per level tablespoon. Ditto for mayonnaise, Russian dressing, and tartar sauce.

Mind over Platter

204. Examine Your Conscience

Being fat is often the symptom, not the problem, says Barbara Jacobson, coauthor of *Weight, Sex, and Marriage: A Delicate Balance.* Weight gain can often mask a psychological problem.

"We never start obesity treatment by telling people to eat less. We start by helping them find other ways to satisfy their psycholog-ical hunger." For example, eating can be an oasis in a boring or stressful life. Dr. Jacobson suggests keeping a journal to help sort out your feelings about obesity and weight loss. Without this self-understanding, she believes, weight-loss efforts are doomed to failure.

205. Avoid Self-Defeating Thoughts

Even after you identify your problem, little negative thoughts are likely to keep repeating in your mind: "I'm unattractive. I'll never lose weight. It's unfair that I can gain weight on celery, when my friend stays skinny on ice cream and cheesecake."

You can stop this no-win self-talk with a little retraining. Start by taking note of the thoughts that are tripping you up. Joyce Nash, Ph.D., author of *Maximize Your Body Potential*, suggests periodic thought-inspection breaks. "Put stick-on dots from the stationery store on places you typically glance throughout the day—watch, mirror, dashboard. Whenever you see a dot, examine your self-talk. If you find yourself being critical, replace this talk with accepting, supportive, and encouraging thoughts."

206. Accept Responsibility for Your Weight

Do you tend to blame others for your weight problems? Is it your spouse's fault for bringing candy home? When Mom offers a third helping, do you think she's the cause of your weight-loss failure?

The fact is, if you *think* of yourself as a victim, you *will* be a victim. But if you realize that you have some control over the situation, you'll tell your husband or your mom you're on a diet and ask for help in keeping temptation out of your path.

207. Lose Weight for You and No One Else

Don't set out to lose weight to please your spouse, your parents, or your friends. You can only succeed at weight loss when it's something *you* want to do.

208. Stand Up for Your Weight-Control Rights

Learn that it's okay to say an assertive, "No, thank you," when other people coax you to eat food you don't really need.

Learn to communicate. Express your needs and don't be afraid to say no. Be aware of how other people are feeling. Seek out friends who will support you and be there when you need them.

209. Picture the Worst

Visualization can suppress an unruly appetite. Every time you think of a favorite forbidden food, sit quietly, close your eyes, and relax. Picture the tempting food with ugly bugs, mold, or something equally unappetizing covering it. By concentrating on such unattrac-

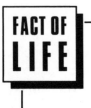

FACT OF LIFE

Women Are the Fatter Sex

A survey of 17,294 adults in Finland showed that both men and women tend to gain weight until age 40. At that point, men level off, but women keep gaining for another 20 years. In the United States and Canada, weight gain peaks about a decade later—at age 50 for men and age 64 for women. So, generally, middle-aged women are more likely to be overweight than middle-aged men.

tive versions of food, you'll find yourself less hungry and better able to fend off any attack to your willpower.

Another way to use this technique involves imagining yourself 10 pounds heavier. Then add a few more pounds. Ask yourself if you still really want to eat. Close your eyes and imagine yourself at your ideal weight.

Successful Strategies for Shedding Pounds

210. Set Reasonable Goals

If your weight-loss goal is too high, you're bound to fall short. That's when you'll start to criticize yourself and feel like a failure. Avoid this cycle of failure by setting realistic, concrete goals, says Dr. Nash. Instead of setting abstract goals like "I want to lose 30 pounds," think in terms of day-to-day: "I'll work to increase my exercise to 30 minutes every other day," or "I'll cut butter from my diet this week."

211. Get a Grip on Yourself

Speaking of concrete goals, here's one way to grasp the challenge ahead: Find an object that weighs what you want to lose and carry it around for a while. You'll quickly realize what a burden this excess weight is to your body. Even 10 pounds means a significant amount of stress.

212. Dodge Your Diet Demons

One of the simplest ways to lose weight is to put temptation out of your path, says Kelly Brownell, Ph.D., a weight-loss specialist at the University of Pennsylvania. All you have to do is break the links in the chain that leads to overeating: Don't go shopping when you're hungry. Don't buy food you shouldn't eat. Don't leave tempting food out on the kitchen counter (or bags of potato chips on top of the refrigerator). Don't put yourself in overeating situations, such as meeting your friends in a restaurant. Break any of these links, and you're on the way to controlling overeating.

213. Keep a Food Diary

Many people gain weight because they honestly don't realize how much they eat. They don't remember the bag of chips that disappeared while they worked at their desk or watched TV or engaged in other "automatic" eating. So record what you taste when you cook, everything you eat, what you were doing at the time, how you felt. Not only will the diary tell you something important about yourself (your temptation times, the emotional states that encourage you to snack), but it may also help you curb unconscious eating patterns once you become aware of when and why they are happening.

214. Get Off the Couch, Potato

Watching television can grow on you—in ways you don't want. One study of 6,138 men found that those who watched TV for more than 3 hours a day were more than twice as likely to be obese than those who watched TV less than 1 hour a day.

215. Freeze Temptation

If the pie on the counter—or anything else, for that matter—is just too great a temptation, and you don't want to throw it away, freeze it. Cut the pie in small pieces and take them out of the freezer only one at a time.

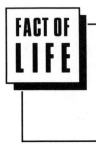

FACT OF LIFE

Prosperity Breeds Obesity?

A report published in the *American Journal of Public Health* found that a higher percentage of Americans are obese than Canadians or Britons. The researchers suggest that affluence may contribute to overweight.

216. Make Dining the Main Event

Doing two things at once, like eating dinner and catching the news, might seem like an efficient way to use your time, but it's not. It can lead to what some weight-loss specialists call "eating amnesia." You don't pay attention to what you're eating, meaning you can eat too fast and too much without even realizing it.

Always eat at the table, with the television off. Concentrate on eating every mouthful slowly and savoring each morsel. Chew everything 10 to 20 times. And count. The idea is to enjoy every morsel.

217. Eat Your Salad First

Europeans may consider it odd to eat a salad before the meal, but salad (topped with a low-calorie, oil-free dressing) will dull your appetite before the entree arrives.

218. Eat Light at Night

Adjust your eating habits so you eat most of your calories early in the day and a light meal in the evening. Studies indicate that people who eat the majority of their calories earlier in the day lose more weight than those who eat the same amount at night. Food consumed early in the day has a better chance of being burned off through daily activity than an evening meal, which is digested while you're sleeping.

219. Water Your Diet

Drink six to eight glasses of water a day. Water itself will help cut down on water retention because it acts as a diuretic. It also dulls the appetite when you drink it before meals, because it gives you the feeling of being full. Also, keep a glass of water by your bed to help quiet the hunger pangs that wake you up.

220. Try the Forklift Diet

Here's a unique strategy that will automatically disqualify some of the most damaging foods from your menu: Eat only foods you can consume with a fork. (Better yet, use a cocktail fork.) You'll find yourself shying away from calorie powerhouses like potato chips, pudding, ice cream, candy bars, pistachios, and yogurt-covered raisins.

221. Try a Little Mood Music

Before sitting down to eat, put on some slow, relaxing tunes. You may find yourself eating less.

That's what researchers at the Johns Hopkins Health, Weight, and Stress Clinic in Baltimore observed when they watched people eat to both fast and slow music.

When slow classical music was playing, people took fewer bites per minute, chewed more, and swallowed before taking another bite. Even though their meals were about 15 minutes longer, they ate less. They also apparently had a happier time, for they talked more with their dinner companions and were more likely to say they'd enjoyed the meal.

222. Soup Slows the Appetite

Eating soup can help suppress your appetite. When researchers at Baylor College of Medicine and Arkansas Department of Health included soup at least once a day in the diet of a group of would-be weight-losers, the soup group wound up considerably slimmer after one year than a group instructed to eat the same number of calories but without soup.

Why? Soup helped them to eat more slowly, allowing them to feel more satisfied than the soupless dieters. Other studies have backed up this theory—people who eat more soup seem to eat less food and gain less weight.

223. Take Time Out for Tea

To break your eating momentum and cut consumption, establish a time-out routine halfway through your meals. Put a large pot of water on the stove when you sit down to eat. When it boils in about 10 or 15 minutes, get up and make yourself a pot of tea. When you go back to the table, you probably won't feel like eating much more.

224. Grocery Shop after Dinner

You already know not to shop on an empty stomach. The best time to do your shopping is when you have a full stomach—like right after dinner.

225. Plan Your Next Dinner after Your Last Dinner

Plan meals on a full stomach, and you'll find less of an urge to think big. A weekly meal plan is even better.

226. Use Diet-Friendly Dinnerware

Eat food from gray, green, or brown plates. Studies show those colors make you eat less. Blue and green are less stimulating to the eye than orange or yellow.

Two other hints from the world of decorator psychology:

• Put your food on smaller plates. It will look like more.
• Eat from your own special plate, on your own special place mat, and adopt the Japanese art of food arranging to make your meal, however spartan, look lovely. This trick helps chronic overeaters and bingers pay attention to their food, instead of consuming it unconsciously.

227. Cheat—Just a Little

Believe it or not, a little cheating can help you stick to your weight-loss plan. Eating too few calories or abandoning your favorite foods will make you feel terrible and may drive you back to your overeating habits. Have ice cream, if you must, but just a little. And be content with a slower weight loss. Remember, you're less likely to gain back what you lose slowly.

228. Stay Out of the Kitchen

Make the kitchen off-limits at any time other than mealtime. Balancing your checkbook at the kitchen table will put you closer to the refrigerator and will make you go way over your calorie budget.

Sneaky Tricks to Trim Calories in the Kitchen

229. Put on the Pressure

If you own a pressure cooker but use it only occasionally (if ever), dig it out and dust it off. Pressure-cooked vegetables, beans, and rice cook up fast and tender in a pressure cooker, with no added fat or loss of moisture.

230. Defat Soups, Stews, and Sauces

When you cook lean ground beef for homemade soups, tacos, chili, or casseroles, pour off all the fat before adding the remaining ingredients. Similarly, after making soups, stews, pot roast, chili, or spaghetti sauce containing meat, refrigerate them and skim off the layer of fat that forms on the surface. (A gravy skimmer does this best.) For every tablespoon of fat you remove, you'll save about 100 calories.

231. Thicken with Potatoes

Don't thicken soup with flour or cream. Instead, cook a potato or two, mash it, and stir it into the broth.

232. Poaching Is Perfection

As a low-fat cooking method, poaching is hard to beat. Simmering fish or poultry in water or seasoned stock over gentle heat is the leanest way to prepare these foods while still retaining moisture.

233. Vegetables Go for Steam Heat

For lean, pristine, stove-top vegetables, cook with steam. You'll conserve flavor and nutrients and dispense with butter or other cooking fat. Steamers and steaming baskets make this low-calorie cooking strategy a snap. For peak flavor, steam *lightly*—vegetables should be a tad crunchy, not soggy—then toss with lemon juice or a favorite herb such as thyme.

234. Zap Calories in a Microwave

Microwaves save time *and* calories. They do a fabulous job on high-moisture, low-fat, low-calorie foods such as fish, poultry, vegetables, and fruits. And since microwaves retain moisture, there's no need to use butter or oil to prevent food from sticking to dishes. Flavor is enhanced, foods stay moist, and you save calories. In fact, a U.S. Department of Agriculture study found that microwaved meats had less fat and fewer calories than meat cooked by electric broiling, charbroiling, roasting, convection heating, or frying.

235. A Smarter Way to Sauté

Sautéing is often the technique of choice for softening onions, mushrooms, or peppers, and it's also a standard method of cooking lean meats like boneless chicken breasts, fish, and veal fillets. The problem is that most directions for sautéing call for a tablespoon or two of butter, margarine, or cooking oil, and that adds 100 to 200 calories worth of pure fat to an otherwise respectable dish.

The next time you take your sauté pan in hand, substitute chicken broth for butter, margarine, or oil, and "steam sauté" the food at hand. You'll produce flavorful results without the unwanted calories.

236. Stir-Fry with a Twist

Stir-frying is a well-known technique from the Orient that cooks foods like chopped beef, chicken, pork, or vegetables quickly as they're whisked around in a film of hot oil. To cut calories, skip the oil. Instead, add a little juice, water, or stock to a well-seasoned pan and proceed as usual.

237. Hot Oil Goes Further

If you do sauté or stir-fry with fat, make sure the cooking oil is hot before adding the food. Reason: Foods soak up cool oil faster than hot oil. One extra tablespoon of absorbed oil can add 120 calories to your meal.

238. Roasting Made Lean

Roasting is a traditional method for cooking large cuts of beef, pork, veal, or poultry. Yet tradition also calls for larding roasts generously and basting them frequently with fatty meat drippings to prevent the meat from drying out during its long stint in the oven.

To cut fat and calories, break with tradition:

• Choose only the leanest cuts of meat and trim off all visible fat. Then set the meat on a wire rack, so the fat can run off.
• Baste with broth rather than meat drippings.
• Cook accompanying vegetables, like carrots, onions, or turnips, on the roasting rack beside the meat, not in the pan, so they don't soak up fat from meat drippings.

Some special tips for turkey:

• To keep turkey lean but moist during roasting, baste with orange juice instead of butter or pan drippings.
• Bake turkey stuffing separately. If baked in the turkey cavity, stuffing acts like a sponge, absorbing fat released from the meat as it roasts.

239. Bag Your Roast

Oven bags are a no-fuss means of cooking moist, low-calorie roasts when you don't have time to baste. For use in both conventional and microwave ovens, these specially made, heat-resistant bags create a moist environment to keep lean meats and poultry from drying out during cooking with no added fats.

240. Make Spare-the-Fat Ribs

You can remove a fair amount of fat from spareribs by boiling them for 20 minutes before you grill or broil them. Fat will separate in the water. Remove and drain on paper towels before grilling. Drain again before serving.

241. Broil Away Fat and Calories

When you broil, place meat on a ridged broiler pan or broiling rack: It will actually lose fat and calories as it cooks! As meat cooks, fat liquefies and drips into the pan, away from the meat. Result: You end up with far fewer calories than you started out with. As with roasting, you can prevent meat from drying out by brushing it with clear broth two or three times while it broils.

242. Marinate Meat for Flavor-Plus

Another way to conserve moisture and flavor when you broil, bake, grill, or spit-roast meat or poultry is to marinate it for an hour or more in a no-oil marinade of juice, mustard, herbs, or other acidic, savory ingredients. Example: In a glass baking dish, combine 2 tablespoons coarse mustard, ½ teaspoon crushed mustard seed, 3 tablespoons apple cider vinegar, and ½ cup chicken stock. Add chicken parts and marinate in the refrigerator for 1 hour. Bake as usual.

243. Bake It Light

Baking is a perfect method for cooking potatoes, squash, and low-fat vegetable casseroles because it requires no added fat (such as butter or margarine) to keep the food moist. Just cover the pan and forget about it.

244. Make No-Fry Home Fries

To make low-calorie home fries, slice potatoes into slabs ⅛ inch thick. Spray the potato slices lightly with cooking oil and bake on a cookie sheet for 20 minutes at 450°F. Turn once during baking.

245. Spray and Save

Instead of greasing loaf pans with thick gobs of vegetable shortening or butter, spray with Pam or other no-stick spray cooking oils.

(Even nonstick pans can benefit from a quick spritz of no-stick spray.) Made from lecithin, no-stick spray can grease a pan with just 7 calories, compared to a tablespoon of oil or butter at about 100 calories.

246. Try Exotic Oils

Keep an array of exotically flavored cooking oils like olive, peanut, or sesame oil on hand and use them sparingly.

"In one experiment, we found that people who used olive, peanut, or sesame oil consumed fewer calories via fat than people using blander vegetable oils," says Susan S. Schiffman, Ph.D., director of the weight-loss center at Duke University's Department of Psychology. Probable explanation: Any kind of oil is teeming with calories, but using highly flavored oils may encourage you to use less of them.

247. Butter Taste without the Calories

If you use Butter Buds Sprinkles or Molly McButter (two brands of butter-flavored powder sold in stores) on cooked vegetables, baked potatoes, or noodles, you'll consume only a fraction of the calories of regular butter.

Butter substitutes are made of maltodextrin, a sweet-tasting cornstarch, with natural butter flavor and other ingredients. They have only 4 calories per ½ teaspoon, compared to 18 for real butter. Butter substitutes are best sprinkled on hot, moist foods like cooked cereal, hot noodles, or steamed vegetables, or mixed into cake batters, casseroles, or sauces. But butter substitutes can't be used for frying.

248. Peel Your Butter

If you want to use butter or margarine on corn on the cob, mashed potatoes, or cooked vegetables, peel a sliver off a stick of spread with a potato peeler. You'll get about 12 calories worth of fat, compared to 36 in a pat.

249. Herbed Vinegar Does Butter One Better

Splash some herb or malt vinegar on fish or vegetables instead of tartar sauce or butter. You'll easily save 100 calories per meal.

250. Fruit Glaze Can Stand In for Butter

Instead of buttering cooked carrots, squash, and onions, brush them with a glaze made of fresh orange juice and honey.

251. Yogurt: the Sour Cream Substitute

Sour cream has 26 calories per tablespoon; plain low-fat yogurt has 10. So if you use a tablespoon of plain low-fat yogurt and chopped chives instead of sour cream on a baked potato, you'll save 16 calories. And if you use plain low-fat yogurt instead of sour cream in a recipe, you'll save 349 calories per cup.

Some special handling tips:

- Be careful with hot dishes. If you cook yogurt, it'll curdle. So if you use yogurt in stroganoff, whisk it in just before you serve, to heat it through without cooking it.
- Substitute yogurt for sour cream in a dip recipe. Let it drain first in a fine-meshed strainer lined with cheesecloth for an hour, to give it a firmer consistency. Or mix half plain low-fat yogurt and half low-fat cottage cheese and combine with dill, garlic powder, or other herbs.

252. A Low-Calorie Trick for Big Dippers

Here's another low-calorie way to prepare dips that are tasty to your lips but easy on your hips: Blend canned pinto beans with taco seasoning and a little chopped onion. Perfect low-calorie partners: fresh, crisp vegetables like celery and zucchini sticks, red pepper strips, and cauliflowerets.

253. Choose White Meat instead of Dark

Chicken and turkey are versatile meats, and packages of lean, boneless, skinned chicken or turkey breast make great low-calorie "convenience" foods. Dice them and toss in soup, cut into slivers and toss into a stir-fry, or pound them thin for a quick scallopini.

Three ounces of dark turkey meat contain 6 grams of fat and 159 calories; the same amount of white turkey meat contains 3 grams of fat and 133 calories. Also, 3 ounces of dark chicken meat contain 8.6 grams of fat and 174 calories, while 3 ounces of white chicken meat contain 4 grams of fat and 147 calories. So you cut calories if you routinely choose white poultry meat over dark.

254. Go Wild

Look for quail, pheasant, rabbit, and free-range chickens in the supermarket. Game birds and unpenned chickens are leaner than run-of-the-slaughterhouse birds because they're allowed to run around and build muscle instead of being confined, where they fatten up. The same goes for wild game, like wild turkey or venison. These meats are best cooked by braising or other moisture-conserving methods already described. And marinating these meats helps conserve flavor and moisture, too.

255. Hold the Yolks

Most of the fat in eggs, and hence the calories, are contained in the yolk. So you can cut calories by subtracting one yolk in recipes for muffins, quick breads, quiches, and frittatas and replacing it with an additional egg white.

Or use egg substitutes for omelets and frittatas.

256. Weigh and Measure Your Food

A kitchen scale, calibrated in quarter-ounces, is indispensable when trying to keep your calories in check. Otherwise, you could easily end up eating a 400-calorie portion of chicken when you think you're getting 250.

Also measure recipe ingredients like butter, margarine, oil, and sugar, to make sure you don't go overboard on fat.

257. Skimp on Sugar in Baked Goods

Most recipes calling for sugar taste almost the same with slightly less sweetener. So you can cut calories by skimping when you measure sugar. If the recipe calls for 1 cup of sugar, for example, cut back to ¾ cup. Or use 1 tablespoon less each time you make the recipe until you find the minimum amount needed to maintain taste and texture. You can make up for some of the missing sweetness by adding a teaspoon or so of almond or vanilla extract to the recipe.

258. Baby Your Taste Buds

If you have a hard time cooking without tasting too much as you go, keep an infant feeding spoon handy. Use the baby spoon instead of a ladle or teaspoon. It really helps cut down on calories, and you taste enough to tell you if you need to adjust the seasoning but not enough to give you a lot of calories.

The Battle of the Binge

259. Fake Out Your Fat Tooth

Often when people think they're suffering from a sweet craving, what they're actually craving is fat. Treats like ice cream and candy bars are high in sugar, but they're also loaded with fat. To combat this craving, plan snacks that are low in fat and high in carbohydrates. When you do get that 4 o'clock yearning, have a glass of skim milk with an apple, for example. The high-carbohydrate apple can help you ward off fat cravings for several hours.

Carbohydrates will help keep away the after-dinner munchies, too. At dinnertime, the first thing you eat should be a starch or carbohydrate. Soups that contain noodles, potatoes, rice, barley, or legumes are excellent choices. Low-fat whole-wheat bread is another perfect food. Then try to stretch out the meal. Eat slowly and take time between courses so it lasts for at least 20 minutes. That gives the carbohydrates time to activate the hormones in your intestinal tract, liver, and brain so you won't feel as much of a craving for fat as you go on with the meal.

FACT OF LIFE

Mood Swings Lead to Bingeing

Psychologists at Kent State University have found that binge eaters experience greater mood swings—that is, bouts of anxiety, depression, or hostility—than nonbinge eaters. This confirms what many overeaters have known for a long time: "Negative mood states" can easily trigger or perpetuate a food binge.

Life-Extension Tools

The Fat Finder

Medical experts say that keeping your daily intake of dietary fat below 30 percent will help prevent heart disease and cancer. But how do you figure out how fatty a food is? One way is by using an inexpensive ($3.95), ingenious device called the Fat Finder. This hand-held disk calculates the percentage of fat in calories from nutritional data printed on the labels of food items like milk, cereal, crackers, soup, sandwich meats, entrees, salad dressing, and countless other packaged foods.

Say you want to determine the percentage of calories from fat in a packaged frozen dinner, for example. You simply look for the number of calories and grams of fat per serving shown on the box. Then line up those two numbers on the Fat Finder wheel, and read the percentage of calories from fat.

The Fat Finder is available from some hospitals and in a few stores, but you can also buy one through the mail from Vitaerobics, 41–905 Boardwalk, Suite B, Palm Desert, CA 92260.

Compucal

This more sophisticated, more expensive device can help you find the percentage of fat in nonpackaged food items such as cheese, ground beef, or avocados. A cross between a scale and a simple computer, Compucal reveals close-to-exact counts for the amount of calories, carbohydrates, fats, sodium, protein, and cholesterol in foods from abalone to zwieback. Available in retail stores for approximately $135 (not including batteries or an AC adapter), Compucal is yet another tool to help you keep your fat intake under the recommended 30 percent level.

The Futrex–1000

So much for measuring the fat in your food. You also want to keep tabs on the fat in your body. In fact, your percentage of body fat may be a more realistic gauge of your fitness level than the bathroom scale: People who are fit and muscular may be overweight according to standard height/weight charts, but not overfat. On the other hand, some people who are the proper weight according to the charts are overfat.

(continued)

Life-Extension Tools—*Continued*

Low body fat means a decreased risk of coronary heart disease, adult-onset diabetes, high blood pressure, kidney disease, and cancer of the breast, ovaries, prostate, and intestine.

The Futrex–1000 is a hand-held flashlightlike instrument you can use to measure body fat. You simply place it against various parts of your body—underneath your upper arm, your thigh, your abdomen—and enter your age, sex, height, and weight into the built-in computer. The light spectrum will change according to the amount of fat the instrument detects. The instrument analayzes the change and calculates your percentage of body fat, which is displayed within 10 seconds on an LCD window.

Although there is no established standard for recommended percentage of body fat, many medical experts have reason to believe that men's level of body fat should be between 6 and 23.5 percent and women's should be between 9 and 30.8 percent, depending on age. (The younger you are, the lower your body fat should be.)

The Futrex–1000 gives a more accurate measure of body fat than either skinfold calipers or immersion in water, traditional methods of estimating body fat. The device costs $299 and is available from Futrex, Inc., P.O. 2398, Gaithersburg, MD 20879. Or you can call toll-free at 1–800–255–4206 for the name of the Futrex dealer nearest you.

---

260. Avoid the Sugar Trap

Try to avoid sugar. It tends to make you crave even more food, according to experts at the Johns Hopkins Health, Weight, and Stress Clinic in Baltimore.

261. Be Prepared for a Snack Attack

Make sure you have plenty of foods like raw vegetables and air-popped popcorn on hand at home and at work for those times when the hungries hit without warning. They're high in fiber, satisfying, and filling, the perfect combination to quell a snack attack.

262. A Toothsome Idea

Tempted to eat a candy bar? Brush your teeth. The sweetness of the toothpaste may take away your craving.

263. Pick and Peck a Pickle or Pepper

If you feel a powerful urge to overeat, suck on a pickle or sourball. Or eat a hot pepper. The jolt to your taste buds may eliminate your craving.

264. A Sip Can Stop a Splurge

If you crave something sweet, try eating a piece of fruit or have a little fruit juice. Its sweetness may be enough to get you through the crisis.

265. Feed Your Head, Not Your Face

When a craving hits, go for a walk, play solitaire, or start a crossword puzzle. But do something that'll keep your mind off food. This is especially helpful if you eat out of anger or boredom.

Boredom can drive you into a feeding frenzy. It's scientific fact: One researcher isolated a colony of rats with little to see or do, and before long the rodents were bored to tears and nervous wrecks—they nibbled constantly. Eating is not an instant solution to the blahs.

266. Take a New Way Home

If your usual route takes you too close to a tempting sweet shop or by your favorite hot dog vendor, blaze some new, nonfattening trails.

267. Relationships Are Important

Companions and confidants are the best substitute for comfort foods. If you feel happy, loved, and content, you'll be less inclined to overeat.

268. Meet Temptation Halfway

If you find yourself giving in to temptation, eat only half the treat and throw the rest away.

Don't ever put a food on a pedestal and make it a forbidden food, because you'll just go crazy for it, warn weight-control experts. There's nothing in the world you can't eat if you keep to reasonable amounts.

But watch out for what size portions you take. Eating half means half of a reasonable portion, not half a pie.

Strategies for Dining Out

269. Don't Eat the Whole Thing

Until a few years ago, most people regarded dining out as a special treat, a rare chance to splurge. But now, 41 percent of all food dollars is spent on meals consumed outside the home. For many people, restaurant fare accounts for a significant portion of the week's food consumption. The problem is, the typical restaurant portion is designed with an average 5-foot 8-inch active man in mind.

FACT OF LIFE

Lone Diners Are Better Off

Do you hate to eat alone? Well, listen to this: A study conducted at Georgia State University found that people ate 44 percent more food when they dined with others than when they ate alone, regardless of how much time had elapsed since their last meal. Yet the same diners felt 30 percent *less satisfied* when they ate with others than when they ate alone. "This suggests that if people were encouraged to eat alone, they would eat less and include a smaller proportion of fat, yet obtain a greater amount of satiety per calorie of energy ingested," say the researchers. In plain English: When you eat alone, you're less likely to overeat, and you'll enjoy your food *more*.

Other people don't necessarily need that much food. So don't feel guilty about leaving food on your plate.

270. Eat the Bread but Not the Spread

Restraint begins with the bread and butter of a meal. Don't butter your rolls. And don't eat roll after roll just for something to do while you wait for the rest of your meal to arrive.

271. Order What's Not on the Menu

Since a lot of restaurant food is made to order, you may have more choice than you think when it comes to ordering. Some helpful strategies follow.

- Ask for sauces or dressing on the side, so you can control the amount you eat.
- Ask for plain steamed vegetables instead of those that are deep-fried, mayonnaise-laced, or dripping in butter or cheese sauce.
- Order meat or poultry steamed, poached, or grilled rather than sautéed or fried.
- If you aren't sure how a dish is prepared, ask the server. If a sauce doesn't sound familiar, for example, ask for an explanation. Does it have butter, cream, cheese, eggs, or other high-fat ingredients?

272. Hold the Topping

Whether it's a burger or a baked potato, say no to gourmet toppings. Special sauces can push the fat count sky-high. A plain baked potato can swell from 1 percent to 49 percent when topped with things like bacon and cheese.

273. Eat Only What You Order

If you're ordering a sandwich, ask the waiter if it comes "garnished" with anything like coleslaw, French fries, or potato chips. If so, tell the server not to bring them. "It's much easier not to have the

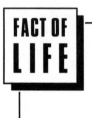

Americans Are in the Chips

Average number of pounds of potato chips eaten by each American every year: 12. Average number of pounds of broccoli eaten: 3. Number of calories consumed eating those chips: 30,912. Broccoli: 435.

chips than it is to sit there with them in front of you," says Mona Sutnick, a registered dietitian and spokesperson for the American Dietetic Association.

274. Eat Your Dressing with a Fork

Here's a strategy that yields good taste without excess fat and calories. "Order your dressing or sauce on the side, then dip your fork into the dressing and stab the food. You get flavor in every bite with considerably less calories," says Darlene Dougherty, a registered dietitian and president of the American Dietetic Association.

275. Buffer the Buffet by Eating First

A visually tempting array of food, combined with industrial-sized serving utensils and an inherent tendency for people to try to get their money's worth, make buffets a minefield for dieters, warns Dougherty. If you must attend a buffet, fill up on salad and vegetables first, then return for the entrees when your appetite is tame.

276. Patronize Diet-Conscious Restaurants

As a general rule, the better the restaurant, the more the kitchen staff should be able to accommodate special requests. You can't expect to visit a hamburger chain and order poached salmon with steamed belgian endive, for instance.

277. Salad Bar Savvy

Steer clear of the mayonnaise-laden coleslaws and potato salads, and don't make the mistake of sabotaging a healthful plate of otherwise innocent greens with a high-fat (100-calorie-per-table-spoon) dressing. Use a reduced-calorie dressing or plain vinegar, if available. Bacon bits (if real), cheese, and egg toppings also can raise a salad's calorie count in a hurry.

278. Be Especially Aware of Specialty Salads

A chef's salad with one packet of Thousand Island dressing at McDonald's gives you 621 calories and 52 grams of fat—even more than in a 570-calorie Big Mac! Opt for the shrimp salad instead.

The taco salad with ranch dressing at Taco Bell comes to a monstrous 1,167 calories and 86 grams of fat. Skipping the taco shell and using salsa instead of the dressing will help cut down on the fat and calories.

279. If You Must Have Dessert, Share

Turning your back on the restaurant dessert cart can be as difficult as passing up a ride to a service station when your car has a flat. Restaurant cakes, pies, and mousses are yummy-looking works of culinary art. If you can't resist the temptation, split dessert with someone else at the table. Or opt for fruit ice or sorbet.

280. Don't Let Fast Food Become a Bad Habit

Your weight-control program may survive an occasional visit to the fast-food counter, but no more. If you have fast food for one meal, you can round out your day healthfully at home with some vegetable dishes, skim milk, and perhaps fresh fruit for dessert.

281. Make Lunch a Picnic

If the only convenient lunch spots near work are greasy cafeterias, fast-food restaurants, and hot dog stands, lean, light food may be hard to find, and the limited choice can break your diet. So pack your own—it puts you in control, so you can make sure it's nutritious.

Be inventive. Pack last night's leftovers, or create a simple pasta salad. Wrap your lunch in pretty paper and use real silverware. To put even more spin on your midday meal, make lunch a relaxing retreat. Enjoy a lunchtime walk to a park and picnic with a friend.

Melting the Fat

282. Exercise Is Essential

There are three good reasons you should exercise when you diet.

- Exercise reverses diet-slowed metabolism and helps burn fat and calories. When you eat a limited number of calories, your resting metabolic rate (RMR)—that is, the number of calories you burn at rest or asleep—drops, canceling out some of your dieting effort. But when you exercise, your RMR increases. In one study, overweight dieters consumed a very low-calorie diet—500 calories a day—for four weeks. They remained sedentary for the first two weeks and exercised 30 minutes a day for the next two weeks. RMR dropped to approximately 87 percent of the prestudy rate while they were inactive but jumped back to normal when they exercised.
- Exercise prevents dieting-induced heart muscle loss. "When you gain weight, you gain muscle and fat. Heart size is also increased to keep up with the extra load," explains Emory University researcher Mary Ellen Sweeney, M.D., who studied 21 obese women. "When you lose weight, the heart's workload is decreased because there is less mass to pump blood to." By increasing that workload through exercise, you can prevent the loss of heart muscle that dieting alone can cause.
- Exercise burns calories. In one study researchers surveyed 141 women aged 34 to 59 and found that the more physically active women were less overweight than those who were inactive.

283. Miles Melt the Pounds

The heavier you are, the harder it may be to exercise, but the more important it is to exercise. Walking is definitely the recommended choice. It's gentle on the joints, yet it still burns fat. A 1-mile brisk walk is worth about 100 calories.

Start slowly and work at your own pace. Put petroleum jelly or talcum powder on your thighs to cut down on chafing. If you're

You Can Avoid Middle-Age Spread

The speed at which your body metabolizes fuel decreases slightly as you age, dropping about 2 percent per decade. This accounts for a weight gain of about 3 or 4 pounds in a given ten-year period. You *can* prevent the resulting love handles, saddlebags, and other middle-age parcels of pudge, though, if you cut daily calorie intake by 2 percent each decade. To trim a daily intake of 1,800 calories by 2 percent, you have to eliminate 36 calories—the equivalent of 1 teaspoon of butter.

extra heavy, consider the extra support of running shoes rather than walking shoes.

Walk for as long as you feel comfortable, even if it seems extremely short at first. Let your breathing be your guide. If a daily 5-minute walk is the most you can bear, then so be it. When you become comfortable with that much, increase it by another 5 minutes. The point is to walk a little every day. You'll see results in good time.

"For someone who gets out of breath just going up a flight of stairs, a walk to the end of the driveway and back is a big deal," says Gail Johnston, the director of the Aerobics and Fitness Association of America's specialty certification program, Fitness for the Overweight. "Give yourself credit for whatever you can do—don't blame yourself for what you can't."

284. Tone Up with Water Walking

Water walking is an enjoyable way for people who are out of shape, overweight, or new to exercise to shape up as they slim down. Water walking requires no special swimming skills, and like road walking, it requires no equipment, not even walking shoes! And you don't have to get your hair wet, either. All you have to do is walk in thigh- to chest-deep water for 20 minutes at least three times a week. It burns up to 460 calories per hour—without sweating or risk of injury.

You shouldn't have to look far to find somewhere to water walk. It's catching on at Y's, health clubs, and private pools nationwide.

285. Take Up Table Tennis

Fast action makes table tennis (a.k.a. Ping Pong) good for 355 calories an hour—more than singles tennis. And you don't waste as much time searching far and wide for stray balls.

286. Go the 300

To lose weight, you should strive for an exercise program that burns about 300 calories or more per session.

Besides walking, you might want to bicycle, swim, or pursue some other activity. Here's a rough guide to a few popular pursuits and how many calories they burn per hour, calculated for someone who weighs 132 pounds and exercises moderately. People who weigh less will burn a few calories less; people who weigh more will burn a few calories more.

Volleyball: 310
Gardening: 345
Bicycling: 370
Stationary bicyling: 375
Swimming (crawl): 375
Aerobic dancing: 395
Calisthenics: 395
Skipping rope: 495
Running: 585

287. Exercise on Empty and Burn More Fat

If you're trying to lose excess fat, don't eat before you exercise. A study conducted at Kansas State University involving two groups of women showed that while both groups burned about the same amount of calories, the amount of fat they used differed significantly. For example, when exercising 90 minutes after eating, the subjects burned 69 fat calories. When doing the same workout on an empty stomach, they burned 94.

Researchers conclude that when you eat before exercise, your body relies more on carbohydrates for energy, and you burn less fat. If you're trying to lose fat, save the meal until after your workout.

288. Buy a Video Rated X-tra Large

Many overweight people are too embarrassed or self-conscious to attend a typical aerobics class. Enter VCRs. But regular workout tapes may be too strenuous for bigger bodies. The answer: Exercise videos for the extra large. That is, workout tapes with safe, gentle routines, with none of the leaping and jumping that can destroy your knees and ankles, or leave you sore and stiff after the first workout.

Some samples of what's on the market include *Women at Large: Breakout* (available from Women at Large, 1020 S. 48th Avenue, Yakima, WA 98908), *Feel Beautiful* (available from B. R. Anderson Enterprises, 5308 Chateau Place, Minneapolis, MN 55417), and *Get Started with Richard Simmons* (available in video stores, by Warner Home Video).

Maintaining Momentum

289. Let the Mirror Be Your Judge

Don't worry about what the scale is telling you about your weight-loss efforts. Let the mirror and your clothes be your guide. Sometimes your clothes may fit better even if you haven't lost weight, due to toning and muscle development resulting from exercise.

290. Avoid the Plateau Panic

If you find yourself staying at the same weight, don't panic—it's your body getting used to the new you. Drink water, increase your exercise, or reduce your calories (but don't eat less than 1,000 calories a day) to give you the boost you need.

291. Take Your Personality into Account

The best method of dieting depends on your personality, says Sarah C. Sitton, Ph.D., formerly of the Texas Higher Education Coordinating Board. She says those who described themselves as emotional "feelers" had best results when dieting in a group such as Weight Watchers; those considering themselves thinking and logical did best when dieting alone.

If you've been having problems sticking to a diet, the problem may be in the social setting rather than in the calories. Social types enjoy the atmosphere of a group, while more goal-oriented people prefer their autonomy.

292. Diet with a Buddy

Many successful weight-loss programs rely heavily on support groups: caring people who help one another succeed. Encourage your spouse or a friend to join you in your weight-control efforts. Or start your own group, even if you team up with just one other person. (You'll feel obligated to work out if someone else is depending on you.)

293. Hang a Gorgeous Outfit on Your Closet Door

Buy something attractive to wear in the size you'd like to be in a few weeks, and look at it when you get dressed in the morning. Try it on once a week to boost your motivation.

In fact, your clothes may be a more accurate gauge of your progress than the scale. It's possible to drop down two clothing sizes and not lose a pound. Plotting your progress by the scale alone may cause you to see yourself unjustly as a failure.

294. Picture Someone Else on the Refrigerator

Forget the demoralizing picture-on-the-refrigerator trick. It will only depress you. Instead, tack up a picture of yourself at your thinnest—or your favorite celebrity whose shape you admire—to give you something to work toward.

295. Dress for Weight-Loss Success

Dress thin *while* you're losing weight, and you're more likely to follow through. Wear clothes that make you feel good—follow fashion and learn what colors work well on you. Clothes that make you look even fatter will only discourage your efforts.

Keep in mind, too, that there are many ways clothing can disguise an undesirable physical feature. Did you ever hear of a diet for short legs? Or broad shoulders? Of course not. Here are some design tips for less-than-perfect female physiques.

- For heavy thighs or hips, choose softly gathered skirts, straight skirts with small slits or kick pleats. Jackets with padded shoulders and wide lapels can help to balance your upper torso with your hips. Avoid pleated skirts or pants with patch pockets at the hips.
- For short legs, choose skirts with hemlines that fall below your knee. Team them with color-coordinated hosiery and shoes for a continuous—and longer-looking—toe-to-hip line. For similar reasons, if you wear boots, be sure your hem covers the tops. Also, choose shirtwaist dresses or coatdresses with vertical seams from neck to hemline. Wear tapered pants, without cuffs. Avoid above-the-knee hemlines, wide, cuffed pants, and boots that reach midcalf or just above the ankle.
- To minimize an ample abdomen, choose pants in woven fabrics such as poplin, gabardine, or wool flannel that hang straight from a tailored waistband. Avoid clingy jersey or polyester knits and elasticized waistbands, which accentuate bulges. Avoid clingy sheaths, belted dresses, and dresses with fitted midriffs. Wear control-top pantyhose for additional support.
- For a large bust or broad shoulders, look for dolman sleeves, blouson sweaters, small collars, vertical necklines, narrow lapels, and wrap fronts in straight-hanging (not clingy) fabrics. Avoid wide necklines, puffed sleeves, ruffles, gathers, padded shoulders, wide belts, and empire waistlines. Be sure garments don't pull across the bustline or shoulder blades. And by all means, wear a good bra with adequate support to minimize drooping.

296. Stop Postponing Life Until You're Thin

"Buy new clothes, change your hairstyle, join that aerobics class *now*," say Linda Crawford and Sadie Drumm, behavioral specialist and exercise physiologist at Green Mountain at Fox Run, a Vermont-based center for weight and health management.

297. Don't Let Age Interfere with Your Aspirations

"You can always improve your body and your health," says Jack LaLanne, "America's Fitness King" for 50 years.

"Your body certainly will try to make you fatter as you get older," says Dr. Miller of the Hilton Head Institute. "But you don't have to put up with it. If you do nothing to fight the effects of age on your metabolism, I can guarantee you will gradually gain weight each year for the rest of your life. But there's no reason you can't weigh the same at 60 as you did at 20."

298. Seek New Rewards

If you usually use food as a reward, establish a new reward system. Buy yourself flowers, an attractive new coffee mug, or a new outfit.

299. Hit the Scales Once a Week

Weigh yourself once a week at the same time. Your weight fluctuates constantly, and you can weigh more at night than you did in the morning—a downer if you've stuck to your diet all day.

300. Beware of Co-Workers Bearing Doughnuts

Notify your family, friends, and co-workers of your weight-loss wishes. Ask them to understand if you turn down their baked goods or dinner invitations.

Words of Wisdom

301. Don't Be Pound Foolish

Many dieters are tempted to simply give up food altogether in order to lose weight as quickly as possible. Don't do it!

"The initial rapid weight loss you get with a starvation diet is caused by water and muscle loss," says Garth Fischer, Ph.D., director of the Human Performance Research Center at Brigham Young University in Utah and coauthor of *How to Lower Your Fat Thermostat.* "But your body metabolism slows down, halting weight loss in a desperate attempt to save your life." So undereating eventually causes a plateau—you don't lose, even though you don't eat.

302. Be Diet Wise

If you cut way back on food, or limit yourself to a few foods (like an all-fruit or rice diet), you're depriving yourself of essential vitamins and minerals. Also, such extreme diets can strain the heart, kidneys, and liver. Any rapid weight loss you might achieve on such a stringent diet can lead to painful gallstones, according to medical literature.

"It's a good thing fad diets are so hard to stick to," says Bryant Stamford, Ph.D., director of the Health Promotion and Wellness Center at the University of Louisville School of Medicine. "Because the longer you pursue them, the more they can harm you. Especially diets that go below 1,000 calories a day."

303. Lose, Gain, Lose: A Dangerous Pattern

Losing the same 20 or 30 pounds over and over is self-defeating. For one, regained fat tends to come back in the belly more than the butt, hips, or legs. So when you gain the weight back, you may appear to be fatter than you were last time you gained.

But yo-yo dieting effects more than your appearance. It can be hazardous to your health. Fluctuating weight eventually causes "dieter's hypertension"—a stubborn form of high blood pressure set

FACT OF LIFE

Eating Less Costs Lots

According to some estimates, 65 million Americans are dieting at any one time. And they spend lots of bucks—over $29 billion a year—to control their weight, according to Marketdata Enterprises. Dieting dollars are expected to swell to $50.7 billion by 1995.

in motion by changes in norepinephrine, a hormone that constricts blood vessels, raising blood pressure. Normally, during starvation, the brain cuts back production of norepinephrine. At first, blood pressure drops. But animal studies show that after a series of yo-yo weight changes, the norepinephrine-releasing cells get stuck in overdrive, and blood pressure remains elevated.

This long-term effect of yo-yo dieting could explain why overweight people are twice as likely to develop high blood pressure than normal weight individuals, according to Paul Ernsberger, Ph.D., assistant professor of medicine at Case Western Reserve University Medical School, who's studied this phenomenon. "Loss/gain cycles make yo-yo dieters especially prone to congestive heart failure."

And the news gets even more distressing. A study conducted on yo-yo dieters at the West Los Angeles Veterans Administration Medical Center found that 80 percent developed diabetes and 25 percent died of heart disease. That's 13 times higher than the rate of premature death for overweight nondieters!

Now for the good news. If you maintain your new weight at one level, yo-yo dieting–induced hypertension eventually subsides, according to Dr. Ernsberger. Insulin levels should also even out.

"The more often body fat is lost and then regained as abdominal fat, the greater the possibility of developing diabetes and of augmenting factors that contribute to heart failure," says Dr. C. Wayne Callaway, associate professor of medicine at George Washington University School of Medicine.

304. You Must Remember This

There is no such thing as a miracle diet. When trying to lose weight, you should follow a good slimming program—one that allows safe permanent weight loss. A good, healthy program is one that:

- Incorporates exercise.
- Keeps daily consumption above 1,200 calories (unless it's medically supervised).
- Produces weight loss of no more than 1 to 2 pounds a week.
- Includes a variety of foods that contain adequate nutrients.
- Encourages dietary and behavior changes that you can stick with throughout your life.

305. Patience Leads to Perfection

Patience is a dieter's best friend.

"Fat takes a long time to go away," says Dr. Stamford. "If you're losing weight rapidly, you're not losing fat. Anything more than 1 or 2 pounds a week is mostly water, carbohydrate, and muscle."

306. Don't Expect Overnight Success

Cold turkey may be good to eat, but it shouldn't be how you approach a diet change. You've been eating the way you have for a long time, so gradually change how you eat over time.

And how much time should you take? Take whatever time you need, says Sonja Connor, a registered dietitian and assistant professor at Oregon Health Sciences University. When she went about changing how she and her family eat, she took five years to do it. "And we're still making changes. It's a constant process."

C H A P T E R · 4

![black bar]

YOUR CANCER PREVENTION PLAN

Do you know someone with cancer? We'll bet that you do. We'll bet that you do because cancer strikes 3 out of every 4 families in the United States and kills about 500,000 men and women every year.

Most cancer victims die from cancer of the lung, breast, colon, or prostate. Breast cancer deaths have held steady over the past 30 years, but prostate cancer deaths have increased 9 percent, colon cancer deaths have increased 22 percent in men, and lung cancer deaths have increased a shocking 161 percent in men and a horrifying 396 percent in women.

Those increases make cancer the nation's second most common cause of death. But what's causing this epidemic of neoplasmic proliferation?

Most of the time it's things we do to ourselves. We take a 3-inch paper-covered cylinder out of a pack, put one end in our mouths, and set the other end on fire—even when we know that 83 percent of all lung cancer is caused by smoking cigarettes. Or we pull up to a fast-food drive-in, order a bacon double cheeseburger, large fries, and jumbo milkshake—even when we know that the risk of dying from breast cancer increases 40 percent for every extra 1,000 grams of fat we eat a month. Or maybe for breakfast we eat the cute little pink-and-white cereal advertised on Saturday morning cartoons— even when we know that a low-fiber diet is a significant factor in the development of colon cancer.

68 Percent Can Be Prevented

All told, scientists estimate, 35 percent of all cancer deaths are caused by bad diet, 30 percent by smoking, 2 percent by a polluted environment, and 1 percent by food additives.

These numbers add up to the fact that more than 68 percent of all cancer deaths are caused by things we do to ourselves and one another. And that means that every one of these deaths is preventable.

Which ones? In large measure, we can prevent bladder, breast, colon, esophageal, larynx, liver, lung, oral, skin, stomach, and uterine cancer by carefully choosing what we eat, drink, and breathe. The following tips will show us how.

Foods to Fight Cancer

307. Eat Bran and Other Fibers

A decade of studies has clearly demonstrated that people who eat a high-fiber diet have a low incidence of cancer—especially colon cancer.

Why? "Fiber appears to dilute intestinal contents and reduces the amount of time carcinogens might spend in your intestines," says the American Cancer Society.

Most people, though, don't eat nearly enough fiber. Current recommendations call for eating 20 to 30 grams a day, while most of us only get about half that.

If you're looking to increase your fiber intake, try eating foods like whole-grain breads, rice, wheat and bran cereals, popcorn, raisins, peaches, apricots, apples with skin, oranges, strawberries, cherries, potatoes, spinach, peas, tomatoes, kidney beans, carrots, and broccoli.

308. Eat Less Fat

"Numerous studies have shown that high-fat diets increase the incidence of breast, prostate, and colon cancer," says the American Cancer Society.

So cut down on your total fat intake and really declare war on the saturated fats—the kind of fat that stays solid at room temperature. Most doctors now agree that the amount of fat you consume should equal no more than 30 percent of your total calories.

Start by eating lean meats, skinned poultry, and low-fat dairy products, and bake or broil rather than fry fish, meat, and poultry.

309. Reach for Vitamin A

Researchers around the world are singing the praises of vitamin A:

- In Canada and India, vitamin A supplements reversed more than half of the oral ulcers that usually lead to oral cancer.
- At the University of Wales College of Medicine, a vitamin A derivative reduced the number of precancerous and cancerous skin growths in 15 patients.
- In China, vaginal suppositories containing another vitamin A derivative reversed precancerous cervical changes in 26 out of 27 women.
- At the University of Colorado Health Sciences Center, researchers found that retinoic acid, a synthetic form of vitamin A, reduced the growth of cancer cells in a laboratory culture.

Those are only a few of the many positive studies that have surfaced. But a word of caution: High doses of vitamin A can be toxic, so it's not recommended that you take supplements to get this cancer-fighting potential. Instead, eat foods rich in vitamin A.

Look for dark green or deep yellow vegetables such as spinach, tomatoes, or carrots, or fruits such as cantaloupes, apricots, and peaches.

310. Eat a Carrot a Day

Beta-carotene is the natural pigment found in fruits and vegetables that your body turns into vitamin A. And like vitamin A, it's also been found to help prevent lung cancer.

Researchers at the State University of New York at Buffalo compared the diets of 450 people with lung cancer to the diets of over 900 healthy people. They found that the people with lung cancer had a significantly lower carotene intake than the people without lung cancer. And men with the lowest carotene intake had an 80 percent greater risk than those with the highest intake.

How much carotene would you need to have in your diet to reduce your risk of cancer? Not much. The researchers found the differences in carotene levels was about 6,750 international units— or about the amount of carotene found in one carrot.

311. Smokers Need Their B's

Since studies show that smokers have lower levels of vitamin B_{12} and folate than nonsmokers, scientists are beginning to suspect that tobacco smoke may deplete these two essential B vitamins from the cells lining the lung.

Researchers at the University of Alabama at Birmingham decided to clear the air and find out just how these nutrients may play a role in preventing cancer. They studied 73 longtime smokers, all with precancerous cell changes in lung secretions. Half of these smokers received supplements of folate and B_{12}; the other half were given placebos (inactive substances).

After four months, the researchers rechecked the smokers' lung fluids. The fluids of those who took vitamins were found to have less severe precancerous changes than the fluids of those who did not.

You can get B_{12} by eating lean beef and other meats and certain fish, such as salmon and oysters. Good sources of folate include kidney beans, soybeans, cowpeas, spinach, brewer's yeast, broccoli, and sweet potatoes.

FACT OF LIFE

Smoking Is Double Trouble for Some

If one of your parents or siblings has lung cancer and you're a woman, you shouldn't even think of smoking. A recent study found that a family history of lung cancer actually *doubles* the odds of lung cancer in women who smoke.

312. Hold the Bacon

Nitrates have been traditionally used as a way of preserving meat because they act as a preventive against botulism. Trouble is, although they may stop you from getting food poisoning, they may contribute to giving you cancer.

According to the American Cancer Society, in parts of the world where nitrates are common in food and water—Colombia, for instance—stomach and esophageal cancers are common.

In addition, there is chemical evidence that nitrates can enhance nitrosamine formation both in foods and our digestive tract. And nitrosamines have been proven to be potent cancer-causing agents in animals.

Nitrates are found in many processed meat products such as hot dogs, bacon, bologna, and ham. It's best to use these foods in moderation—or skip them altogether.

313. Or Make It in the Microwave

Researchers have found that microwaving bacon produces fewer cancer-causing nitrosamines than does frying.

How do they know? They cooked up a bunch of bacon. Forty-five seconds of microwaving—the usual amount of time it takes to thoroughly cook a single strip of bacon—produced no nitrosamines. The same amount of time spent in the frying pan produced a significant amount.

Microwaving doesn't make the bacon less fatty, though, even when it's cooked on paper towels. But if you want to reduce your fat as well as your nitrosamines, choose one of the lower-fat bacon substitutes on the market.

314. Eat Your Bacon with an Orange Juice Chaser

People who eat vitamin C-rich fresh fruits daily have a lower incidence of cancers of the stomach, esophagus, mouth, larynx, and cervix. There is even evidence that it may help prevent colon and lung cancers as well.

The reason vitamin C is so potent against stomach-related cancers apparently is due to its ability to halt the formation of cancer-causing nitrosamines that form in the stomach after eating foods containing nitrates.

Scientists involved in these studies recommend that to get this protective effect you should eat citrus fruits, not take a vitamin C supplement. That's because they found that the nations and groups of people with the lowest incidence of these cancers get their vitamin C by eating lots of fresh citrus fruits. The possibility exists, they speculate, that there could actually be something in citrus fruit other than just vitamin C that's providing cancer protection.

315. Calcium Helps Block Colon Cancer

When researchers at the University of Utah School of Medicine compared 231 people with colon cancer against 391 healthy people, they discovered that the people who were cancer-free ate a diet richer in calcium than those with the disease.

The theory behind the study suggests that calcium may slow colon cancer development by binding with the fats and bile acids that could cause bowel tumors.

316. Open Wide for Vitamin E

Imagine trying to get a hamster to say "Ahhhh." Researchers trying to detect oral cancer at Harvard's School of Dental Medicine spent 28 weeks looking into the gaping jaws of hamsters, trying to detect oral cancer.

What they were doing was treating the hamsters' mouths with a carcinogen combined with a twice-weekly dose of vitamin E. The results after all those weeks? "No evidence whatsoever" of any tumors were found in the hamsters who were given vitamin E. Hamsters given the carcinogen without the vitamin E, though, did show tumor development.

"If vitamin E worked on mouth cancer," says Gerald Shklar, M.D., one of the researchers involved, "you have something that may prevent other cancers as well."

Finnish researchers apparently agree. A ten-year Finnish study that included more than 21,000 men found that those with the highest level of vitamin E had a 36 percent lower risk of cancer than those with the lowest levels of vitamin E.

The reason, they suggest, is that vitamin E is an anti-oxidant, and slower oxidation of body cells may protect against cancer.

"There is good evidence to show that vitamin E can help prevent cancer," concludes Denham Harman, M.D., Ph.D., a vitamin E researcher at the University of Nebraska College of Medicine.

Vitamin E has also been shown to enhance the effectiveness of anticancer drugs used in chemotherapy in rats.

Foods high in vitamin E are wheat germ oil, sunflower seeds and oil, almonds, peanuts, lobster, salmon, soybean oil, and pecans.

317. Go Easy on the Iron

Researchers at the National Cancer Institute in Washington, D.C., have found that people with high stores of the mineral iron in their body are at greater risk of developing cancer.

Do not take extra iron unless you need to, says Elizabeth Applegate, Ph.D., nutrition director of the University of California at Davis Adult Fitness and Cardiac Rehabilitation Program. If you do feel the need for some "insurance," she suggests you take a multivitamin/mineral supplement, which typically contains the U.S. Recommended Daily Allowance of iron—18 milligrams.

Most people can get all the iron they need by eating foods rich in the substance, however. Good sources for iron are foods like lean red meat, dark meat poultry, fish, dried beans, whole grains, dried fruit, enriched grain products, and leafy vegetables.

One last tip: Eat foods rich in vitamin C along with meals. It will improve your iron absorption.

318. Selenium Shows Some Promise

Preliminary studies are showing that too little selenium may increase your chances of getting cancer.

In Finland, researchers found that when 143 men with lung cancer were compared to 264 healthy men, those with the least amount of selenium in their blood were also those who had a higher risk of cancer.

At the University of Bonn in West Germany, scientists wanted to find out if selenium would protect people from the most deadly form of skin cancer, malignant melanoma.

When 101 melanoma victims were compared to 57 cancer-free people, the skin cancer sufferers had lower levels of selenium. People with advanced cancer had the least selenium of all.

None of this means you should go out and buy selenium supplements. Because of the possibility of selenium poisoning, the American Cancer Society advises that "the medically unsupervised use of selenium as a food supplement cannot be recommended."

Instead, get your selenium from foods like seafood (especially tuna fish), kidney, liver, grains, nuts, and rice.

319. Head for the Cabbage Patch

Researchers have been intrigued for years over the possibility that cruciferous vegetables (such as cabbage, brussels sprouts, and broccoli) contain a substance that helps prevent cancer.

At the University of Nebraska Medical Center, for instance, cancer researchers divided a bunch of mice into two groups. One group was given a regular diet, the others were fed diets rich in cabbage or collard greens. At the end of six weeks the mice were injected with breast cancer cells. The result? The mice fed lots of cabbage and greens diet developed fewer tumors.

The evidence is intriguing enough that the American Cancer Society suggests you include cruciferous vegetables in your cancer-prevention diet.

320. Go Heavy on the Onions, Please

In China, researchers say they've found a link between low cancer rates and foods from the allium family of plants, including onions and garlic.

The Chinese compared a group of 564 stomach cancer patients to a group of 1,131 healthy people. What they found was that the people who reported eating the greatest number of allium vegetables had the fewest cases of stomach cancer.

In fact, people who ate these vegetables the most had only 40 percent as great a risk for stomach cancer as did people who rarely ate them.

And in another study—this one at the Department of Oral Medicine and Oral Pathology in the Harvard School of Dental Medicine—onion extract placed in a test tube with cancer cells stopped cancer growth in its tracks. "Tumor growth inhibition began after 24 hours," report the scientists, "and after four days and ten days of incubation, there was a noted decrease in tumor proliferation."

321. Start a Strawberry Patch

Scientists have found that strawberries contain an acid that can kill cancer-causing compounds. Ellagic acid has been shown to destroy hydrocarbons, one of the chemicals found in tobacco smoke that's known to cause lung cancer.

You'll also find ellagic acid in grapes and Brazil nuts.

322. Fish Eaters Have Less Cancer

Scientists looking at the diets of people in 32 countries have found that those who eat fish have less cancer.

In countries where breast cancer rates are high, fish consumption is low. On the other hand, in countries like Japan where fish consumption is high, breast cancer rates tend to be low.

The study was conducted by researchers at the Ludwig Institute for Cancer Research in Toronto, Canada. Scientists there suspect the link between fish and cancer may come about because fish contains omega–3 fatty acids, which have been shown to suppress cancer cells in laboratory tests.

While the results are only preliminary, the school of thought is it wouldn't hurt to try to increase the amount of fish in your diet.

323. Tea for You?

At the National Cancer Center Research Institute in Tokyo, scientists believe that drinking green tea (so named because it's made from green leaves and is unfermented) can inhibit the growth of cancer tumors.

Areas of Japan where green tea is popular have very low cancer death rates. The researchers believe that a compound in the tea—called EGCG—can block tumor-promoting agents.

Rats (not known to actually drink tea) who had EGCG found in the green tea applied to their skin had significantly lower cancer rates than those not treated.

Oriental green tea can be found in stores that sell a wide variety of herbal teas.

324. Watch Where You're Woking

Stir-fry vegetables may be good for you—but apparently only if you're not doing the frying.

The smoky fumes from high-temperature cooking oils could cause lung cancer, according to a study of Chinese women who use oils in wok cooking.

Wok-using Chinese women have the same lung cancer rate as American women, but they smoke tobacco only half as much, leading researchers to suspect the wok as the woeful cause.

If you cook with a wok, try to keep the oil temperatures down and further protect yourself by woking in a well-ventilated area.

325. Practice Safe Grilling

Ah! The smell of sizzling burgers can bring out the carnivore in the best of us. Unfortunately, both the smoke and the char create possible cancer-causing compounds that can be deposited on food. Here are some ways to minimize your barbecue risks.

- Pick low-fat meats for the grill. Fat dripping on hot coals creates harmful smoke and flare-ups that can blacken the meat.
- Cover the grill with foil to protect the meat from the smoke and flames. Punch holes in the foil to let the fat drip out.
- Wrap vegetables and fish in foil to preserve their flavors while at the same time protecting them from the smoke.
- Basting foods while they're cooking will help keep them moist. But don't baste with fat, which can cause flare-ups. Instead use lemon juice, wine, or barbecue sauce.
- Poach or microwave poultry or thick meat until partially cooked, then finish it on the grill. This cuts cooking time and reduces exposure to smoke.
- Trim charred parts before eating.

326. Order Your Ham Fresh

Conventionally smoked foods like hams and some varieties of sausage and fish absorb at least a portion of the tars that rise from incomplete combustion (smoke), according to the American Cancer Society. These tars contain "numerous carcinogens that are similar chemically to the carcinogenic tars in tobacco smoke."

The risk applies primarily to conventionally smoked meats and fish but probably doesn't apply to "liquid smoke" flavoring. If you eat smoked products, the best advice is to do so in moderation.

327. Eat a Safer Hot Dog

If it's just not the Fourth of July without those weenies cooking on the grill, try to buy hot dogs containing the ingredients ascorbic acid, sodium ascorbate, or sodium erthrobate, suggests the American Cancer Society.

Those three ingredients are vitamin C compounds, and they have been added to the food to protect against cancer-causing substances. Look for them in luncheon meats, too.

A Cancer-Free Lifestyle

328. Root for a Smokeless Society

Here's one irrefutable fact that should come as no surprise: Smoking causes cancer.

In fact, "cigarette smoking is the most important known *preventable* cause of cancer," notes Ronald Ross, M.D., a professor in the Department of Preventive Medicine at the University of Southern California School of Medicine and an associate director of the Kenneth Norris/USC Comprehensive Cancer Center.

FACT OF LIFE

Smoke Signals Risk

Someone who smokes two or more packs per day is 20 to 25 times more likely to get cancer than someone who doesn't smoke. Even smokers of low-tar cigarettes are still 11 times more likely to get lung cancer than nonsmokers.

And it's never too late to stop—no matter how long you've been smoking. "A person who begins smoking a pack of cigarettes a day at age 20 and stops smoking at age 60 will, by age 70, have one-half the lung cancer risk of the individual who continues to smoke until age 70," says Dr. Ross.

Make the next cigarette you put out your last.

329. Do It for Her

If none of the other reasons to stop smoking has worked on you, try this one: Wives of smokers are more likely to develop breast cancer than wives of nonsmokers.

An Oregon researcher analyzed information from 50 countries and found that where male death rates from lung cancer are high, female death rates from breast cancer are high, too.

In countries where few men die from lung cancer, breast cancer is also rare. Experts are wondering whether a passive smoking link could explain why breast cancer rates are rising in so many countries.

330. Too Fat Is Too Risky

Being overweight can increase your chances of developing certain types of cancer.

In a massive 12-year study conducted by the American Cancer Society, researchers found a marked increase in cancers of the uterus, gallbladder, kidney, stomach, colon, and breast associated with obesity.

"When data for men and women 40 percent or more over ideal weight were reviewed, the women were found to have a 55 percent greater risk and the men a 33 percent greater risk of cancer than those of normal body weight," reported the study.

331. Drink in Moderation

Alcohol consumption has been linked to 3 percent of the overall cancer rate, with cancers of the liver, mouth, throat, esophagus, larynx, rectum, colon, and breast being implicated.

In a study of 106,203 men and women in northern California, for example, researchers found that people who drank more than three alcoholic drinks a day had a three times greater risk of developing rectal cancer than those who never drank.

And a Harvard Medical School survey of the eating and drinking habits of 89,000 women found that those who drank one or more drinks a day increased their risk of developing breast cancer by 50 percent.

Most scientists, however, are quick to say that the alcohol/cancer link is not 100 proof. For one thing, many of the people studied drank *and* smoked. Their choice of drink also varied greatly.

Nevertheless, there is enough evidence to indicate that excessive use of alcohol is a bad idea.

The best advice? If you must drink, do it in moderation.

332. Get Out and Exercise

Those who exercise most are least likely to get cancer, according to the results of several studies.

In a Harvard study of 17,000 alumni, researchers found that the death rate from cancer was highest in those who exercised the least. Moderate exercisers did better than those who were sedentary, but not as well as the most active alumni.

Even ex-jocks get a benefit from their past life. When 5,398 people were questioned in another study, it was found that former college athletes had a lower lifetime occurrence rate of cancer than nonathletes.

The nonathletes had almost twice the risk of breast cancer and

FACT OF LIFE

Men with Active Jobs Are Less Cancer-Prone

Three separate studies have found that men with physically active jobs—carpenters, plumbers, gardeners, and mail carriers, for example—are much less likely to develop colon cancer than accountants, lawyers, bookkeepers, and other workers who merely shuffle papers and push pencils.

two and a half times the risk of reproductive system cancer as did former athletes.

Another study, this one among 5,138 men and 7,407 women ranging in age from 25 to 74, came to the same conclusion: "Inactive people are at increased risk of cancer."

It's not exactly known why exercise may help you avoid cancer. Some scientists think it may be because exercise reduces obesity. Others think, at least in some women, it may have to do with the fact that exercise reduces estrogen levels. Others feel it make be linked to the simple fact that exercisers generally have a healthier lifestyle.

Whatever the reason, start walking, swimming, riding a bicycle—anything that will get you exercising at least 30 minutes three times a week.

333. Put Your Drive in Park

A 22-year study of more than 3,000 men suggests that Type-A behavior—hard-driving, impatient, sometimes hostile—may increase the risk of death from almost every type of cancer.

Conducted by David Ragland, Ph.D., a researcher at the School of Public Health at the University of California at Berkeley, and his colleagues, the study found that the Type-A male was 50 percent more likely to die from all types of cancer, except lung cancer, than the laid-back Type-B male. Their lung cancer rates were the same.

The researchers say they are not sure why Type A's are more cancer-prone, but they speculate that it has more to do with lifestyle than with personality.

334. Smile, You'll Live Longer

Being depressed could increase your risk of dying from cancer. A study of 2,018 employees at the Western Electric Company near Chicago over a 20-year period reveals that depression may exacerbate cancer—although, fortunately, it doesn't seem to cause it.

Does that mean that happiness will help ensure you'll be around longer? There are plenty of people—including scientists—who say yes. At least, it's the right attitude to have.

Testing Saves Lives

335. Get a Regular Pap Test

A study of 1,500 older women by scientists at the Mount Sinai School of Medicine in New York reveals that most women over the age of 65 don't have regular Pap tests—and that one-quarter of them have never had one at all.

The American Cancer Society suggests that every woman should have the test—once a year until she's had three negative smears, and thereafter on her doctor's advice—no matter what her age. The five year survival rate for uterine cancer—which a Pap test can detect—is over 85 percent when it's caught and treated early.

The test may be particularly important for older women. Other studies have found that women older than 65 have two to three times the incidence of abnormal smears—which may be an early sign of cervical or endometrial cancer—than younger women.

336. Ask the Right Questions

Even though the Pap test is one of the most important medical tests a woman will ever have, the American College of Obstetricians and Gynocologists reports that test results are in error 20 percent of the time. That means one out of every five Pap tests may be wrong.

Half of the errors stem from your doctor's cell sampling techniques, while laboratory problems account for the other half.

How can you fight incompetence? According to the American Cancer Society, you can ensure the best possible work from both your doctor and the lab by asking the following questions:

- Where is my Pap smear going to be sent?
- Is it a licensed and accredited lab?
- Will the laboratory have the test rechecked if the results are abnormal?
- Does the lab provide a full written report?
- Does the lab report poor samples as "inadequate for evaluation" or simply as "negative"?

Your questions are guaranteed to keep your doctor on his toes. And *his* questions to the lab will keep them on theirs.

Life-Extension Tools

Lung Damage Monitor for Smokers

If you smoke, you know that your lungs are vulnerable to cancer. And you probably wonder just how much damage has already been done. Are there precancerous changes that warn of malignancy to come?

Now, a take-home test called the LungCheck can tell you what's going on inside your chest. You or your physician can obtain the test materials by contacting CytoSciences, Inc., 1601 Saratoga-Sunnyvale Road, Cupertino, CA 95014 (1–800–433–8278; in California, 408–966–0600). They'll send you a collection container. For three mornings in a row, you force a cough and spit whatever comes up into the container. Then send the container to their lab. Forty-eight hours later, the lab will send you a report in easy-to-understand terms. Your doctor will receive a more technical report.

The test can detect lung cancer *two to five years* before it would show up on x-rays—early enough, perhaps, for successful surgical treatment. And precancerous changes detected by this test could be a powerful incentive to quit before your lungs get any worse.

Colorectal Cancer Self-Tests

Surveys show that most American men are reluctant to seek regular medical care. Unfortunately, that reluctance often means they don't get regular cancer checkups—which may account for the fact that almost twice as many men as women die of cancer.

But today there's a way for even doctor-phobic shrinking violets to be screened for colorectal cancer, the cancer that kills 30,000 men a year. Two tests—each of which costs under $10 and can be purchased at your local drugstore—have been developed that can be used in the privacy of your home.

Warner-Lambert's Early Detector Test simply involves wiping the anal area with a pad after a bowel movement and spraying the pad with a chemical in the test kit. If the pad turns blue, you may have colorectal cancer. There are a fair number of false-positives with this kind of test, however, so have your doctor confirm the results. The kit is also available by mail from Warner-Lambert, 201 Tabor Road, Morris Plains, NJ 07950.

(continued)

Life-Extension Tools—*Continued*

The other test, the ColoScreen Self-Test by Helena Laboratories, supplies a pad with two test areas on it. Simply toss the pad into the toilet bowl after a bowel movement. If one of the test areas turns reddish-orange, consult your physician. This test is available by mail from Habits for Health, 622 Casas de Leon, Redlands, CA 92373, and from Medical Self-Care, 349 Healdsburg Avenue, Healdsburg, CA 95448.

337. Check Your Breasts Up and Down

Examining your breasts in an up-and-down rectangular pattern is more likely to detect tumors than using the traditional concentric circle pattern women have been taught, studies reveal.

Researchers have found that moving your fingers in straight lines up and down your breast between collar bone and bra line, from armpit to breast bone, is more effective than the concentric circle pattern. The rectangular pattern, doctors say, provides more complete coverage of the area in which tumors generally occur.

In one study, for example, the up-and-down search pattern covered 25 percent more of the breast and 12 percent more of the tumor-prone area than the concentric circle method.

338. Older Women Should Schedule a Mammogram

Women between the ages of 35 and 40 should have a baseline mammogram, doctors suggest, while women aged 40 to 49 should have a mammogram every one or two years. Women over 50 should have one every year. Mammograms are an effective way for doctors

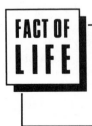

FACT OF LIFE

Breast Self-Exams Are Lifesavers

Don't underestimate your ability to perform a breast self-examination. More than 70 percent of all breast cancers are found by women themselves, not their doctors.

to see even the smallest tumor. If you've had a breast implant, however, take note: Implants obscure from 22 to 83 percent of the breast during a mammogram—making it hard for tumors to be spotted.

The solution? Make sure your mammogram includes "pinched views," says Judy Destouet, M.D., associate professor of radiology at Washington University School of Medicine, St. Louis, Missouri.

A pinched view means the breast tissue is pulled forward and away from the implant and four x-rays are taken instead of the normal two.

339. Test Your Testes

Testicular cancer is one of the most common cancers in men between the ages of 15 and 34. Symptoms—enlargement of one or both testes or a persistent, low back pain—are easily missed, so doctors suggest you regularly examine your testes.

Once a month, when the scrotum is relaxed after a hot shower or bath, roll each testicle between your thumb and middle fingers. If you find a small, hard, usually pain-free lump or area of swelling, see a urologist immediately.

If testicular cancer is treated early, the five-year survival rate is 75 percent. Untreated, it's zero.

340. Have Your Prostate Checked

Cancer of the prostate gland occurs mainly in men over the age of 60. It's the third leading cause of cancer deaths—claiming roughly 25,000 victims a year.

To keep from becoming one of these statistics, the National Cancer Institute recommends that you have your prostate examined every year after the age of 40.

341. Check for Colorectal Cancer

Colorectal cancer is the second leading cause of cancer death in men. Seventy-five percent of those who get it could be saved, however, if the disease were detected and treated at an early stage.

To optimize the chances of detecting colorectal cancer, the American Cancer Society recommends that, once a year, men and women over the age of 50 have a stool sample checked for blood.

Rectal bleeding—frequently undetectable by the naked eye—is an early warning sign of cancer.

The society also recommends a sigmoidoscopy—an internal exam that allows your doctor to look inside the colon—at age 50. Once you've had a satisfactory exam two years in a row, however, you only need to have it repeated every three to five years.

The Skin Care Formula

342. Inspect Your Birthday Suit Every Year

At least 90 percent of all skin cancers are curable if they're discovered early. So get into the habit of giving yourself an annual birthday suit exam—and use a hand mirror along with the full-length one on your bathroom door to make sure you don't miss any nooks or crannies.

What are you looking for? You're looking for a skin growth that has increased in size since your last exam. It may appear pearly, translucent, tan, brown, black, or multicolored. Whatever its color, if it's growing, see your doctor.

But that's not where your responsibility ends. Any spot or growth that attracts your attention between exams—whether it itches, hurts, crusts, scabs, erodes, bleeds, or heals and reopens— should also be checked by a doctor, as should any open wound or sore that persists for more than four weeks.

343. Know a Safe Mole from a Sinister One

The prevalence of precancerous moles has multiplied tenfold in the past decade, reports Los Angeles dermatologist Norman Brooks, M.D.

How can we stop the epidemic? By getting better at spotting dangerous moles, says Dr. Brooks. Look for moles that have an irregular border and exhibit variable colors. Harmless moles have a clearly defined border and are uniformly brown or tan.

If you spot a mole that looks suspicious, see your doctor right away. If caught early, precancerous moles can safely and easily be removed—*before* they turn into a deadly cancer.

FACT OF LIFE

Skin Cancer Is Growing

As air pollution shoots the earth's ozone layer full of holes, the atmosphere's natural protection from ultraviolet rays is diminishing, and the incidence of skin cancer is growing. It's increased 29 percent in men over the past 30 years alone. Now 1 out of every 3 new cancers diagnosed is a cancer of the skin. And some of them are deadly malignant melanoma.

344. Wear a Sunscreen

Overexposure to the ultraviolet rays of the sun is the number one cause of skin cancer.

Light-skinned people—usually redheads and blonds—are at greatest risk because they lack sufficient quantities of melanin, the protective pigment that prevents burning.

Whatever color your skin, the American Cancer Society recommends you wear a sunscreen whenever you go outdoors. And they specifically recommend that you use one with a Sun Protection Factor (SPF) of 15 or more.

Apply the sunscreen at least 15 minutes before you walk out the door. That will give your skin a chance to absorb it. Slather on more every two hours. If you go swimming, however, reapply the sunscreen whenever you come out of the water.

345. Wear Protective Clothing

If your clothes are sheer enough to see through, the sun can shine through, too. So save transparent blouses for the nightclub. Long-sleeved shirts and long pants made of lightweight but tightly woven fabrics are best in the sun. And always wear a hat—preferably one with a wide, wide brim.

346. Schedule Your Sun Time Wisely

Stay out of the sun during the most dangerous period of the day. Ultraviolet rays are strongest between 10:00 A.M. and 2:00 P.M.

(11:00 A.M. to 3:00 P.M. daylight saving time) in most parts of the United States. So plan outdoor activities for the early morning or later afternoon.

And beware of overcast days. Since 85 percent of the sun's ultraviolet rays can penetrate clouds, those rays can be almost as damaging when it's dreary as when it's sunny.

347. Don Quality Shades

Skin cancer can occur on your eyelids. So look for sunglasses that block at least 95 percent of ultraviolet rays, and 75 percent of visible and infrared light. If those numbers aren't on the tag or frame, ask the salesperson or call the manufacturer.

348. Don't Forget Your Lips

Lips get a considerable amount of sun exposure, and they have no protective pigment at all. Yet how many times have you rubbed a sunscreen all over your body and forgotten to do your lips?

Next time you buy the sunscreen for your body, look for an SPF–15 lip balm. Put it on just as often as you put a sunscreen on the rest of you.

349. Avoid the Tan Accelerator

There are some products that claim they can speed up the tanning process, thus reducing the amount of sun it takes to create a golden glow.

Less sun to get a tan? It may sound like a shortcut to cancer prevention, but it's not. It's a rip-off. According to some dermatologists, tan accelerators simply don't work. So save your dough—or invest it in a good sunscreen, instead.

350. Take a Lesson from the Outdoor Worker

Short periods of intense sun appear to put you at higher risk of developing skin cancer than do long periods of gradually more intense exposure.

Research on people in seemingly high-risk professions—outdoor workers such as lifeguards and farmers—shows that they had the same amount or even *less* skin cancer than indoor workers.

Why? Well, one theory is that the indoor worker's sun exposure is less frequent but more severe. A secretary who pounds a type-writer every weekday and then pounds the tennis court on Saturday, for example, is likely to come away from a match with more than a winning serve. She's liable to have a scorching sunburn as well.

In contrast, an outdoor worker has a long period of gradually increasing exposure. A bulldozer operator, for example, is likely to be out in the sun every day from 7:00 A.M. until 5:00 P.M. And since he's always outside, his exposure is essentially controlled by the sea-sonal movement of the earth toward and away from the sun. The result is regular exposure to gradually intensifying ultraviolet rays.

So if you want to be a sun worshiper, take a lesson from the outdoor worker and gradually build up your exposure to the sun.

351. Stay out of Tanning Salons

Tanning salons that claim they're safer than the sun are deceiv-ing their customers, reports the federal Food and Drug Administra-tion (FDA). In fact, an FDA study found that tanning booths which use ultraviolet A (UVA) light actually increase your risk of skin cancer.

Tanning studios that claim their booths use ultraviolet B (UVB) aren't doing you any favors, either. UVB also causes skin cancer. The best approach might be to simply stay clear of any box lined with tubes that glow in the dark.

352. Older Folks Need to Soak Up the Sun

Older folks who regularly use sunscreens can become vitamin D deficient even in the middle of summer, reports a study at Boston University Medical School.

How? Any sunscreen with an SPF of more than 8 will prevent the sun from reaching your skin and combining with natural chem-icals on its surface to make vitamin D, explains Michael Holick, M.D., director of the university's clinical research center.

It's not a serious problem for children or adults who spend lots of time outdoors. Their repeated casual exposure—running in and out of doors many times a day without a sunscreen—ensures vitamin D production. But older folks, who tend to stay inside a lot, need to soak up some sun before they apply a sunscreen.

"If you live in Florida or another sunny area, try to get 5 minutes of exposure two or three times a week," suggests Dr. Holick.

"If you live up north, try to get 10 to 15 minutes of sunshine two to three times a week. After that, put the sunscreen on."

Another way would be to add two or three glasses of milk to your diet every day to take care of your need for vitamin D.

Other Anticancer Strategies

353. Don't Overdo Dental X-Rays

Healthy adults with no signs of cavities should get dental x-rays no more than every 18 months, says George Kaugars, D.D.S., a researcher at the Medical College of Virginia. "Dental x-rays do pose a risk for cancer," he adds. And even though that risk is very small, it should not be ignored.

354. Answer When Nature Calls

Frequent urination may relieve you of bladder cancer. That's the surprising conclusion of an Israeli study that looked at the bathroom habits of 631 randomly chosen rural and urban men.

FACT OF LIFE

Short Guys Finish First

Short men are less likely to get cancer than tall men—at least that's what the statistics show. According to the National Cancer Insitute, short men—those who measure less than 5 feet 6½ inches tall—are at a reduced risk of getting cancer. A study of more than 12,000 adults over a ten-year period found that the shortest 25 percent of the men developed about one-third less cancers than the other 75 percent.

Rural men—who generally suffer from bladder cancer far less often than their urban brethren—urinated an average of six times a day, researchers found, while urban cowboys urinated only five times a day.

Why the difference? Rural men drink more liquids, reported the researchers. And—as most urban men will confirm—it's easier to find a tree in the country than a public restroom in the city.

Since prolonged retention of urinary waste may be a cause of bladder cancer, some scientists theorize that urban men are more likely to suffer from bladder cancer because they're more likely to put their bladder on hold as they search for a restroom.

355. Watch Birds from Afar

Dutch researchers have discovered that people who keep birds have almost *seven times* more risk of developing lung cancer than those who live bird-free.

No one knows why, but one theory is that people with pet birds inhale excessive amounts of allergens and dust particles—either of which can lead to a pair of ailing lungs.

If you're a bird lover, you might be better off putting a feeder in your yard. It will attract plenty of feathery company, and you never have to clean the cage. If you already have a pet bird, however, keep the cage as clean as possible. And wear a dust mask when you clean it.

356. Join a Cancer Registry

If two or more of your close relatives have been diagnosed with ovarian, thyroid, breast, brain, bone, or childhood cancer, you and other family members might be at increased risk of the disease. That's because these particular cancers—plus malignant melanoma, a skin cancer, and familial adenomatous polyposis, a hereditary tendency to form intestinal polyps that may become cancerous—seem to have a genetic basis.

What can you do about this potentially deadly inheritance?

Enroll in a cancer registry. Once enrolled, you can either be tested for the genetic abnormality that causes the type of cancer that runs in your family, or you can be screened for early warning signs on a regular basis.

Ask your doctor or call your local hospital for more information on how you can join a cancer registry. Or contact the Hereditary Cancer Consultation Center at Creighton University School of Medicine in Omaha, Nebraska.

357. Go Back to School

The more you know about cancer, the more you can prevent it. That's why a number of colleges around the country have begun offering courses in cancer biology. And you don't have to be a third-year medical student to take them.

Of students who have taken such courses already, scientists report, nearly half have cut their intake of fat and increased their fiber consumption—two great cancer preventives.

358. Use Barrier Contraceptives

A study at the University of Southern California found that women who regularly used contraceptive jellies or foams, with or without a diaphragm, over a ten-year period—or who had partners who regularly used condoms—cut their risk of cervical cancer by 75 percent. Those who used them over a two- to nine-year period cut the risk by half.

"These findings add strong evidence to the growing belief that most cervical cancer is caused by a sexually transmitted agent," says Ruth Peters, Sc.D., the study's main researcher. "Barrier contraceptives keep such agents as viruses from reaching the cervix, while spermicides may kill anything that's alive."

C H A P T E R · 5

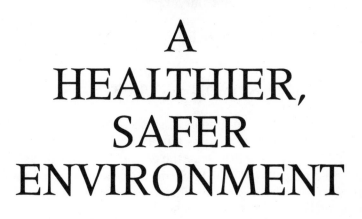

A
HEALTHIER,
SAFER
ENVIRONMENT

Every day we eat plenty of fresh fruits and vegetables because scientists have found that we can reap a bounty of health benefits, like protecting ourselves from cancer. Yet every day millions of acres of our fresh fruits and vegetables are doused with chemical pesticides, many of which, scientists have found, can threaten our health, even to the extent of causing cancer.

Every week we make it a practice to eat more ocean-roaming fish, because scientists believe their oils possess a substance that can keep our hearts healthy. Yet in any given week we hear newscasters throw around terms like PCBs, mercury, and industrial wastes, all harmful elements that are polluting our ocean waters.

We quit smoking because there's more proof than ever before that nicotine causes cancer, only to find that the smoke from someone else's cigarette is still threatening our lives.

Years ago we sealed our home windows, insulated the attic, cemented the foundation, and bought airtight doors in an effort to help save the world's fuel. Now we're threatened by an odorless, invisible, naturally occurring gas called radon that can build up in a tightly insulated environment and give us cancer.

We've hit the roads in our jogging shoes and on our bicycles to feel good and look good, only to find that the fumes we breathe along the way are damaging our lungs.

It's a catch–22—the "yes, but" price we pay for living in a modern world. However, it's by no means a no-win situation.

It's Everywhere, It's Everywhere

For the first time in human existence, every person on earth is exposed in some degree to some kind of chemical danger. For many of us, it happens every day. Since the production of the first synthetic pesticide during World War ll, chemical components and products have been so widely distributed that today they exist virtually everywhere, notes the U.S. Environmental Protection Agency (EPA).

And they're resilient. According to the EPA, a pesticide placed in the soil dozens of years ago can still be found in trace amounts in animals that forage that same ground today. Pesticides have the ability to seep into soil and water, permeate the air, and penetrate the food chain from plant to people. And while only trace amounts of toxins may show up in our food, air, and water, over time they can accumulate in body tissues, where they can jeopardize our health.

Every year in the United States, over a billion pounds of pesticides are applied to crops, forests, lawns, and dwellings. It's not done without reason—chemicals save crops from being damaged by fungi and insects. They're also used to prevent disease. "If grapes weren't sprayed with fungicides, for example, they'd be contaminated with a dangerous type of mold known as aflatoxin," says Joseph Hotchkiss, Ph.D., associate professor of food science at Cornell University. "Aflatoxin is one of the most potent carcinogens [cancer triggers] known."

Pesticides aren't the only pollutants we must deal with day to day. Consider these facts. If you live, work, or dine in the vicinity of people who smoke, you're exposed to more than 4,000 compounds—43 of which are believed to cause cancer—every time they light up. A study conducted by researchers at the Roswell Park Cancer Institute found that nonsmokers carry traces of nicotine byproducts in their urine, a result of breathing other people's cigarette smoke.

If you exercise outdoors, especially along heavily traveled roads, you breathe at least twice as much carbon monoxide and other

FACT OF LIFE

Pesticides Are Popular

A lot of human exposure to potentially hazardous pesticides occurs right in the "safety" of our own homes. The EPA reports that 91 percent of all households in the United States use pesticides.

harmful pollutants from auto and truck exhaust as casual strollers—an ironic price to pay for keeping your lungs in powerful shape.

If you live in a geographic area rich in uranium, radon may be leaking into your home. As you breathe, radon decay products can become trapped in your lungs. As these decay products break down further, they release small bursts of radioactive energy, which can damage lung tissue and lead to lung cancer. Radon gas that enters homes from underlying soil is responsible for an estimated 5,000 to 20,000 cases of lung cancer per year, say scientists. Yet relatively small changes made to your house can cut radon levels—and the inherent health risk—significantly.

Indoor levels of toxic gases run two to five times higher than outdoor levels. Fumes from household products like paints, paint strippers, wood preservatives, aerosol sprays, cleansers, disinfectants, moth repellents, air fresheners, stored fuels, automotive products, and hobby supplies accumulate in an invisible, odorless toxic cloud right inside your home. Gases from household products can damage the kidneys, liver, and central nervous system and are even suspected of causing cancer.

You Can Deal with Reality

Add it up, and the environment can appear to be a mine field of toxic pollution. But it doesn't have to cloud your future. There may be a limit to what you as an individual can do to reduce global pollution, but there's plenty you can do to limit, or at least minimize, the pollution in the little world that is yours.

The EPA issues this sage bit of advice: If we are going to eat, drink, and sleep with environmental chemicals, we need to be wise to their powerful nature. Yes, you *can* reduce your exposure to potentially harmful toxins. Here's how.

Pesticide Patrol

359. Buy Domestically Grown Produce

Imported produce is twice as likely as domestic produce to contain traces of risky pesticides, according to the Food and Drug Administration (FDA). That's because foreign growers often use pesticides banned in the United States, or they use more than the legal amount of FDA-approved pesticides. Imported cantaloupes, for instance, are seven times as likely to contain pesticide residues as domestic cantaloupes. So ask the produce manager at your supermarket where the produce is grown and buy fruit and vegetables from California, Florida, New Jersey, or other areas of the United States.

360. Discard Outer Leaves

Discarding the outer leaves of lettuce and cabbage may also help reduce your exposure to pesticides. So will trimming the leaves and tops off celery. Celery's vascular system acts like a wick, drawing pesticides up the stalk. According to the Natural Resources Defense Council, one study found that trimming celery reduced residues of methomyl, an insecticide believed to cause cancer, by 50 to 90 percent.

361. Peel What You Can

Peeling thin-skinned produce, like carrots and apples, can help, too. Although peeling sacrifices some nutrients, it can significantly remove pesticides that exist in soil and penetrate root vegetables. Peeling will also remove the fungicide-laced wax on produce like cucumbers, apples, eggplants, parsnips, turnips, and squash. Wax, which gives produce that high-gloss look, is being used by fewer growers nowadays, however.

362. Husks and Rinds Are Protective Shields

Domestic produce is not pesticide-free, of course. Partly because consumers shy away from spotty peaches, wormy apples, and moldy grapes, growers use pesticides to successfully produce a reliable supply of good-looking fruit. But produce with tough, removable

FACT OF LIFE

What's Your Pleasure?

Your taste buds have a lot to do with the amount of pesticides you'll consume in your life. Corn, bananas, watermelons, and cauliflower are least likely to contain residues of potentially harmful pesticides, according to reports from the National Resources Defense Council. Strawberries, peaches, celery, cherries, and cucumbers have the most.

skins—like citrus fruit, watermelons, bananas, and corn—generally contain significantly fewer pesticide residues than "naked" or thinner-skinned produce. So does cauliflower, to some extent. Their tough outer coverings act as shields against pesticides. So by buying fruits and vegetables with husks and rinds, you can reduce the amount of pesticides you consume.

363. Scrub the Sturdy

Not all produce can be easily husked or peeled, of course. The U.S. Department of Agriculture (USDA) and the EPA advise people to scrub sturdy produce like celery with a vegetable brush, preferably under running water. Both agencies note, though, that no amount of scrubbing will remove pesticides absorbed by the plant during the growing process.

364. Be Tender to the Tender

Some fruits and vegetables, like grapes, can't be scrubbed easily. The USDA advises consumers to dunk produce like grapes in a bowl of water, then rinse in a colander, so any pesticide residues drain off.

The National Resources Defense Council goes one step further and advises consumers to wash produce in a mild solution of dishwashing detergent and water and then rinse thoroughly.

As for waxed fruit, the International Apple Institute recommends scrubbing waxed apples in detergent and *hot* water (to soften the wax), then rinsing the fruit thoroughly in fresh water.

The FDA cautions, however, that dish detergent is approved for use on eating utensils only. So make sure you rinse produce *thoroughly*.

365. Trim the Fat from Meat and Poultry

Residues of some pesticides in food and water concentrate in fatty tissues of animals and can be passed on to you when you eat beef, pork, or poultry. So cutting away the fat has yet another health benefit (in addition to protecting against heart disease and some forms of cancer), notes the Environmental Protection Agency: It helps cut down any health risks associated with pesticides.

366. Hold the Gravy

Here's another fat- and pesticide-reducing tactic: Skim the fat off broth made from meat or poultry. Discard pan drippings and don't use rendered fat to make gravy. You'll sidestep pesticides and save calories, too.

367. Buy Organically Grown Food

Gone are the days when the only organically grown produce you could find were vegetables like dusty, uninviting carrots in even dustier, out-of-the-way stores. Now you can buy organically grown fruits and vegetables that look and taste as appealing as their chemically-nurtured counterparts. And you don't have to go out of your way to find it. More and more stores and supermarkets now offer food grown without the use of pesticides.

Chemical-Free Gardening

368. Test Your Garden Soil for Lead

If your garden is near a major roadway, you should have the soil checked for lead, a highly toxic mineral. Possible consequences of lead poisoning include blood, nerve, and kidney disease, and exposure to high amounts of lead can be fatal.

You should also check for lead in the soil if you live near a busy airport, battery factory, or metal smelter, or if your garden plot was once used for trash disposal. (If an old, discarded window has been sitting on the soil, for example, lead from paint could have seeped into the ground.) And lead arsenate, sometimes used on fruit trees, can contaminate garden soil.

As a matter of fact, lead is so ubiquitous, it's probably wise to test your soil for lead regardless of what you know (or don't know) about the location. Check with your county agricultural extension service agency. Or contact Woods End Laboratories, Mt. Vernon, ME 04352.

369. Getting the Lead Out

If your garden soil has high levels of lead, you can still cultivate it safely. Truck in clean, lead-free soil—enough to build up a garden bed about 8 inches deep. Be careful not to mix new, uncontaminated soil with the problem soil below. You can ensure this by putting a layer of plastic between the old soil and the new. Your county agent should be able to assist you with any questions or concerns.

370. Scout Out a Pesticide-Free Plot

Growing some of your own food is another way to reduce your exposure to pesticide residues. But chemical-free gardening takes some special planning, beginning with careful site selection. Here are some tips from the EPA for selecting your garden site.

- Avoid sites where pesticides used by a neighbor might drift or run off into your plot.
- Find out how the previous occupants used the land you intend to cultivate. Did they use chemical pesticides? If you're going to convert part of a lawn to garden space, find out if the lawn was sprayed with chemical weed killers or fertilizer. Residues can remain in the soil for years and can leach through the root systems of newly planted crops.

 FACT OF LIFE

Children at Special Risk

Researchers at the University of Southern California found that children whose parents use pesticides inside the home have a 3.8 greater risk of developing childhood leukemia than those who don't. In homes where garden sprays are used, children have a 6.5 times greater risk.

371. Detox Your Garden Plot

Importing clean soil is also an option if your garden plot has been treated with pesticides. But you don't have to go to the expense—you can banish these chemicals yourself, says the EPA. Here's how.

- Before the growing season, turn over the soil often—two or three times a week—for two weeks. Sunlight breaks down some pesticide residues.
- Sow rye grass, clover, alfalfa, or some other nonfood cover crop, then discard the plants you harvest. Don't work them back into the soil. The dense, fibrous root systems of these cover crops will take up some of the lingering pesticide residues.
- Once you begin gardening in earnest, alternate food crops with nonfood cover crops in the off season. They will draw out even more residue.

372. Learn the Secrets of Successful Organic Gardening

Certain strategies can reduce your need for pesticides without sacrificing crop yields. Here are some suggestions from the EPA:

- Healthy soil grows healthy plants, so enrich your garden soil with compost and manure.
- To keep weeds in check and retain moisture in the soil, mulch your garden with leaves, hay, shredded or chipped bark, or seaweed. Grass clippings are fine too, as long as you don't spray your lawn with pesticides.
- Select disease-resistant varieties of seeds and seedlings. You'll get hardy plants that will survive and flourish without pesticides.
- To discourage pests that thrive on one type of plant or another, plant a different kind of vegetable in each row, instead of corralling all the tomatoes in one area, for example, and all the broccoli in another.
- Rotate your crops. If, for example, you plant tomatoes in one spot this year, plant them somewhere else next year. Rotated plants will be less susceptible to pests that survive the winter.
- Remove and destroy diseased plants, tree prunings, and fallen fruit that might harbor pests.

- Control pests further by introducing enemies of plant pests, like purple martins, praying mantises, and ladybugs, or pest-killing organisms like bacteria or viruses (such as *Bacillus thuringiensis*).

As for where to buy nonchemical gardening aids, you can send a postcard with your name and address to Natural Gardening Research Center, Highway 48, P.O. Box 149, Sunman, IN 47041. Ask for their catalog.

373. Grow a Chemical-Free Lawn

You *can* have an attractive lawn without resorting to toxic weed killers, says Warren Schultz, author of *The Chemical-Free Lawn*. But much depends on your idea of what constitutes a good-looking lawn. If you want your backyard to look like a golf green, then all weeds and undesirable grasses must go. But if all you want is a pleasant place to play Frisbee or have a barbecue, you can probably live with a few weeds and avoid powerful herbicides. (A herbicide is a chemical that kills weeds.)

In fact, your lawn is better off without weed killers, even if you're not concerned about toxic exposure, says Schultz. In the long run, weed killers actually aggravate a weed problem: Besides killing weeds, they slow down the biological activity of the soil. That weakens grass plants and encourages plant disease.

Here are some guidelines on pesticide-free lawn care from Schultz's book.

- Decide which weeds you hate the most and attack them. If you have just a few weeds, pull, dig, or cut them. Reseed with grass and water thoroughly until the grass germinates.
- Don't mow too closely. Give your grass a crew cut and wild weeds take over.
- Loosen compacted soil and correct drainage problems. Grass struggles to survive in soil that's wet or dense, while weeds thrive in soggy, heavy turf.
- Fertilize with organic matter early in the spring to give grass a fair chance to get established before cool-season weeds germinate.
- Choose grass seed appropriate for the soil and conditions in your yard. Certain grasses do well in shady areas, for ex-

ample, nudging out weeds that thrive without direct sunlight. If you live in a dry climate or want to conserve water, choose varieties of grass that do well without frequent watering. Still other varieties of grass do well under heavy foot traffic and are smart choices for backyard play areas.

• Dig up weed-infested areas, then reseed.

Above all, be patient, says Schultz. Chemical-free techniques won't produce an attractive lawn overnight, but they're better for your lawn—and you.

If You Must Use Pesticides . . .

374. First, Follow Directions

According to the EPA, the most important safeguard you can take when using pesticides at home is to thoroughly read and carefully follow the label directions and precautions. For starters:

• Don't use more pesticide than the label recommends. You won't kill any more bugs, but you will certainly expose yourself, your family, and your pets to unnecessary risk.

• Use pesticides only at the time, under the conditions, and for the listed purpose the manufacturer specifies.

• Store all pesticides in their original containers. Never transfer a product to an empty soft drink bottle or other container. And make sure containers are clearly marked if the labels start to wear off.

375. Foremost, Use Common Sense

The following caveats may *not* appear on the label, says the EPA, but are equally important to limiting your exposure to the chemicals.

• Avoid applying pesticides outdoors in windy weather (that is, when the wind exceeds 10 miles per hour). Close the windows to your house and don't stand facing the wind.

• Use pesticides indoors only when absolutely necessary, and then use only in recommended amounts. Remove food, dishes, pots, pans, and toys from the area.

• Apply spray as close to the target as possible, using a coarse droplet nozzle to reduce misting.

The Message behind the Label

By law, manufacturers of pesticides must indicate the potential toxicity of their products. Look for these terms:

Danger. This signifies that the product is highly toxic.

Warning. This indicates that the product is moderately toxic.

Caution. This means that the product is only slightly toxic.

Symptoms of pesticide poisoning vary with the type of products inhaled, swallowed, or absorbed through your skin. But if you experience any unusual discomfort (like blurred vision, diarrhea, giddiness, headache, or confusion) after being around a pesticide, call a poison control center or get medical attention immediately (or both). And take the container of the substance in question with you to the doctor or emergency room, to help identify the poison and determine what action is appropriate.

376. Choose the Spray to Fit the Pest

You wouldn't try to remove a paper staple with a crowbar. The same principle applies to pesticides. To avoid unnecessarily exposing you and your family to their toxic effects, the EPA says you should choose a pesticide designed to destroy only the particular pest you're trying to control. "The stronger, the better" is only dangerous thinking.

A product label will tell you what kind of pest the compound is formulated to control: mites, flies, Japanese beetle grubs, whatever. The label will also tell you where a product is to be used: lawns, swimming pools, roses, specific vegetable crops, and so forth.

377. Wear Protective Clothing

If a chemical is powerful enough to kill weeds and insects on contact, imagine what it might be doing to your skin, eyes, or lungs. The EPA says you should always wear protective clothing and take measures to avoid inhaling the pesticide or absorbing it through your skin. Check the label. If the manufacturer recommends you wear long sleeves and pants, vinyl or rubber gloves (not canvas or leather gloves), footwear, a hat, safety goggles, or a respirator, do it. You can find everything you need in a building supply store or hardware store.

378. Don't Smoke and Spray

Some pesticides are flammable, so if you light up when handling these chemicals, you could start a fire and get burned. Aside from the risk of flames, you could easily transfer the toxic material from your hand to your mouth as you smoke. And since you breathe more deeply when you draw on a cigarette, you inhale twice the amount of toxic fumes if you smoke while mixing pesticides.

379. Clean Up Spills Pronto

If you spill a pesticide, clean it up immediately. Don't try to wash away the spill, though. It'll only end up in your well water or soil. Instead, sprinkle the area with an absorbent material like sawdust, vermiculite, or kitty litter to wick it up, then sweep the spill into a plastic garbage bag and dispose of it with other trash.

380. Hit the Showers

The EPA recommends that you shower and shampoo thoroughly after using a pesticide, even if you haven't spilled any chemicals. Rinse your boots or shoes, too, and wash any other protective clothing separately from the family laundry.

381. To Air Is Humane

Pesticide fumes dissipate more slowly indoors than outdoors. So if you've applied a pesticide indoors, air out the house thoroughly and often. To speed up the exchange of outdoor air (which is generally fresher and purer) for indoor air, open doors and windows, and switch on overhead or whole house fans.

382. Ask the Pros about Nonchemical Warfare

Some jobs, such as termite control, are best left to professional bug busters. If you hire a pest control firm, ask the crew to use the least toxic—or chemical-free—pest control method available. Some home pest control companies, for example, offer an electro-gun technique to control termites and similar infestations by penetrating trouble areas and zapping the pests without using *any* chemicals.

383. Discard Carefully

Don't leave empty or half-empty containers of chemicals around the basement or garage—remember, they're *poisons*. Don't pour leftover pesticides down the sink or toilet—they can contaminate the water supply. And don't burn pesticide boxes or sacks outdoors or in apartment incinerators—burning can create poisonous fumes or gases (or an explosion).

Unless the product label states otherwise, you should secure the cap to prevent leaks, then wrap the container in several layers of newspaper and tie it securely. Then place the package in a *covered* trash can for routine collection.

Natural Pest Control

384. Use Cedar Chips for Winter Woolens

Many mothballs and moth crystals contain p-dichlorobenzene, a chemical suspected of causing cancer, says the EPA. And they smell bad, too.

Housekeepers have found that natural repellents, like cedar chips or sachets of dried lavender, pennyroyal leaves and stems, or a sprinkling of dried, ground pyrethrum flowers, can do the job just as effectively.

As with chemical moth repellents, these natural alternatives work best if you clean the clothes thoroughly, then store them with the repellent in airtight containers.

385. Roaches: Search and Destroy

Boric acid reportedly can kill cockroaches just as well as some more expensive, commercial antiroach powders. In her book *The Healthy Home*, Linda Mason Hunter recommends the following Anti-Roach Recipe, a tasty last supper for these resilient pests: Combine 1 cup borax, ½ cup flour, ¼ cup confectioners' sugar, and 1 cup cornmeal. Sprinkle the powder in the dark, warm places roaches love: under sinks and stoves, behind the refrigerator, and in cabinets and closets. (Keep this mixture out of reach of children or pets. If eaten, it could make them sick.)

From time to time, sweep or vacuum the powder and replace with a fresh batch. Continue until you've eradicated the roaches.

386. Give Your Houseplants a Sponge Bath

If you notice bugs such as aphids and mealybugs on your houseplants, there's no need to reach for a powerful chemical assault weapon. Instead, wipe the stems and leaves with a mild soap-and-water solution, such as Safer's soap spray.

387. Give Rover a Cedar Chalet

Is your outdoor pet hounded by fleas? Line his dog house with an enclosed bed of cedar shavings or pine needles. It's a natural repellent that's worth a try.

388. Wash Your Pets' Bedding Often

If your pets sleep on a doggie blanket or kitty quilt, wash the bedding often in hot water and soap or detergent. Veterinarians say it's an effective way to discourage fleas from infesting your pets and your house.

389. Put Fleas in a Vacuum

Frequent, thorough vacuuming of carpeting, furniture, and other areas your pet frequents is another helpful antiflea measure. To vacuum thoroughly, move the wand in slow, overlapping strokes, covering each area with six or seven strokes.

390. Make the Earth Move

Diatomaceous earth is a fine-textured silica derived from a form of algae, and some claim it makes a very effective nontoxic flea powder. (Regular dirt doesn't work.) Sprinkle it on carpeting, woodwork, and your pet's bedding. Diatomaceous earth kills fleas by drying them out. And it won't harm your pet. Be forewarned: It can be a little messy.

You can find diatomaceous earth at garden centers that carry natural products or order it from Nitron Industries, Inc. Be sure to buy an unprocessed brand, because kinds sold for use in swimming pool filters are harmful if inhaled. For a catalog, write to P.O. Box 1447, Fayetteville, AR 72702–1447, or call toll-free 1–800–835–0123.

Safer Fish

391. Go for the Young and Lean

Fish least likely to be contaminated by PCBs, DDT, and other contaminants include cod, haddock, and pollock, according to the Center for Science in the Public Interest. Fish most likely to be tainted are catfish, carp, bluefish, striped bass, and swordfish. Here's why.

- Predators, like bluefish, accumulate toxins when they consume smaller, contaminated fish.
- Fatty fish, like carp, store toxins in their fat.
- Older fish have more time to accumulate pollutants.

This only holds true for fish taken from potentially polluted waters, though. A fatty fish from a clean stream in Idaho, for example, will be safer to eat than a lean fish from a dirtied water such as Boston Harbor.

392. Fish Fresh from the Farm Is Best

Aquaculture is a burgeoning industry in which certain species of fish, most notably catfish and rainbow trout, are raised on commercial fish ranches in uncontaminated ponds and beds.

The advantage to the fish farmer is the ability to harvest seasonal varieties on demand and make them available fresh to the customer. The advantage to the consumer, however, is twofold: top quality fish that is almost certain to be toxin-free. Striped bass, oysters, and mussels are also being farmed in some parts of the country.

393. Buy from a Market You Trust

If you don't have a local fishmonger you can get to know and trust, your best bet is to buy from a large commercial market. They

---

Fish Oil Is Safe

If the oil in your fish-oil capsules came from fish contaminated with PCBs or some other pollutant, would your capsule end up polluting you? Interesting question. Or at least researchers at the Toxic Chemicals Laboratory at Cornell University and the New York State College of Agriculture and Life Sciences found it intriguing enough to look for an answer. In a pilot study, the researchers analyzed four major brands of fish-oil supplements. Although minute amounts of PCBs and other harmful contaminants were detected, the researchers concluded that most of the toxic residue was removed during purification. (The question was probably posed in the first place because fish store toxins in their fat.)

The researchers say that while this was not an extensive, in-depth study, they're fairly confident that fish-oil capsules—believed to help lower levels of blood fats and thus protect against heart disease—don't pose a health threat. "Probably the advantages of taking the capsules outweigh the disadvantages of any harmful effects from contaminants," says Joseph G. Ebel, Jr., Ph.D., who was one of the researchers for the study.

---

sell mostly open-water fish from a variety of sources, which are generally safe waters, according to Usha Varanasi, Ph.D., of the National Marine Fishery Service.

"I think you have to balance the small risk of toxins against the fact that fish and shellfish are healthy and highly nutritious," says Dr. Varanasi. "It would be very unwise to conclude that because some rivers and bays are polluted, you should back away from fish completely."

394. Leisure-Time Fishermen, Take Note

Sport fishermen who eat their catch from rivers, bays, and coastlines near urban industrial areas are at greater risk of contamination than people who buy fish at retail outlets. Some places where high toxic levels have been found include Long Island Sound, parts of Puget Sound, San Francisco Bay, Boston Harbor, the Chesapeake Bay, the Hudson River, and the Great Lakes.

Some states neighboring the Great Lakes, for example, advise people living nearby not to eat fish taken from the lakes more than once a week in order to keep intake of toxins to a minimum.

Until scientists know more about the potential health effects of toxic substances in fish, this is probably a good rule for anyone who eats fish caught in waters near industrialized areas. But it's especially important for pregnant or nursing women.

395. Cook Away Contaminants

Fatty fish are more pollution-prone than lean fish because pollutants such as PCBs have an affinity for fat—they concentrate in fatty tissues. You should also grill or broil fatty fish on a rack, so the fat and juices—and any contaminants it may contain—can drain away.

Clean Air Action

396. Don't Jog in the Smog

When you exercise hard, you inhale more deeply, taking in about five to six times the amount of air you breathe while at rest. So if you jog or cycle in a city or roadside park, you can breathe in unhealthy car exhaust and toxic fumes. But that's not all. The ultraviolet rays of the sun turn these fumes into a cloud of pollutants known as ozone, a potent and hazardous form of oxygen. The cloud can travel for miles.

Time your workout to avoid peak pollution periods: Exercise in the morning during the summer, and in the evening during the winter. In summer, ozone levels build during the day, peak in late afternoon, and trail off by nightfall. In winter, ozone is less of a problem, but cold air can trap a layer of carbon dioxide, nitrogen dioxide, sulfur dioxide, and other pollutants overnight.

397. Avoid Rush-Hour Running

Avoid running or biking along main roads during rush hour, when traffic—and exhaust fumes—are heaviest. Also avoid running in place or standing at intersections, where carbon monoxide tends to build up.

398. Take Your Workout Indoors

When newspapers or broadcast media issue pollution warnings, forgo plans to run or bike outdoors. Instead, head for a gym, pool, health club, or other indoor activity. The air inside may not be mountain fresh, but pollution levels in most gyms and pools are half what they are in traffic—even less if the building is air-conditioned.

399. Check Out an Old Flame

The flame on all gas appliances (including water heaters) should be blue. If there's a trace of yellow (or an irregular shape) to the flame, you may be breathing carbon monoxide and other harmful by-products of inefficient gas combustion. Call the gas company and schedule a service call as soon as possible.

400. Have Your Oil Burner Serviced Annually

Clean, properly maintained oil heaters burn fuel more efficiently. But yearly tune-ups save you more than money; they also cut down on air pollution inside your home. One study showed that after tuning up an oil burner and replacing nozzles and filters, smoke was reduced by 59 percent, carbon monoxide by more than 81 percent, gaseous hydrocarbons by 90 percent, and filterable particulate (soot) by 24 percent.

Some other hints:

- Ask the service technician to vacuum the unit, if necessary. (You should have this done every one to five years, depending on how smoky your system is.)
- Check air filters monthly for soot and replace them at least twice during the heating season. Dirty filters mean dirty air and can reduce furnace efficiency.

401. Replace Your Old Oil Burner

If no amount of tuning and tinkering can make your oil burner operate efficiently, consider replacing it. (Anything less than 70 percent efficiency is below par.) The savings in fuel cost will eventually offset the cost of a new burner—and you'll breathe easier as a result.

FACT OF LIFE

Thousands Dying to Stay Warm

About 3,800 people a year are accidentally killed from the buildup of carbon monoxide, an odorless, colorless gas that is emitted when a faulty or poorly ventilated heat source consumes precious oxygen. Potential indoor sources include gas appliances, oil burners, wood stoves, and kerosene heaters.

402. Make Sure Your Wood Stove Is Certified

Residential wood stoves, whether freestanding or as fireplace inserts, are one of the largest sources of indoor air pollution. Wood smoke contains significant amounts of carbon monoxide, hydrocarbons, and many other compounds that are known triggers for respiratory and cardiovascular problems.

The EPA now requires manufacturers to equip wood stoves with catalytic combustors and other design features to improve fuel efficiency and reduce pollution.

To gauge how efficiently your wood stove burns, go outside and check your chimney: If you see little or no smoke after the fire has been burning for an hour, the stove is operating efficiently.

403. Forget about Kerosene Space Heaters

Kerosene space heaters are designed to be used with a copious amount of ventilation—wide-open windows. But few people do that. (After all, they want to stay warm.) And without lots of fresh air, kerosene heaters quickly consume oxygen—*your* oxygen. They also give off a laundry list of potentially harmful gases, including carbon monoxide. So your best—and safest—bet is to avoid using kerosene space heaters altogether.

404. Test Your House for Radon—Twice

Outdoors, radon emitted by soil and rocks is diluted to such low concentrations that it poses no threat to health. But once radon seeps inside an enclosed space (like many of today's well-insulated

Life-Extension Tool

Radon Detectors

Radon is a potentially cancer-causing gas that can seep into your home and threaten your health. You can't see it or smell it, but you can detect it. If you want to find out whether you're breathing unhealthy levels of the gas, you can install a radon detector in your home. The two most popular commercially available types are the charcoal canister and the alpha track detector.

Charcoal canisters cost $10 to $25 each and are kept in place for three to seven days. Alpha track detectors cost $20 to $50 each and are kept in place for two to four weeks or longer. (Other types of radon detectors are available, but they're more expensive, and they must be operated by trained personnel.) To get an accurate measurement, be sure to keep the device in place for the period of time specified by the manufacturer. Then take the detection device to a laboratory for analysis.

To locate a radon-testing laboratory near you, consult your telephone directory. For reliable results, look for a lab participating in the Radon Measurement Proficiency Program. Or call or write to your state radiation protection office or regional EPA office for the name of a participating laboratory.

The lab will report the results of the radon test in one of two ways. Results from devices which measure radon decay products are reported as working levels (WL). Results from devices that measure concentrations of radon gas itself are reported as picocuries per liter (pCi/l).

If the results show radon levels greater than about 1.0 WL or 200 pCi/l, you should consider taking immediate action to reduce the radon levels in your home. Radon is blamed for about 5,000 to 20,000 cases of cancer a year.

homes), it can accumulate to unhealthful levels, putting you at risk for developing lung cancer. And your risk increases as the level of radon and the length of time you're exposed to it increases.

For about $25, you can have your home tested for radon. Radon detectors are available from your state or local government, or from private firms. Call your state radiation protection office or EPA regional office for details.

FACT OF LIFE

Radon: The West Has Less

States with highest levels of cancer-causing radon include Rhode Island, Connecticut, Pennsylvania, Indiana, Michigan, Kentucky, Tennessee, Missouri, Kansas, Colorado, Wyoming, North Dakota, Minnesota, and Wisconsin.

The two most popular commercially available radon detectors are the charcoal canister and the alpha track detector. Both are exposed to the air in your home for a specified period of time and sent to a laboratory for analysis.

The EPA suggests that you have your home tested more than once, in different locations, to get a good estimate of the average radon concentration to which you and your family are exposed.

Your basement will probably have more radon than the rest of the house—partly because it's nearer the ground, and partly because basements tend to be poorly ventilated. The firm that conducts the test will let you know if your house has unhealthful levels of radon gas.

405. Give Radon the Boot

If tests show you do indeed have a radon problem, don't panic. But the higher the radon level, the quicker you should act. Here are some effective options recommended by the EPA.

- Whenever practical, open all windows and turn on fans to increase the air flow into and throughout the house. If you use exhaust fans, be sure to open windows evenly on all sides of the house. Otherwise, you'll draw more radon into the house than you get rid of.
- If your home is built above a crawl space, open the crawl space vents on all sides and keep them open year-round.
- Seal cracks and other openings in basement floors.
- Ask your local plumber or plumbing supply dealer about special basement floor drains designed to allow water to drain while they seal out radon gas.
- Don't sleep in a below-ground room. Since radon concentrations tend to be greater on the lower levels of a home, any-

one who sleeps in a basement bedroom—or consistently sacks out on the rec room couch for hours while watching TV—is at greater risk than those who sleep upstairs.

• Don't smoke and ask guests who smoke to step outside. Studies show that smoking exacerbates the risk of exposure to radon.

406. Initiate Air-to-Air Combat

You can improve the quality of your indoor air by installing a heat-recovery ventilator, commonly known as an air-to-air heat exchanger. It increases ventilation by drawing purer, outside air into the home and exhausting more polluted, indoor air to the outdoors. A heat exchanger, installed in windows or as part of a central air system, can significantly reduce levels of radon and other toxic gases.

407. Let Your Plants Clean the Air

Aside from adding a decorative touch to your home environment, houseplants help reduce trace amounts of formaldehyde, benzene, and trichloroethylene, which are all indoor pollutants, say researchers at the National Aeronautics and Space Administration (NASA).

"Fifteen to 20 potted plants of the right variety in an average-sized home would do the work of a good high-efficiency air cleaner," says Bill Wolverton, Ph.D., senior research scientist for the NASA environmental research lab at John C. Stennis Space Center in Mississippi.

"We've identified several varieties that are *very* beneficial indoors," says Dr. Wolverton. "They absorb formaldehyde fumes released from new carpeting and building materials and clear substances like benzene [a carcinogen in cigarette smoke] and carbon monoxide out of the air."

The best species? "Spider plants are very good at this, but philodendrons are even better—and they're very easy to grow because they require little light and care," says Dr. Wolverton. "If you can't grow philodendrons, you can't grow anything."

You don't necessarily need to line every window sill in your house with potted plants, though. Vines like heart-leaf philodendron and golden pothos can be trellised to cover a large area.

"In my office here at NASA, there's just one golden pothos vining its way around," says Dr. Wolverton. "With just one pot, I've got a jungle here!"

Aloe vera, peace lilies, corn plants (and other kinds of dracaena), snakeplant, potted ivy, and flowering bananas also work well.

Healthier Housekeeping

408. Ammonia Is a Solo Performer

Certain household cleaners, most notably ammonia and chlorine bleach, are fairly harmless when used by themselves but become hazardous to your health if combined. Together they give off chloramine, a toxic gas which can cause irritation to your air passages.

Combine either with a toilet bowl cleaner, and you end up with mixtures that release either free ammonia or free chlorine, both of which are harmful to breathe. Even products that contain ammonia are harmful when mixed.

Should you notice a strong, offensive odor or suffer eye, nose, or throat irritation when using household products, stop what you're doing and open all the windows. Get as much fresh air as you can. If you don't feel better within 30 minutes, call your nearest poison control center, listed in your telephone directory.

But play it safe in the first place: Don't mix *any* household products.

409. Get Back to Basics: Baking Soda and Borax

Sodium bicarbonate (baking soda), a simple compound added to baked goods to help them rise, and sodium borate (borax) are all-around cleaners that are virtually harmless to your health. These two housecleaning basics can take the place of scouring powder, fabric fresheners, carpet deodorizers, air fresheners, and tub, tile, and toilet bowl cleaners. (They're inexpensive, so they save you money, too.)

Friends of the Earth, an organization based in Ontario, Canada, dedicated to environmental research and education, suggests the following uses for baking soda and borax.

Scouring powder. Sprinkle baking soda or borax on kitchen sinks, bathtubs, tile, counters—wherever you would normally use a scouring powder. Scrub with a damp cloth or a plastic mesh scrubber. Washing soda (sodium carbonate) works well, too.

Fabric freshener. For cleaning things like dirty diapers, mix ½ cup baking soda with 2 gallons of water. Soak the soiled items for 2 hours or longer, then launder using borax.

Carpet and rug deodorizer. Sprinkle baking soda liberally on a dry carpet or rug. Let stand for at least 15 minutes, then vacuum thoroughly. (You may want to test this on a small, hidden section of carpeting first, to be sure the carpet won't discolor.)

Drain cleaner. Pour ¼ cup of baking soda and ½ cup of vinegar down a sluggish drain and cover tightly for a minute by stuffing a rag into the drain. The bubbling action should loosen the debris. Then flush the drain with boiling water.

410. Use Methylene Chloride with Care

Fumes from certain household chemicals and cleaners can accumulate into a toxic cloud if you don't take appropriate precautions. This is especially critical when using household products containing methylene chloride, commonly found in paint strippers, adhesive removers, aerosol spray paints, and pesticide "bombs." Methylene chloride causes cancer in animals and is converted to carbon monoxide in the body.

To reduce exposure to this potentially dangerous gas:

- Buy only as much of a product as you will use soon and follow the manufacturer's directions.
- Use hobby and fix-it products outdoors if at all possible, or in a well-ventilated area.
- Throw away unused or little-used containers, like cans of spray paint containing small amounts of leftover paint.

411. Pump, Don't Spray

Aerosol cans of hairspray, furniture polish, and other grooming, cleaning, and hobby products deliver powerful and often toxic chemicals in a fine mist.

Normally, your nose and cilia can filter out large particles in the air, but aerosol mists can sneak by your body's natural filtering mechanisms and lodge deep in the lungs, where they put you at possible risk for cancer. A safer bet: non-aerosol, pump versions of the same products.

412. Soil and Vinegar

Dilute acetic acid—plain old white vinegar—is more than just a low-fat salad dressing. It's a housecleaning staple that can also be used as a nontoxic household cleaner. Here are some ideas.

Mold and mildew remover. Wipe down tile grout, shower curtains, and other mold- and mildew-prone surfaces with a cloth moistened with vinegar. You can also use an old toothbrush to scrub tile grout.

Fabric softener. When doing laundry, add ¼ cup of white vinegar to the final rinse cycle.

Carpet stain remover. For pet stains and odors in carpeting, first soak up as much moisture as you can with dry paper towels. Then mix 2 cups of white vinegar in a gallon of cold water. Apply the vinegar mixture to the spot with a clean cloth or paper towels and gently blot out the stain. (Test this first on a small, hidden spot of carpeting, to be sure the color doesn't fade.) Clean all spills immediately—they're harder to remove after they set.

Glass and mirror cleaner. In a 16-ounce spray bottle, mix 1 cup vinegar with 1 cup water. Spray on windows and mirrors and dry with a cloth or paper towel.

413. Use Elbow Grease to Free a Drain

For stubbornly clogged drains, use a plunger or mechanical (wire) snake, available at hardware or department stores. To use a plunger, fill the sink or tub with 3 or 4 inches of water (if water isn't already backed up). Then, holding a rag in the overflow outlet, repeatedly move the plunger up and down forcefully over the drain.

To use a mechanical snake to break up a clog, push the snake into the drain, and move it up and down.

This should eliminate your need to use potent household drain cleaners, which can be deadly if accidentally swallowed.

414. A Safer Bowl Cleaner

To clean and deodorize your toilet bowl without resorting to harsh chemicals, try this: Sprinkle baking soda into the water, then splash a little vinegar against the inside of the bowl and scour with a toilet cleaning brush.

If the toilet is really stained, try this alternative: Pour about ¼ cup of bleach in the bowl. Let it stand unflushed all day, then brush and flush. Stains should disappear with little or no effort.

415. Clean Your Oven without Getting Gassed

Baked-on oven grease is about the stubbornest kind of dirt in the house. So it's not surprising that commercial oven cleaners contain some powerful chemicals, some of which can give off toxic fumes. You can avoid oven cleaners entirely, though. Friends of the Earth suggests the following oven cleaning strategy: Clean up after spills using a paste of baking soda and water. Or mix 2 tablespoons of phosphate-free dishwashing soap with 1 tablespoon borax in a spray bottle filled with warm water. Spray the solution in the oven and leave for at least 20 minutes. Then use fine steel wool or a plastic kitchen scrubber for tough spots.

416. Give Your Clothes a Good Whiff

When clothes come back from the dry cleaner, smell them for any trace of chemicals. The smell is a sign that the dry cleaner didn't adequately remove perchloroethylene (the most commonly used dry cleaning chemical) from the garment, says the EPA. In laboratory studies, perchloroethylene causes cancer in animals, and people who wear drycleaned garments or store them in their homes are exposed to breathing low levels of this chemical if the clothes are not properly cleaned. If you detect an odor, use another cleaner.

417. You Can't Can Freshness

Commercial artificial air fresheners do not remove odors so much as cover them up with an even stronger chemical scent. For a chemical-free freshener, simmer lemon rind or pleasant-smelling herbs like peppermint in a pot of water on the stove. Or leave a potpourri of herbs in an open jar on a shelf or toilet tank. To freshen closets, hang a cloth bag filled with cedar chips or dried herbs such as lavender.

418. Unbleached Paper Is Safer

Environmental groups like Greenpeace warn that bleached paper products, like coffee filters, contain too much of the toxic chemical dioxin. Now consumers can buy unbleached coffee filters from Melitta, the world's largest manufacturer of coffee filters. Melitta spokesmen say coffee brewed with the new filters may taste pleasantly milder than with the bleached filters. As concern over environmental pollutants grows, manufacturers of other commonly used paper products, like milk cartons and paper towels, are expected to offer consumers unbleached products as an alternative.

Effective Smoke Screens

419. Fight the Smoky Flight Syndrome

Booking a seat in the "nonsmoking" section on an overseas flight (smoking on domestic flights was banned in early February of 1990) doesn't always guarantee you a smoke-free flight—especially if you're in the last nonsmoking row, or you have to pass through the smokers on the way to the rest room, or it's a very *long* flight with *lots* of smokers. Then there's also the poor ventilation (opening vents uses up extra fuel) you frequently find in the cabin.

To help get you a smoke-free flight, here's what to do.

- When you book your flight, ask for a seat assignment in the middle of the no-smoking section, preferably in coach class. The first-class section is so small that the air in the seats neighboring the no-smoking rows may be worse than the air in no-smoking seats in coach. And seats toward the front or back of the no-smoking section in coach are too close to the smoking sections to assure you of smoke-free air.
- Complain. "The captain can increase the amount of fresh air entering the cabin—*if* you complain enough," says Donald

FACT OF LIFE

All Work and No Smoke

The winds of change are definitely blowing in the workplace—and the air that's blowing is fresh. It's currently estimated that half of all U.S. workplaces have nonsmoking policies—and the number is growing daily.

Stedman, Ph.D., professor and chairman of the Department of Environmental Chemistry at the University of Denver.

- "Send word to the cockpit that you'd like to speak with the flight engineer. Explain that you're having difficulty breathing and would like more fresh air in the cabin." And be polite—courtesy is usually more effective than rudeness.
- Be prepared to report your dissatisfaction. Ask the flight engineer for his or her *full* name, and have pen and paper in hand, ready to write it down. "Crew members know that if you send a letter of complaint to the airline, it stays in their file," says Dr. Stedman. "Most airline employees will go to a good deal of trouble to avoid a bad [letter about them]."

420. Go to Restaurants with No-Smoking Sections

By law, many cities and states require restaurants to offer no-smoking seating areas. And some restaurants have voluntarily banned smoking entirely. When dining out, call ahead to find out if the restaurant has a no-smoking section and request a table there.

421. Dine Early

Smoke gets thicker as the night wears on, and in some restaurants, smoke from diners in the smoking section can drift into the nonsmoking section. So try to arrive early in the evening.

422. Use Gentle Persuasion

If you've steered your way to a no-smoking area and someone lights up anyway, your first instinct may probably be to cough, wave your hands, fan away the smoke, and otherwise try to shame the smoker into putting out the cigarette. But behavioral psychologists say that's the worst strategy: Instead, confront the smoker, offering an alternative that *saves* face. Barry Lubetkin, Ph.D., director of the Institute for Behavior Therapy in New York City, suggests you try the following lines.

- "I would appreciate it if you blew your smoke in another direction."
- "I understand that you want to continue to smoke, but could you hold your cigarette in your other hand?"
- "We'll be leaving in 10 minutes. If you can hold off smoking until then, we'd appreciate it."

If those entreaties don't work, escalate your request, says Dr. Lubetkin.

- "Would you mind putting out your cigarette? This is a no-smoking area."
- "Excuse me, I'm allergic to cigarette smoke" (or, "I have trouble breathing cigarette smoke") and "I must ask you to put out your cigarette."

Virtually all smokers will comply with these last two requests, says Dr. Lubetkin. If they don't, and you're in a restaurant, ask your waiter or waitress to make the request. In the rare case where all efforts fail, ask to be seated at another table.

423. Throw a Nonsmoking Party

If you like to entertain but prefer people not smoke in your home, here are some suggestions to help you discourage guests from lighting up.

- When you telephone smokers to invite them to your home, say warmly, "We are so eager to see you; I hope you can attend. You should know, however, that this will be a no-smoking party." You could also say, "We are expecting several guests who, like us, have trouble tolerating cigarette smoke."
- Put a no-smoking sign on the door or in the entry hall.
- Remove all ashtrays.
- Offer an area where guests can smoke—ideally, outdoors on a patio or well-ventilated porch.

424. Negotiate a Smoke-Free Zone

If your spouse or roommate smokes, don't nag about it. Begging and pleading may only make him more obstinate. Instead, work out a compromise—try to persuade him to smoke outdoors only or in a well-ventilated room with the door shut.

Water Fit to Drink

425. Safeguard Your Well Water

If you draw your drinking water from a well, you can take these steps to avoid contaminating the supply:

- Be sure your well is deep enough to reach an aquifer that is below and isolated from surface waters, and be sure the well shaft is tightly sealed.
- Before applying a pesticide outdoors, check with your EPA regional office to find out if it will leach into ground water. Avoid pesticides that leach.
- Never use or mix a pesticide of any kind near your wellhead.

426. Test Your Water

Take a sample of your water to a lab and have it analyzed. Compare the results with the standards established by the EPA (see "National Primary Drinking Water Safety Standards" on the opposite page). If it's contaminated, one of the following procedures might help.

- If your well water contains dangerous levels of pesticide residues, you can install a reverse osmosis water-treatment system.
- If your well water contains radon, you can aerate or filter it through granulated activated charcoal.
- If your water contains toxic organic chemicals—like trihalomethanes (THMs), which are potential causes of cancer—activated carbon can do the job.
- If your water contains heavy metals like lead, reverse osmosis or a point-of-use distiller will reduce lead levels.

National Primary Drinking Water Safety Standards

This is a partial listing. For more complete data, contact the U.S. Environmental Protection Agency, Office of Drinking Water, 401 M Street SW, Washington, DC 20460.

Contaminant	Possible Health Effects	Quantity (mg/liter)	Sources
Inorganic Chemicals			
Arsenic	Skin problems; nervous system toxicity	0.05	Geological; pesticide residues; industrial waste and smelter operations*
Barium	Circulatory system effects	1.0	Source not indicated
Cadmium	Kidney effects	0.01	Geological; mining and smelter operations*
Chromium	Liver or kidney effects (or both)	0.05	Source not indicated
Lead	Central and peripheral nervous system damage; kidney effects; highly toxic to infants and pregnant women	0.05†	Leaches from lead pipes and lead-based solder pipe joints
Mercury	Central nervous system disorders; kidney effects	0.002	Used in manufacture of paint, paper, vinyl chloride; used in fungicides; geological
Organic Chemicals			
1,1-Dichloro-ethylene	Liver or kidney effects (or both)	0.007	Used in manufacture of plastics, dyes, perfumes, paints
1,1,1-Trichloro-ethane	Nervous system effects	0.2	Used in manufacture of food wrappings, synthetic fibers

(continued)

National Primary Drinking Water Safety Standards—*Continued*

Contaminant	Possible Health Effects	Quantity (mg/liter)	Sources
Organic Chemicals —continued			
1,2-Dichloro-ethane	Possible cancer‡	0.005	Used in manufacture of insecticides, gasoline
2,4-D	Liver or kidney effects (or both)	0.1	Used as herbicide to control broad-leaf weeds in agriculture; used on forests, ranges, pastures, bodies of water
2,4,5-TP Silvex	Liver or kidney effects (or both)	0.01	Herbicide (banned in 1984)
Benzene	Cancer§	0.005	Fuel (leaking tanks); solvent commonly used in manufacture of industrial chemicals, pharmaceuticals, pesticides, paints, plastics
Carbon tetrachloride	Possible cancer‡	0.005	Common in cleaning agents and industrial wastes (from manufacture of coolants)
Endrin	Nervous system or kidney effects (or both)	0.0002	Insecticide used on cotton, small grains, orchards
Lindane	Nervous system or liver effects (or both)	0.004	Insecticide used on seed and soil treatments; foliage application; wood protection
Methoxychlor	Nervous system or kidney effects (or both)	0.10	Insecticide used on fruit trees, vegetables
p-Dichloro-benzene	Possible cancer‡	0.075	Used in insecticides, mothballs, air deodorizers

(continued)

National Primary Drinking Water Safety Standards—*Continued*

Contaminant	Possible Health Effects	Quantity (mg/liter)	Sources
Organic Chemicals —continued			
Total trihalo-methanes (TTHM) (chloroform, bromoform, bromo-dichloro methane, dibromo-chloro-methane)	Cancer§	0.1	Primarily formed when surface water containing organic matter is treated with chlorine
Toxaphene	Cancer§	0.005	Insecticide used on cotton, corn, grain
Trichloro-ethylene (TCE)	Cancer§	0.005	Waste from disposal or dry cleaning materials and manufacture of pesticides, paints, waxes and varnishes, paint stripper, metal degreaser
Vinyl chloride	Possible cancer‡	0.002	Polyvinylchloride pipes (PVC) and solvents used to join them; industrial waste from manufacture of plastics and synthetic rubber

SOURCE: U.S. Environmental Protection Agency, Office of Water, Washington, D.C.
*Geological sources means the element or compound is found in rocks, soil, and other components of the earth's surface.
†Agency is considering substantially lower number.
‡There is reasonable belief, but no substantial scientific evidence, that this chemical can cause cancer.
§There is substantial scientific evidence that this chemical can cause cancer.

427. Run Your Tap Water

Any time a faucet hasn't been used for 6 hours or longer, flush the cold water pipes by running the water until it gets as cold as possible. It can take anywhere from 30 seconds to 5 minutes. Running the tap will flush out stagnant water that may have collected lead from the plumbing overnight.

428. Save the Hot Water for Your Bath

Never drink or cook with hot water from the tap, advises the EPA. Hot water is more likely to dissolve lead from lead pipes or lead solder than cold water is, especially in areas where drinking water is soft and acidic.

Homes less than five years old are at greatest risk of lead contamination because the water pipes don't have the protective buildup of magnesium and calcium salts that keep lead from the water.

429. Bottled Isn't Always Better

Many people assume bottled water is 100 percent pure and free from potentially harmful elements. Not so, says Raymond Gabler, Ph.D., in his book *Is Your Water Safe to Drink?* There is currently only one rule governing bottled water. It must be as safe as tap water. Some states apply stringent regulations for bottled water, others do not. The only way to find out for sure what your bottled water contains is to have it tested.

To get the purest water possible, Dr. Gabler suggests you follow these guidelines.

- Buy bottled water in glass containers, not plastic. Organic toxins (like plasticizers used to keep bottles flexible) can leach into the water. So can the plastic itself.
- Ask the bottling company to send you an analysis of their water from an accredited laboratory. (Or you can take a sample to a lab and have it tested yourself.)

C H A P T E R · 6

CONTROL YOUR BLOOD PRESSURE— PERMANENTLY

The ominous link between high blood pressure and death is irrefutable: The higher your blood pressure, the more likely you are to die before your time.

Why? Because, day by day, the physical force exerted by high blood pressure insidiously damages your nervous system, overworks your heart, and mercilessly speeds up atherosclerosis—the process by which arteries are narrowed and hardened—until blood streaming to your major organs to keep them alive is reduced to a life-threatening trickle. And that sets the stage for heart disease, kidney failure, and stroke—each of which can kill you 15 or 20 years before your time. It's no coincidence that half of those having a first heart attack and two-thirds of those having a first stroke also have high blood pressure.

Those most at risk for high blood pressure seem to be people who are black, obese, older, have a family history of the disease, have a high salt intake, or consume excessive amounts of alcohol. Yet even though high blood pressure—or hypertension, as doctors call it—kills an estimated 250,000 Americans every year, for the most part no one knows what really causes it.

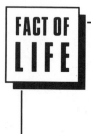

FACT OF LIFE

The Mercury Goes Up as Your Age Goes Up

High blood pressure can affect people of all ages, but most people with the problem seem to be over the age of 40. Two-thirds of those between ages 65 and 74, and three-quarters of those over 75 have high blood pressure.

About 5 percent of all cases of high blood pressure are triggered by an underlying but clearly identifiable problem such as kidney disease, adrenal gland malfunction, tumor, or birth control pills. But what causes the rest is still a mystery. Leading suspects, however, are the overproduction of an as-yet-unidentified salt-retaining hormone, chronic high salt intake, increased secretion of an enzyme in the kidney, a specific group of overactive nerves, congenital abnormalities of various blood vessels, or a lack of naturally occurring body chemicals that dilate blood vessels.

The Silent Killer

Unfortunately, high blood pressure is difficult to detect no matter what its cause. That's because there are no symptoms—no bruises or tremors or lumps that you can point to and say, "Aha! That means I have high blood pressure!"

The lack of symptoms also explains why more than half of the 60 million Americans with high blood pressure don't even know they have it. Unfortunately, the only way to tell if you have high blood pressure is to slap a blood pressure cuff around your arm, pump the mercury up the glass column of a manometer, and listen through a stethoscope as you watch the mercury fall.

The manometer literally measures the pressure inside your arteries. A normal blood pressure, for example, is usually 120/80 or a little bit less. The first, or top, number is your "systolic" pressure—the pressure created when your heart contracts to pump out blood—and the second, bottom number is your "diastolic" pressure—the pressure created when your heart is filling with blood for the next beat.

What the Numbers Mean

A blood pressure reading of 120/80 is a textbook-perfect reading, but what does it mean if the numbers indicate you aren't so perfect? The following should give you an idea of what those numbers mean.

Blood Pressure Reading	Evaluation
Systolic (top number)	
Less than 140	Normal blood pressure
140–159	Borderline hypertension
More than 159	Hypertension
Diastolic (bottom number)	
Less than 85	Normal blood pressure
85–89	High normal blood pressure
90–104	Mild hypertension
105–114	Moderate hypertension
More than 114	Severe hypertension

The Joint National Committee on the Detection, Evaluation, and Treatment of High Blood Pressure cautions that the term *mild* should not be interpreted as "unimportant." Even mild hypertension requires medical attention.

If your numbers are 140/90 or higher, you are usually diagnosed as having high blood pressure. But don't decide to forget about your blood pressure if it's wandering around in the no-man's land between the normal of 120/80 and the high of 140/90.

Bringing It Back to Normal

"Research shows that there's a progressive increase in cardiovascular risk as systolic pressure rises above 130 and diastolic pressure goes above 85," cautions Aram V. Chobanian, M.D., chairman of the Joint National Committee on the Detection, Evaluation, and Treatment of High Blood Pressure.

"Even people with diastolic pressure as low as 85 to 89 should act to bring their pressures under control, especially since a significant number of these people eventually become severe hypertensives," he says.

Fortunately, the good news is that high blood pressure can be both prevented and controlled. "Thirty years ago relatively few people with hypertension could control their blood pressure," says Dr. Chobanian. "But now practically everyone can achieve some degree of control, and most people can bring their pressures down to the normal range."

Here are the tips you need to do it.

High Nutrition, Low Pressure

430. Get Plenty of Calcium

A study of nearly 2,300 people conducted at Erasmus University in the Netherlands discovered that the more calcium in your diet, the lower your blood pressure. Another study at the same university revealed that young people with mild hypertension—a blood pressure in which the bottom number is between 90 and 104—also benefited from calcium supplementation. Diastolic blood pressure dropped significantly in people who took 1,000 milligrams of calcium a day as compared to people who took only a placebo (fake pill).

Moreover, when researchers at Harvard Medical School checked into the health and dietary habits of over 58,000 nurses, they found that women who consumed the Recommended Dietary Allowance (RDA) for calcium (currently set at 800 milligrams) decreased their risk of high blood pressure by 22 percent.

But other equally well-respected studies have found that extra calcium can also raise blood pressure. So what gives?

Apparently, calcium lowers blood pressure *only* if you're sensitive to salt, says Lawrence Resnick, M.D., a researcher at the New York Hospital–Cornell Medical Center. In fact, studies show that getting extra calcium has no benefit whatsoever if you're not salt sensitive. And, interestingly, a sensitivity to salt seems to correlate with groups which are more likely to develop hypertension. "Young people tend not to be salt sensitive," Dr. Resnick points out. "Blacks and older people are. And, in general, calcium seems to make a bigger difference as you get older."

Foods high in calcium include dairy products, salmon, and mackerel, as well as collard and beet greens.

431. Learn to Dig Potatoes

Potatoes are a potent source of potassium, and research is showing that blood pressure drops in people who get a fair amount of that mineral on a regular basis. That's because potassium helps regulate your blood pressure by helping your body excrete more sodium and water. Too much of either one can send your blood pressure soaring. Potassium encourages both salt and water to head for the nearest exit.

At Duke University, for example, a group of patients with high blood pressure was given high doses of potassium while another group received a placebo. After two months, blood pressure in the potassium-supplemented group had dropped significantly. And in another study, researchers used potassium with basically the same result: The participants' blood pressure was lowered an average of 10 percent over a 15-week period.

People with the highest salt intake seemed to benefit most from the extra potassium, scientists reported. They figure you need three times as much potassium as you do salt. Just make sure you get your potassium from dietary sources. (See "Pack in the Potassium" on page 176 for a list of foods high in the nutrient). With this particular nutrient, supplements can be toxic. And the heavy-duty kind used in studies is sold only by prescription.

432. Magnesium Is Magnificent

Researchers who work with the Honolulu Heart Program examined 61 different factors in the diets of healthy, older men and found that people with the highest magnesium intake had the lowest blood pressure.

Researchers at Kobe University School of Medicine in Kobe, Japan, also studied the relationship between magnesium and blood pressure. They gave patients with mild hypertension—diastolic between 90 and 104—600 milligrams of magnesium a day (the RDA

Pack in the Potassium

Most of us should eat three times as much potassium as we do salt to keep our blood pressure low. Salt sends blood pressure up; potassium brings it back down. To help get the potassium you need, eat one to three helpings of potassium-rich foods each day. Here is a list of the best sources.

Food	Portion	Potassium (mg)
Potato, baked	1 medium	844
Avocado	½	602
Raisins	½ cup	545
Sardines	3 oz.	501
Flounder	3 oz.	498
Orange juice	1 cup	496
Banana	1	471
Apricots, dried	¼ cup	448
Squash, winter, cooked	½ cup	445
Cantaloupe	¼ medium	413
Skim milk	1 cup	406
Sweet potato, baked	1 medium	397
Salmon filet, cooked	3 oz.	378
Buttermilk	1 cup	371
Whole milk	1 cup	370
Round steak, trimmed, broiled	3 oz.	352
Cod, baked	3 oz.	345
Sirloin, trimmed, broiled	3 oz.	342
Apricots, fresh	3	313
Beef liver	3 oz.	309
Haddock, fried	3 oz.	297
Pork, trimmed	3 oz.	283
Tomato, raw	1	279
Chicken, light meat, roasted	3 oz.	210
Broccoli, cooked	½ cup	127

is 350 milligrams) for one month and found that the patients' blood pressure plummeted.

You don't necessarily have to stock up on magnesium supplements, however. Whole grains, beans, leafy greens, pumpkin seeds, and fruits and vegetables are good sources of magnesium.

433. Steam Your Vegetables

Boiling vegetables leaches away a good part of their potassium and magnesium and allows sodium—which elevates blood pressure in some people—to be picked up more easily by the food. It's even worse, of course, if you salt the cooking water. So, as part of your own antihypertension campaign, steam or microwave your vegetables.

434. Reach for the Carbs

Tryptophan is an essential amino acid found in carbohydrates that can lull people to sleep. But it may also lull your blood pressure to new lows.

German researchers gave tryptophan to people with high blood pressure and found that it helped lower their pressure.

Tryptophan is converted in the brain to serotonin, a chemical messenger that's used to relay nerve impulses. It's the serotonin, scientists believe, that actually lowers your blood pressure.

As little as 1 to 2 ounces of carbohydrates such as bread, crackers, pasta, potatoes, rice, corn, and cereals can stimulate your production of serotonin.

435. Fill Up on Fiber

Danish researchers have found that 7 grams of supplemental fiber—about the amount found in a single bowl of bran cereal—significantly reduced blood pressure in a group of people with high blood pressure.

Daily fiber supplements were given to 21 people with blood pressure that ranged from 140/95 to 195/110. After three months, their average systolic pressure fell by 10 points, while diastolic pressure fell by 5 points. And study participants received an extra bonus: Their cholesterol levels fell by 5 percent.

What effect can you expect from a lifetime commitment to fiber? Well, one study found that female Seventh Day Adventists who eat only fiber-rich vegetables have an average blood pressure of 98/65, while their Mormon counterparts who eat meat have an average blood pressure of 103/73.

436. Get Hooked on Mackerel

A diet rich in mackerel can apparently lower blood pressure in people with mild hypertension.

Researchers from the West German Central Institute for Cardiovascular Research gave cans of mackerel flavored with tomatoes to men with mild hypertension who normally didn't eat fish.

The men ate two cans of mackerel a day for two weeks, then tapered off to three cans a week for the following eight months. After that they returned to a normal diet for another two months.

The result? Everyone's blood pressure plummeted from their first bite of fish and didn't increase until they went back to their old habits—a diet low in fish and high in cold cuts.

437. Olive and Peanut Oils Are Golden

A Stanford University study indicates that each tablespoon of monounsaturated fat you eat per 1,000 calories will drop your systolic pressure by 10 points.

The best sources of monounsaturated fat? Olive oil or peanut oil. Sprinkle the mild-tasting olive oil liberally on salads, vegetables, and pastas, or substitute it for the oil in baked goods such as zucchini bread and carrot cake. Use the peanut oil to stir-fry vegetables and chicken when you want to add some zip to a bland entree.

FACT OF LIFE

The Caffeine Connection

Contrary to common belief, caffeine does *not* cause high blood pressure. The caffeine in a single cup of coffee, however, will increase your blood pressure 2 to 4 points for up to 3 hours.

438. Avoid Licorice

Licorice contains glycyrrhizic acid, a naturally occurring chemical that can have a potent effect on your blood pressure—especially if you come from a family that has a lot of high blood pressure. One woman who was sensitive to the chemical recorded a blood pressure of 240/110.

Shake Your Salt Habit

439. Stop at a Teaspoon

Not everyone with high blood pressure is affected by dietary sodium, the main ingredient in salt. But most are. And excess sodium, experts say, will cause many of these people to retain excess fluid, which can raise blood pressure.

If salt makes you retain fluid, the joint national committee on high blood pressure recommends that you reduce your daily intake to 1,500 to 2,000 milligrams—about the amount you'd find in 1 teaspoon of salt. That amount may be enough to drop you out of the high blood pressure club. Or prevent you from joining up.

440. Check Your Salt Sensitivity

Some people are so sensitive to salt that even a small amount can result in large leaps up the blood pressure gauge for someone who would otherwise have normal pressure.

How do you know if you're one of them? There really isn't any easy medical test to check for salt sensitivity, but experts suggest the following strategy: Go on a salt-free diet for one month to see if your blood pressure goes down. If it does, then you can assume you're salt sensitive and will probably benefit from keeping salty foods permanently off your table.

441. Put the Salt Shaker on the Table

To shake the salt habit, you may have been advised to take the salt shaker off the table. Now a study at the Monell Chemical Senses Center in Philadelphia suggests that you leave it there—but take it away from the kitchen counter.

Eleven college students were fed meals prepared with half the usual amount of salt. They were allowed to salt their food at the table. Although one of the students restored all the eliminated sodium via the salt shaker, ten replaced less than 20 percent of it.

This suggests that low-salt cooking coupled with salting "to taste" at the table may be a way to cut sodium consumption and yet retain a palatable diet, say the researchers.

The key, of course, is to give free rein to the salt shaker *only* when low-sodium or no-sodium meals are being served.

442. Cook without Salt

Adding salt to cooking water is more of a habit than a necessity. Break the habit, and while you're at it, cut down or eliminate the salt in every recipe you prepare. Remember, in 99 cases out of 100, salt is merely a flavor enhancer. It's not a major—or even necessary—ingredient. And don't forget to eliminate the salt in baked goods. The American Heart Association suggests that you try sodium-free baking soda and powder in everything you bake.

443. Use Herbs and Salt Substitutes

Fill your salt shaker with your favorite herbs and/or a nonsodium substitute, then shake away. But check with your doctor before you use a salt substitute or mix it with your herbs. The American Heart Association says that some substitutes contain the chemical potassium chloride, which may be harmful to some people.

444. Choose Your Herbs Carefully

Switching from salt to herbs is a good idea, but make it even better by choosing herbs naturally low in sodium.

Lowest of all, with 10 milligrams of sodium per 100 grams (3½ ounces) of herb, are black pepper, white pepper, hot red pepper, chili pepper, cinnamon, nutmeg, mustard powder, garlic powder, dill seed, sage, poppy seed, turmeric, and cardamom.

Next lowest, with 20 milligrams of sodium per 100 grams, are bay leaves, caraway, oregano, paprika, and savory.

Herbs with 30 milligrams per 100 grams include ginger and ses-

Sizing Up Sodium

The following guide will help you keep the sodium level between 1,500 to 2,500 milligrams a day—the amount recommended by the Joint National Committee on the Detection, Evaluation, and Treatment of High Blood Pressure. If that sounds difficult, remember that your taste for salt is an acquired one. You should lose whatever cravings you have for it in just a few weeks.

Food	Portion	Approximate Sodium Content (mg)
Vegetables		
Canned or frozen, with sauce	½ cup	140–460
Fresh or frozen, cooked without added salt	½ cup	Less than 70
Fruit		
Fresh, frozen, or canned	½ cup	Less than 10
Dairy Products		
Buttermilk, salt added	1 cup	260
Cottage cheese, regular and low fat	½ cup	450
Milk and yogurt	1 cup	120–160
Natural cheeses	1½-oz. serving	110–450
Processed cheese and cheese spreads	2-oz. serving	700–900
Meat, Poultry, Fish		
Cured ham, sausage, luncheon meat, frankfurters, canned meat	3-oz. serving	750–1,350
Fresh meat, poultry, finfish	3-oz. serving	Less than 90
Fats, Salad Dressings		
Oil		None
Prepared salad dressings	1 tbsp.	80–250
Salted butter	1 tbsp.	117
Salted margarine	1 tbsp.	133
Salt pork, cooked	1 oz.	360
Unsalted butter or margarine	1 tbsp.	4
Vinegar	1 tbsp.	Less than 6
Condiments		
Catsup, mustard, chili sauce, tartar sauce, steak sauce	1 tbsp.	125–275

(continued)

Sizing Up Sodium—*Continued*

Food	Portion	Approximate Sodium Content (mg)
Condiments—continued		
Salt	1 tbsp.	6,000
Soy sauce	1 tbsp.	1,000
Snacks, Convenience Foods		
Canned and dehydrated soups	1 cup	630–1,300
Canned and frozen main dishes	8-oz. serving	800–1,400
Deep-fried pork rind	1 oz.	750
Salted nuts, potato chips, corn chips	1 oz.	150–300
Unsalted nuts and popcorn	1 oz.	Less than 5

ame. Basil, rosemary, and onion powder have 40 milligrams per 100 grams.

To help you visualize those amounts, the American Spice Trade Association says that 100 grams of ground black pepper would be enough to sprinkle on breakfast eggs every day for the next seven years.

445. Spritz On the Soy

A single tablespoon of soy sauce contains a whopping 1,029 milligrams of sodium, almost a full day's allowance. To get the taste of soy without blowing your low-sodium resolve, use this tip: Fill a mister, like those used for ironing or spraying plants, with soy sauce and spray it sparingly on foods. Diluting it first with a little water will lower the salt content even more.

446. Read Labels

You're not the one putting most of the salt in your food. Seventy-five percent of the salt in your diet is put there by food processing plants.

As a result, salt is a major, hidden ingredient in the most unexpected foods. Cured meats such as bacon, hot dogs, and sausage are loaded with it, for example, as are canned soups, canned tuna, prepared pancakes, and TV dinners.

How can you avoid eating all this salt? Get in the habit of reading the labels on every food that you are going to buy. Then avoid any food with a label that features the word "sodium" anywhere but at the *end* of the ingredient list. Or, better yet, shop for foods that don't have sodium on the ingredient list at all.

447. Buy Low-Sodium Products

If you really want to limit your sodium intake, the American Heart Association advises that you look for labels stating that the food product is "low sodium" or "no salt added."

You'll be amazed at the range of products available: low-sodium breads, cheeses, crackers, cereals, soups, canned vegetables, and bouillon cubes, among others.

448. Make a Pit Stop at Your Local Salad Bar

Eating too much fast food can be a fast way to increase your blood pressure. A McDonald's Big Mac has 950 milligrams of sodium, for example, while a Burger King Whopper with cheese has 1,164. And either one can come close to exceeding a whole day's allowance of salt for those on a sodium-restricted diet!

Yet you still can have a meal on the run. When looking for a quick bite, try making a pit stop at the salad bar. McDonald's Garden Salad has only 160 milligrams of sodium. But skip the bacon bits, pickled vegetables, cheese, olives, croutons, and fancy dressings. They're all high-sodium "wolves" dressed in low-sodium "clothing."

449. Hold the Pickle

Next time you visit a restaurant for lunch, order your sandwich without the pickle. That innocuous little slice of salty cucumber has a whopping 93 milligrams of sodium, say experts at the National High Blood Pressure Program.

And add only small amounts of ketchup and mustard—both have 60 milligrams of sodium per teaspoon—and hold the cheese. A single slice of cheese adds 200 to 400 milligrams of sodium to your sandwich.

450. Cook by the Book

Several cookbooks are now devoted to helping you cook without salt. The books include a wide range of recipes that will satisfy any appetite, even those of a gourmand. Pick up a copy of *The New American Diet* by Sonja L. Connor and William E. Connor, M.D., or *Healthy Microwave Cooking* by Judith Benn Hurley. Then give your kitchen a workout on salt-free cooking.

451. Have Your Drinking Water Tested

The water you drink every day could be adding more sodium to your diet than a handful of pretzels. Studies have shown that municipal water supplies can contain from 4 to 1,900 milligrams of sodium per liter (a liter is 34 ounces). And water from private wells can be even worse. In some parts of the country, wells contain between 100 and 1,000 milligrams of sodium per liter.

Not yours, you say? Keep in mind that water loaded with sodium doesn't necessarily taste salty. So the only way to find out how much sodium is in your water supply is to have it tested.

If you're hooked up to the muncipal water system, call your local water department and ask if they've already had it done. If they haven't, or if you have a private well, you might want to have a local water test company come out and sample your water. Check your telephone directory for the company nearest you.

If you do have a problem, an under-sink water filtration device can remove the excess salt.

FACT OF LIFE

The West Is the Best

Westerners are one-third less likely to have high blood pressure than other Americans. The reason? Scientists suspect it may be because westerners are more physically active, don't smoke as much, and are less likely to be overweight than people who live in other parts of the nation. They also eat more fruits and vegetables and less red meat and salt.

452. Bypass the Water Softener

Most water softeners replace calcium and magnesium—the minerals that make water "hard"—with sodium. If you use a water softener but want to avoid the added sodium, run a line from your water pipe to a special spigot on your sink that bypasses the softener. Use that water for drinking and cooking.

Get Your Body Moving

453. Exercise Is Critical

Research shows that regular aerobic exercise—the kind that gets your heart pumping, such as brisk walking—can lower your pressure by 4 or 5 points.

How? Two ways. It reduces the amount of blood pumping through your arteries by reducing the amount of salt in your blood—your sweat is salty, right?—and it reduces blood levels of "fight or flight" biochemicals that cause blood vessels to constrict and raise pressure.

How much exercise is beneficial? Most of the studies that reported blood pressure decreases were studies on people working out 30 to 60 minutes, three times a week. Don't start out at that level, though. Get your doctor's approval, then start out slowly, increasing your time and distance gradually.

454. Eat and Run

A low-sodium, high-potassium diet will usually lower blood pressure. As will moderate exercise. So it's no wonder that Florida researchers have found that the two combined can really knock blood pressure for a loop.

The researchers divided a group of normal-weight adults with mild hypertension in half. One half went on low-sodium, high-potassium diets, while the other half followed individually tailored aerobic exercise programs. After about four weeks, blood pressure had dropped 10 points or more in both groups.

The two groups merged and went on a combined diet and exercise program for four more weeks. The result? Their blood pressure dropped an *additional* 4 points, putting many of the study's volunteers into the normal range.

"This clearly indicates that a combination of the two is more effective than either one alone," says James Mitchell, Ph.D., the scientist who conducted the study.

455. Pedaling Can Put Your Pressure in Low

Japanese researchers have discovered that gentle bicycling can lower your pressure and keep it low. They conducted a study in which a group of middle-aged men and women with moderately high blood pressure rode bikes for 60 minutes three times a week.

At the end of ten weeks, their blood pressure had dropped an average of 13 points, putting some into the normal range.

456. Walk Your Pressure Down in Less than an Hour

A brisk 40-minute walk significantly reduced the blood pressure in a group monitored at the University of Massachusetts Center for Health and Fitness. Moreover, the reduction lasted for at least 2 hours after the walk.

457. Don't Walk with Hand Weights

Carrying hand weights on your walks may increase your blood pressure.

Researchers at the University of Florida found that "people who are hypertensive . . . may be negatively affected" by using hand weights on their walks.

Their verdict emerged after the scientists measured the effects of carrying 1- to 3-pound weights on 12 healthy volunteers as they walked at varying speeds on a treadmill. At all speeds, the energy demands on their bodies increased in direct response to the amount of weight carried. That's good for weight loss and cardiovascular endurance, but bad for blood pressure—it goes up.

Working with hand weights at 75 percent of their maximum capacity, the systolic pressures of the volunteers averaged 9 points higher than when that same 75 percent capacity was reached without the weights.

FACT OF LIFE

Watch Out for Mornings

Your blood pressure is usually lowest at 3:00 A.M., but it rapidly rises to peak between the hours of 6:00 A.M. and noon—precisely the hours when heart attacks, strokes, and heart failure most frequently occur.

458. "Wanna Lift?" Don't Hold Your Breath!

Holding your breath while lifting weights can increase blood pressure because of temporary constriction of your blood vessels.

If you want to lift weights for exercise, says Gary Sforzo, Ph.D., assistant professor of exercise physiology at Ithaca College, try any kind of rhythmic breathing to counteract the rise in pressure. Exhaling as you lift, for example, will actually cause a decrease in pressure.

Try it next time you lift a set of barbells—or a box of china.

459. Some Drugs Block Exercise Benefits

Some beta-blockers that are commonly prescribed to lower blood pressure and slow your heartbeat may actually block the blood pressure–lowering effects of exercise.

In a study of 30 people with high blood pressure, 10 participants were given the beta-blocker propranolol, 10 others were given the beta-blocker metoprolol, and another 10 took a placebo.

The blood pressure of those on propranolol did not drop a millimeter even after ten weeks of strenuous exercise. The researchers say that even though propanolol itself effectively lowers blood pressure, the drug apparently blocks the additional blood pressure–lowering effect of regular workouts. In the group who took metoprolol, blood pressure dropped as expected.

So the scientists say that if you exercise and take propranolol, you should check with your doctor to see if you might achieve better results from metoprolol or some other drug. And if you keep exercising, says Philip Ades, M.D., who headed the University of Vermont School of Medicine study, you may be able to taper off or eventually discontinue your drug therapy.

Caution: Drugs

460. Drug Cuts Mortality Rate in Half

The anti-hypertensive drug metoprolol prevents more deaths in people with high blood pressure than other medications. According to a report in the *Journal of the American Medical Association*, a study of 3,200 middle-aged men with high blood pressure found that those who used metoprolol had a 48 percent lower chance of dying than did those who used a diuretic.

461. Take Acetaminophen Instead of Ibuprofen

Ibuprofen, a common headache remedy sold as Advil or Nu-prin, can cause a significant increase in blood pressure, reports a study conducted at the University of Cincinnati.

The study also found that when people were given acetaminophen for pain relief, their blood pressure stayed where it was. Acetaminophen is sold under the trade names Tylenol, Anacin–3, Excedrin, and Panadol.

462. Aspirin Can Block the Help of Medication

Diuretics, which are frequently used to treat high blood pressure by reducing the volume of fluid in the blood, can be kept from doing their job if you also take nonsteroidal anti-inflammatory agents such as aspirin, reports the joint national committee on high blood pressure. If you're on any medication to lower your blood pressure, check with your pharmacist or physician before you take any other drug—even one that's available without a prescription.

463. Ulcer Medication Can Cause Interference

Cimetidine, a popular ulcer drug sold under the trade name Tagamet, may prevent your body from effectively using beta-blockers, a type of drug which is frequently prescribed to lower blood pressure, says the joint national committee on high blood pressure. If you have any leftover cimetidine in your medicine cabinet, make sure you either ask your doctor if it's compatible with any medicine you're taking now, or throw it away.

464. The Pill Pumps Up Pressure

Oral contraceptives slightly increase blood pressure in 95 percent of those who take them. It increases blood pressure significantly in the rest.

If you want to take oral contraceptives, ask your doctor about using a preparation with low estrogen/progestogen content. Low-dose formulas will raise your blood pressure less than pills with a higher estrogen/progestogen combination.

465. Diet Pills Can Increase Pressure

If you're thinking about using diet pills to help you lose weight, do so with caution. Many diet pills, both prescription and over the counter, contain a substance called phenylpropanolamine (PPA).

PPA is believed to depress the part of the brain that controls appetite. But in some people it also raises blood pressure.

466. Watch Out for Nose Drops

Even nose drops can contain the ingredient PPA, says Steven Dilsaver, M.D., director of the psychopharmacology program at Ohio State University College of Medicine. So read the ingredient labels on nose drops or sinus medicine to make sure that all they're going to do is open your clogged nose—not increase your blood pressure.

A Low-Key Lifestyle

467. Stop All That Racket

The louder the noise to which you're exposed, the higher your blood pressure, says a study conducted in Japan.

When researchers at the Department of Public Health and Industrial Hygiene Research Center of the Kaohsiung Medical College studied shipyard workers, they found that people exposed to noises over 85 decibels were twice as likely to have high blood pressure as those who worked in an environment under 80 decibels.

How loud is 80 decibels? It's about as loud as a vacuum cleaner

(70 to 80 decibels), or an alarm clock (80), or even the sounds of busy traffic (75 to 85). If you can't avoid loud noise, think about picking up a pair of earplugs at your local drugstore.

468. Keep the Radio On

Some music-therapy experts think that tuning into tunes may help lower your blood pressure. The experts suggest that the music most likely to soothe the savage breast is quiet, instrumental, with slow, predictable rhythms.

469. Two Are Enough

Limit your drinking to two alcoholic drinks a day—tops, experts say. That's 24 ounces of beer, 8 ounces of wine, or 2 ounces of liquor. Drink more and you risk boosting your blood pressure. Drink less— or lower your glass altogether—and your blood pressure will probably drop several points.

470. Lose Weight If You're Overweight

People who are overweight seem to have a tendency to develop high blood pressure. Maybe that's why dropping a few pounds is one of the surest ways to drop your blood pressure. In fact, most people lose 1 point on the blood pressure gauge for every 2 pounds they shed. Losing 20 pounds, for example, can lower your blood pressure by a good 10 points—which is enough to knock some of us right out of the high blood pressure category and back to normal.

471. Cigarettes Make the Problem Worse

Cigarette smoke constricts your blood vessels, which makes your heart work harder to force blood through your arteries and veins. Smoke also weakens the ability of some drugs to lower your blood pressure, while it increases your tendency to develop brain hemorrhages and the worst kind of high blood pressure possible— what doctors call malignant hypertension. Smoking cessation, says the joint national committee on high blood pressure, is strongly recommended for everyone who wants to control their blood pressure.

FACT OF LIFE

A Tall Tale

Yep. The taller you are, the higher your blood pressure can be without it actually being labeled hypertension. The reason? The more there is of you, the more pressure required to pump the blood all the way up to your brain.

472. Avoid Smokeless Tobacco

Smokeless tobacco—otherwise known as chewing tobacco—contains large amounts of sodium to enhance flavor and help your body absorb nicotine. It has no place in any kind of pressure-lowering lifestyle.

473. Take Charge of Your Work Life

Job dissatisfaction can cause high blood pressure, report researchers at the University of Pittsburgh. At greatest risk: those who have poor working relationships and little opportunity to contribute to decision making, as well as those who feel uncertain about their future and see little chance for promotion.

The solution? Take charge of your work life. Sit down with a career counselor—one *not* employed by your company—and decide whether or not your job can be altered to suit your needs. Is there a way for you do an end run around the supervisor who blocks your best ideas? Is there a way for you to delegate the client relations that are not your forte? Can your job be expanded to include more responsibility? Or is it less responsibility that you really want?

The bottom line is that you're in charge of your work life. Either turn your job into one that makes you leap out of bed every morning—or find another one that does.

474. Write Down Angry Words

Keep an anger diary. Both habitually holding in anger or lashing out without trying to solve a problem can lead to erratic increases in blood pressure, experts say.

Keeping track of your anger in a diary, however, helps you identify and understand the causes of your anger. Your diary should monitor what made you angry, what you did about it, and how you felt at the time and later. Then you can reflect and develop strategies for defusing anger constructively.

475. Sleep Problems May Lead to Pressure Problems

Do you suffer from both high blood pressure and insomnia? The reason could be that while you're asleep, you periodically stop breathing, report researchers at the Laboratory for the Diagnosis of Sleep Disorders at the Technion-Israel Institute of Technology. Just for a moment or two, of course, but it can be just long enough to nudge your blood pressure into the stratosphere.

A study conducted by the Israeli research team examined a group of people with high blood pressure and found that 28 percent of them suffer from sleep-related breathing disturbances. Compared with the general public, study participants stopped breathing more frequently—as much as seven times more—than other people studied during the course of a night's sleep. Breathing problems, suggests laboratory director Peretz Lavie, may actually cause high blood pressure in these people.

If your spouse notices that *you* stop breathing for a moment or two during the night, mention it to your doctor. Depending on what he finds, the solution to your high blood pressure may be as simple as learning to control your snoring.

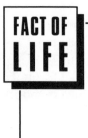

FACT OF LIFE

Profile of a Patient

Researchers have found that people with high blood pressure share a distinct psychological profile defined by three specific characteristics: They have difficulty expressing anger, resentment, and hostility; they are fearful of relating to and communicating with others; and they deny or repress problems.

How does this affect longevity? Suppressing your emotions when you have high blood pressure, researchers say, increases your risk of premature death fivefold.

476. Learn to Relax

Being uptight can send your blood pressure up. But the joint national committee on high blood pressure reports that various relaxation techniques can counteract that effect and produce modest long-term reductions in blood pressure.

What's a good technique? Well, one used by scientists for many years is called Progressive Muscle Relaxation. If you want to give it a try, sit or lie in a comfortable position, then tense and relax the muscles of your body in sequence.

Start by clenching your fists for 3 or 4 seconds, concentrating on how the tension feels. Then relax your hand muscles, letting go of the tension. Continue tensing and relaxing all your major muscles—those in your neck, shoulders, back, arms, abdomen, buttocks, thighs, calves, and feet.

Try this exercise for 10 minutes, twice a day. Eventually you'll learn how to relax your muscles without having to tense them first.

477. Laugh Out Loud

A hearty laugh causes a small but fleeting decrease in blood pressure, experts say. So do it as much as possible. Go to a funny movie. Be with people who make you laugh rather than with people who debate your every word.

478. Pet Your Pet

Stroking a dog, rabbit, cat, or any other animal that's soft and cuddly can lower your blood pressure. "The minute you start talking to and petting your dog, your blood pressure goes down and stays down during the interaction," says Aline Halstead Kidd, Ph.D., a professor of psychology at Mills College in Oakland, California.

"Human-to-human interactions make certain demands," explains Dr. Kidd. "A pet allows you to interact with another living being that makes no demands and loves you without regard to anything." But it's important that the animal be yours, says Dr. Kidd. Meeting a strange pet can entail the same cautious social interplay as when you meet a strange person.

479. Watch the Flames Flicker or the Fins Flutter

"Anything that holds your attention so you're looking and listening but not thinking and worrying reduces blood pressure," says Aaron Katcher, M.D., a psychiatrist at the University of Pennsylvania. Suggested activities? Watching a fireplace, going bird-watching, or watching fish in an aquarium.

Doing any of these things twice a day may be an effective treatment for mild hypertension, says Dr. Katcher.

Measure Your Pressure

480. Check Your Pressure

"Most people should have their blood pressure measured at least once every two years," says Edward Frohlich, M.D., who is a blood pressure specialist at the Ochsner Clinic in New Orleans.

"Individuals at increased risk (those who are black, obese, have a family history of high blood pressure, use an oral contraceptive, or consume excessive amounts of alcohol) should have their blood pressure measured at least once a year."

481. Get an Accurate Reading

Lots of little things can apparently affect a blood pressure reading, doctors say. So make sure your blood pressure is taken after you've been seated for at least 5 minutes. And take off your shirt rather than roll up the sleeve. A rolled-up sleeve will constrict your arm and distort the blood pressure reading.

Two or three measurements should be taken, doctors suggest, with at least 2 minutes between readings.

482. Tell Your Doctor Not to Do It

Anxiety over having your blood pressure taken by a doctor can cause your pressure to rise. It's called white coat hypertension—a reference to the white lab coats that many doctors wear—and it could contribute to a high blood pressure reading.

FACT OF LIFE

It's All in the Family

The longer you've been married, the closer your blood pressure will be to that of your spouse. A study of more than 1,200 couples in Connecticut found that even after discounting the influence of age, obesity, exercise habits, smoking, and salt intake, there was a remarkable similarity between the blood pressure levels of a husband and wife. The reason? Shared stress, or, possibly, poor communication. When communication is a problem in families, researchers say, everyone's blood pressure goes up.

"About a third of people have a significantly lower blood pressure when they're at home or on the job than when they are in the doctor's office," says Richard Reeves, M.D., a professor at the University of Toronto.

This phenomenon, Dr. Reeves adds, could mean that as many as 20 percent of those who've been told they have high blood pressure really don't. How can you avoid it? Have your blood pressure measured by a nurse instead of your doctor to see if there's a difference in the readings.

483. Lower Your Pressure by Taking It Frequently

One of the easiest ways to lower blood pressure may simply be to regularly measure it more frequently than your doctor's annual exam.

In one study of 40 people with mild cases of high blood pressure, for example, blood pressure readings were lower in the group in which blood pressure was checked at nine-week intervals than in a group of people with high blood pressure who were not checked.

Monitoring may serve as its own form of biofeedback as people get to observe their blood pressure on a regular basis, explains Margaret A. Chesney, Ph.D., the study's director. Or there may be a placebo effect as they begin to expect monitoring to lower pressure. And there's always the possibility that the person simply learns to become more relaxed during the actual measurement process.

Life-Extension Tool

Home Blood Pressure Monitor

Studies have shown that buying a home blood pressure monitor and using it regularly makes you more aware of your problem and more apt to do something about it.

When it comes to the purchase of a home monitor, you'll find three different types available. The mercury sphygmomanometer, which ranges in price from $25 to $75, is the standard against which all other blood pressure monitoring devices are measured. It has a long glass measurement column that's filled with mercury, and it comes with an inflatable blood pressure cuff and stethoscope. It gives accurate and consistent readings and does not need readjustment, but it is bulky and heavy to carry, the glass can be broken, and it must be kept on a flat surface while readings are being taken.

An aneroid blood pressure monitoring device is the kind doctors use and is very portable. It is also the most inexpensive, ranging from $15 to $25.

The aneroid equipment consists of a blood pressure cuff connected to a small round gauge, and a stethoscope. The gauge is easy to read but is fairly delicate and can be easily damaged. The gauge must also be checked at least once a year to make sure it is accurate.

Another type of home monitor is the digital model, which is also the most expensive. Digital blood pressure monitors can cost from $70 for a model that requires you to inflate the cuff yourself to over $100 for a model that automatically inflates and deflates when you put on the cuff.

484. Do Your Homework!

Measuring your blood pressure with an at-home monitor for a week (see "Life-Extension Tool" above) can give you a more accurate picture of your blood pressure than having it checked in the doctor's office.

"Compared with in-office measurements," reports Brent Egan, M.D., a blood pressure specialist at the University of Michigan Medical Center, in the journal *Modern Medicine*, "out-of-office readings are more accurate in defining average blood pressure and are espe-

Digitals are very easy to use. They require less manual dexterity than other devices, and the gauge and stethoscope are contained in one unit—which makes it a good choice for those who are hearing-impaired.

Digitals have very sophisticated electronic components, however, so they need to be frequently checked for accuracy. Any adjustments need to be made by the manufacturer. Also, the accuracy of the reading may be influenced by body movements, noise, and other factors in the environment.

The best way to decide which one is best for you is to try out all three devices before you buy them. The American Heart Association has some other advice you should use while making your selection.

- Make sure the cuff is big enough for your arm. The wrong size cuff could result in inaccurate readings.
- If you have to put the cuff on by yourself, consider getting a cuff with a closing and tightening device known as a D-ring. The D-ring will let you fasten the cuff tightly with one hand.
- The numbers on the gauge should be easy to read.
- Check to see if you can hear through the stethoscope. The round diaphragm-type is usually easier to hear with than the bell model. Try both kinds and pay particular attention to how comfortable the ear tips are.
- Look for a unit that has clear, simple instructions about how to use and care for it.
- Make sure you have a medical professional show you how to use any monitoring equipment.

cially useful in making treatment decisions in cases of borderline and mild hypertension."

But how and when you take your blood pressure is important. "Ideally, obtain four readings daily for seven days preceding your visit," suggests Dr. Egan. And take them in the early morning, mid-morning, midafternoon, and late evening. You should be seated with your arm supported at approximately heart level.

It's very important that you make sure your home blood pressure monitor is accurate, however, so take it with you to your doctor and have him test it.

485. Measure Your Pressure at Work

Studies indicate that blood pressure readings at work may be different than those you get at home. Your blood pressure may be hovering around normal when you lean back in front of the TV, for example, but soaring into the stratosphere when you're hunched over a computer keyboard. So if you're trying to monitor your blood pressure, make sure you take it at work as well as at home.

486. Keep a Log

If you have high blood pressure, jot down each blood pressure reading in a log kept especially for that purpose. Also include the date and time. Then bring the log with you to your doctor so that he'll be able to accurately track your progress.

487. Do It Together

Whatever you do to help keep your blood pressure under control, don't do it alone. Get your family to help. Experts say that you are much more likely to stick with any anti-hypertensive regimen if you enlist your whole family in the effort.

Go bicycling with your kids, take a walk with your spouse, buy foods that you and everyone else can eat. It's as healthy a lifestyle for them as it is for you.

C H A P T E R · 7

YOU
CAN
PREVENT
A STROKE

In the time it takes you to blink, your life could be forever changed. Your ability to talk, gone. Your ability to think coherently, gone. Your ability to move freely, gone.

Devastating strokes strike about half a million Americans a year, killing upwards of 150,000 of them. It's the third leading cause of death in the United States, outranked only by heart disease and cancer. Three times as many people die in the United States from stroke as are killed in motor vehicle accidents.

But even of those who survive, two-thirds carry a cross in the form of some sort of disability—inability to walk, impaired speech or vision, memory loss, lack of comprehension, loss of bodily functions, even paralysis of one side of the body. And one out of every ten survivors is disabled so badly that he never returns to work.

What is a stroke? Doctors call it a cerebral emergency, and that description is just about perfect. Cerebral means brain; emergency means sudden—a stroke is the sudden interruption of the blood flow through the arteries in the neck to the brain. This stoppage can be caused by a blood clot, or a rupture in the wall of the artery. Without blood, the brain gets no life-sustaining oxygen; without oxygen, the brain suffocates, and precious cells are killed or seriously damaged. In fact, it only takes 4 or 5 minutes for irreversible damage to occur.

If the affected cells happen to be the cells that control your left arm, or your memory, then those functions become impaired. If too many of your brain cells die, so will you.

The Slow Development of a Stroke-Prone Brain

Strokes, however, don't "just happen" to healthy arteries. They occur in arteries that have been damaged or strained through the years. In many instances, deposits of cholesterol and other substances build up on the inner walls of your arteries, causing them to narrow and inhibit the free flow of blood. This is called atherosclerosis, or hardening of the arteries, and it is the main cause of strokes. High blood pressure can also damage arteries. The stress and strain of elevated pressures can cause them to become scarred, inelastic, and hard. And just time—simple aging—can weaken arteries.

Life-Extension Tool

Balloon Implants

In pioneering surgery, tiny balloons are being permanently placed inside arteries in an attempt to stop life-threatening blood sacs known as aneurysms from bursting.

The procedure, which can be done under local anesthesia, eliminates the need for high-risk brain surgery to repair or remove an aneurysm from one of four major arteries leading to the brain.

Aneurysms that burst cause strokes that kill or incapacitate 1,500 Americans every year.

The balloon implants effectively stop the blood flow in the artery, ending the risk of rupture, explains Jafar J. Jafar, M.D., a neurosurgeon at the University of Illinois at Chicago. Since the brain has four major arteries, stopping the flow of one generally is not a problem.

In the procedure, the deflated balloons are pushed into arteries on the end of thin plastic tubes called catheters. After being positioned in the artery just below the aneurysm, the balloons are then inflated with fluid, effectively blocking off the vulnerable artery.

FACT OF LIFE

The High Cost of Stroke

The cost of caring for stroke victims in the United States each year is a staggering $13.5 billion. That includes physician, nursing, lost productivity, medication, and institutional care charges.

The result is arteries that are more vulnerable to a blood clot getting lodged between their walls and blocking the blood supply. If this happens to one of the arteries feeding blood to the heart, you have a heart attack. If it happens to an artery leading to the brain, you have a stroke.

Death Rate Is Down

If a stroke is scary, the news about strokes isn't. Your chances of surviving a stroke are better today than they ever were. Over the last 40 years, the death rate from strokes has been slashed by more than half—from almost 89 deaths per 100,000 in 1950 to 34 per 100,000 currently.

Why has it gone down? *Prevention.* Smart people—people like you who are concerned about their health—are taking steps to assure stroke doesn't happen in the first place.

"The most important factor to be recognized is the treatment and control of high blood pressure," says James Halsey, M.D., director of the Stroke Research Center at the University of Alabama in Birmingham. High blood pressure is present in 40 to 70 percent of the people who have thrombotic (caused by a blockage) or hemorrhagic (caused by a rupture) types of strokes. People are also doing a lot to prevent heart disease through improved lifestyle and diet. Plus, diagnostic testing and treatment have also improved.

A stroke, says Paul Whelton, M.D., of the Johns Hopkins School of Medicine, doesn't have to happen to anybody. "Strokes aren't like some other diseases that we *think* can be prevented. We're *sure* we know how to prevent strokes."

Make sure you know how to prevent them, too.

Nutritional Self-Healing

488. Go for the Low

The best way to avoid artery-clogging cholesterol is to reduce the amount of fat and saturated fat in your diet.

The American Heart Association recommends that you eat no more than 30 percent of calories from fat (most Americans get around 50 percent) and only 10 percent of those calories from saturated fat. You can do this by eating less red meat, eating only lean meats, avoiding lunch meats, high-fat dairy products, fried foods, and butter. (For specific tips on cutting cholesterol from your diet, see the section "Conquering Fat and Cholesterol" in chapter 2.)

489. Have Just One More Helping

One more helping of fruits and vegetables, that is.

Scientists studied 859 people for 12 years and found that those who ate fruits and vegetables daily developed fewer risk factors for stroke than those who didn't. They say that just one extra serving of fresh fruit and vegetables a day can reduce your risk of having a fatal stroke by 40 percent.

490. Get Protection from Potassium

One reason fruits and vegetables protect you against stroke is that you get the mineral rights of each harvest. Fruits and vegetables are loaded with the mineral potassium, and an increase of just 400

FACT OF LIFE

Seizures Can Signal a Stroke

Studies indicate that there may be a correlation between epilepsy and stroke. In one report published in the British journal *Lancet*, researchers found that 4.5 percent of 176 patients experiencing their first stroke were epileptic. The scientists went on to say that "seizures can be a warning sign for a future stroke."

milligrams of potassium a day (the amount in half a baked potato) can drastically reduce your risk of stroke.

In her study published in the *New England Journal of Medicine,* Elizabeth Barrett-Connor, M.D., chairman of the Department of Community and Family Medicine at the University of California at San Diego, found that "a high intake of potassium from food sources may protect against stroke-associated death."

For her study, Dr. Barrett-Connor divided people into three groups, acording to low, medium, and high intakes of potassium. The group consuming the most potassium suffered *no* deaths from stroke during a 12-year period, compared to 2.4 deaths in the other group.

Foods high in potassium include potatoes, avocados, oranges, dates, cantaloupes, tomatoes, artichokes, carrots, and mangoes.

491. Take a Tip from the Eskimos

Eskimos eat a high-fat diet, yet they still manage to have very few cases of stroke. What's their secret?

Fish. Eskimoes get most of their dietary fat from fatty *fish.* Fatty fish is a great source of omega–3 fatty acids, which have been found to reduce cholesterol and other harmful fats in your blood. It's also been shown to reduce the risk for developing blood clots.

What does all this means in your quest to avoid a stroke? Researchers now say that eating fish just twice a week can play a significant role in preventing a stroke.

Fatty fish are higher in omega–3's than lean fish, and saltwater fish generally contain more than freshwater fish. Finfish rated highest in this nutrient include herring, mackerel, salmon, bluefish, tuna, whitefish, sturgeon, lake trout, and sardines. Anchovies are also high, but aren't recommended because they contain so much salt. Other fish rated as good sources include shark, bass, halibut, cod, flounder, perch, haddock, sole, and swordfish.

492. Take the Landlubber's Route

If you hate fish but like the benefits of omega–3's, try eating soybeans, walnuts, or wheat germ, all of which contain omega–3's. Also, some vegetables like spinach, broccoli, and cauliflower contain very small amounts of the fat.

493. Block Clots with Vitamin E

Here's the antistroke logic of vitamin E, according to R. V. Panganamala, Ph.D., a professor in the Department of Physiological Chemistry at the Ohio State University College of Medicine.

Vitamin E helps prevent a biochemical event called platelet aggregation, or clumping. This happens when platelets—small plate-shaped units of blood—become sticky and form a clump. Clumping can cause a clot. And clots can lead to strokes. Therefore, vitamin E can help prevent a stroke.

Dr. Panganamala explains that vitamin E works in two ways against clumping. It *blocks* the production of a fatty acid the body uses to form a substance called thromboxane, which makes the platelets sticky. And it *stimulates* the production of prostacyclin, a chemical that helps keep platelets slippery and less able to clump.

Good sources of vitamin E include wheat germ (sprinkle it on your cereal or eat it plain), sunflower seeds, almonds, dried pecans and peanuts (just make sure you go for the low-salt variety), and sunflower, corn, and soybean oils (all doubly good because they're high in polyunsaturates, another stroke-beater).

494. Choline Gives Added Protection

A form of the B vitamin choline, called CDP-choline, has been successful in helping victims recover from a mild to moderate stroke.

In a Japanese study of 272 patients, 52 percent of the group who took the CDP-choline showed improvement as compared to only 26 percent in a group who did not take the vitamin.

In a follow-up study done 18 months later, researchers found that the patients who received the CDP-choline had suffered fewer fatalities. The researchers suggest that choline may help to repair damaged cell membranes.

495. Table Your Desire for Salt

Too much salt in your system causes your kidneys to get rid of it by releasing hormones—the same hormones that raise blood pressure and put you at risk for stroke.

Studies show high blood pressure is not a problem in countries where little salt is consumed. In the United States, where blood pressure *is* a problem, the average diet contains too much salt. But all that salt isn't necessary for enjoyable eating. A study conducted by the University of Pennsylvania showed that after five months on a low-salt diet, the people involved actually *preferred* food with much less salt than they had before starting the diet.

The best way to cut back on salt is to eliminate it in cooking and avoid overdoing it on overly processed foods. (For a complete list of low-salt ideas, see the section "Shake Your Salt Habit" in chapter 6.)

496. Develop Two New Food Habits

Out-of-sight, out-of-mouth—that should be one of your new habits. Put stroke-causing foods—those fatty, cholesterol-loaded snacks and goodies—where you can't see them and feel tempted. The *back* of the refrigerator is where they belong. Move the fruits and vegetables up front.

Your second new habit: Eat more slowly. You may be eating too much—and that might mean too much fat—simply because you eat too fast. Be the last to finish at the dinner table. Enjoy your food—and maybe you'll enjoy a lot more years of good eating.

Reducing Your Risk

497. Keep Tabs on Your Blood Pressure

If your blood pressure rises, so does your chance of getting a stroke. The Joint National Committee on Detection, Evaluation, and Treatment of High Blood Pressure recommends that you try to keep your blood pressure level below 140/90, the so-called safe normal range.

Have your blood pressure checked by your doctor or other health professional at least twice a year, so you can be sure your level is in a healthy range.

498. Keep Your Cholesterol below 200

As with blood pressure, the higher your cholesterol level, the greater your chance of developing a stroke.

Cholesterol is the fatty substance that travels through your

Know Your Own Risk

You are at risk for having a stroke if any of the following apply to you.

- You are over 55.
- You have a history of strokes in your family.
- You have high blood pressure.
- You have a high cholesterol level.
- You suffer from heart disease.
- You smoke cigarettes.
- You drink alcohol excessively.
- You are overweight.
- You have diabetes.

---

bloodstream and contributes to the development of atherosclerosis. Health professionals say that keeping cholesterol below 200 should be the goal of all adults.

It takes a blood test to determine what your cholesterol level is, but you need not have it done by your doctor. Awareness of the dangers of high cholesterol has made "on the spot" cholesterol testing available at health fairs held at schools, shopping malls, or churches.

If the results show that your level is high, you should see your doctor, who will be able to run a much more sophisticated and revealing test to accurately determine your risk level. (For tips on how to lower your cholesterol, see the section "Conquering Fat and Cholesterol" in chapter 2.)

499. Chalk One Up for Estrogen

The members of Leisure World retirement community in Laguna Hills, California, may have provided a stroke-prevention clue. A study of the 8,882 women living there, conducted by the Department of Preventive Medicine at the University of Southern California School of Medicine, discovered that "estrogen replacement treatment (ERT) protects against death due to stroke."

The researchers found that among the women who had estrogen replacement therapy after menopause, 20 had died from a stroke. But among the women who did *not* take estrogen after menopause, 43 died from stroke—double the number.

The study determined that women who had used estrogen replacement treatment had a risk of dying from stroke that was 47 percent lower than women who had never taken menopausal estrogens.

The researchers believe estrogen's benefits are probably due to its dilating action on blood vessels, and its ability to favorably alter the levels of blood fats.

500. Reconsider the Birth Control Pill

Oral contraceptives have been linked to an increased risk of stroke in women.

However, low-dose pills are now an option for some women up to age 45. Risks of heart attack and stroke—major complications with the old pills—have been reduced by as much as 80 percent with oral contraceptives containing under 50 milligrams of estrogen.

Still, they are not for everyone, especially those with any risk factors for stroke, like smoking, diabetes, or high blood pressure. Talk to your doctor about which type of contraceptive is best for you.

501. Don't Ignore a TIA

Suddenly you feel weak or numb in your face, arm, hand, or leg. You lose your ability to speak clearly. Your vision blurs, and you feel dizzy and unsteady. Then, within minutes, the sensations go away.

If you've experienced these symptoms, see a physician. It's possible that what you've experienced is a transient ischemic attack (TIA), commonly called a mini-stroke.

About 40 percent of those who have a TIA go on to have a stroke within a week. A major stroke. People who have had one or more of these TIAs are ten times more likely to have a stroke than those who are TIA-free.

And you need to see a doctor *right away.* "The greatest risk is in the first week after a TIA happens," says Harold P. Adams, Jr., M.D., professor of neurology and director of the Cerebrovascular Diseases Division of the University of Iowa Hospital and Clinics.

If you think you have had one of these attacks a while ago, you

Risks Rise with Age

Seventy percent of all strokes occur in those age 65 and older. Men have more strokes than women, and blacks more than whites. Evidence also suggests that the poor are more prone to stroke than the affluent. Overall, your chance of getting a stroke doubles for each decade after age 55.

should still seek medical attention as soon as possible. Studies have shown that some people can go five years after a TIA before they have a major stroke.

502. Diabetics Should Be Doubly Careful

If you have diabetes, your risk for having a stroke is double that of someone without the disease. Although both sexes are at risk, women are at greater risk when it comes to a diabetes-associated stroke.

Why would having diabetes put you at risk for also having a stroke? Experts believe diabetes may contribute to heart disease and atherosclerosis, possibly by causing damage to arteries and allowing them to absorb fatty cholesterol deposits. As deposits build, arteries become prime candidates for clotting, which is a leading cause of stroke.

But having diabetes doesn't mean a stroke is inevitable. "The good news for diabetics," says Robert D. Abbott, Ph.D., head of the Division of Information and Biostatistics at the University of Virginia School of Medicine in Charlottesville, "is that if you can keep your diabetes well controlled, it's likely you can reduce your risk of stroke."

503. Don't Ignore Severe Headaches

Severe headaches are a major symptom of an impending stroke. In fact, 99 percent of subarachnoid hemorrhagic strokes have a severe headache as their major symptom. Many strokes are preceded by a mini-stroke, and the most common symptom of that is typically a severe headache. Beware the onset of severe headaches after the age of 35.

Another sign that your headache might not be the normal take-two-aspirin-and-call-me-in-the-morning type is if it is brought on by exertion or is accompanied by dulled senses and a feeling of being sedated, however slight.

Should you have any of these symptoms, you should see your doctor right away. Treatment may avert a stroke.

The Low-Risk Lifestyle

504. Avoid Gaining Weight

Is that belt of yours getting snug? Are your toes slowly disappearing when you look straight down? When it comes to a stroke, you don't have to be a sumo wrestler to be classified as a heavyweight.

According to a report from the the Framingham Heart Study, people who are more than 10 percent over their desirable body weight are at increased risk for having a stroke.

Ten percent means your shirt buttons no longer close as easily. Ten percent means you see less of the chair seat around you when you sit down.

For a medium-framed 6-foot-tall man, 10 percent means weighing in at 180 instead of 164. It's not that much different, but every pound adds up when it comes to being at risk for stroke.

505. Potbellies Add to the Risk

Another way to reduce your risk of having a stroke is to make sure that your stomach doesn't come into view before you do.

Swedish researchers found that potbellied people are at a much greater risk of getting a stroke than people whose fat settles on their arms or legs or bottom.

506. Booze Can Be Bad for Your Brain

If your cocktail hours are getting to be a daily habit, and you're starting to linger longer at the bar, you could be setting yourself up for a stroke. In a study conducted in England and reported in the *New England Journal of Medicine,* researchers reported that the risk of

FACT OF LIFE

Snorers Are Stroke-Prone

Men who are habitual snorers are more prone to stroke than men who don't snore at all. At least that's what researchers at the University of Helsinki in Finland found when checking the hospital records of more than 4,000 men. All those who suffered a stroke or developed heart disease were snorers. But there were no cases of stroke among the nonsnorers, which lead the researchers to the conclusion that "snoring seems to be a potential determinant of risk for stroke."

stroke in male heavy drinkers was four times higher than in non-drinkers.

An American study of more than 100,000 Californians at Kaiser Foundation Hospital in Oakland, California, revealed that drinking three or more drinks a day increased the risk of hemorrhagic stroke by 3.6 times.

Men, the studies revealed, were most affected when it came to stroke and alcohol. In fact, the London researchers reported, "No excess risk was observed in women, but this may be because of their generally lower alcohol consumption."

If you don't want to stop drinking alcohol, at least cut down on the amount you drink. Light drinking (less than three drinks a day), reported the California researchers, did not increase the risk of stroke.

507. Be Active

Need a reason to go to the gym? Here's one. In a study done in the Netherlands, researchers found that people who had active leisure-time pursuits had only 40 percent of the stroke risk of people who just sat around.

Need more incentive? The University of North Carolina at Chapel Hill tested the fitness level of 3,000 healthy men between the ages of 30 to 69. Eight years later the researchers looked at those same men and found that the ones with the lowest fitness levels had

a 3.4 times greater risk of dying from a stroke than the me
highest fitness levels.

Then there's Harvard University's massive study of 17,000
alumni that found that physically active men lived the longest. The
study defined physical activity as anything that burns extra calories
and raises the pulse rate.

508. Walk on the Prevention Path

You don't have to become a marathon man or woman to reap
the advantages of exercise. Research done at Stanford University
School of Medicine discovered that brisk walking can reduce your
risk of stroke about 80 percent as effectively as jogging.

All it takes is walking briskly for 30 minutes three times a week,
says Barry Franklin, Ph.D., director of Cardiac Rehabilitation and
Exercise Laboratories, Beaumont Hospital Rehabilitation and Health
Center, Birmingham, Michigan.

And what's briskly? Dr. Franklin says it's about four miles an
hour or 15 minutes to the mile.

509. Butt Out

Compared to nonsmokers, studies show cigarette smokers have
two to three times the risk of stroke.

In fact, the more you smoke, the more you're at risk. One study
in the *New England Journal of Medicine* reported that the risk of stroke
in heavy smokers (more than 40 cigarettes per day) was twice that
of light smokers (fewer than 10 cigarettes per day).

But there is good news. When you stop, your risk stops, too.
Stroke risk decreased significantly by two years and was at the level
of nonsmokers by five years after cessation of cigarette smoking.

510. Join the Antidrug Force

Experts have known for a long time that cocaine use can cause
cerebral hemorrhage, but the increased use of the drug over the last
several years has made it a significant cause of stroke, especially in
young adults.

Cocaine use increases a person's blood pressure and heart rate, among other things, with the acute effects lasting from 20 to 60 minutes, depending on how the drug was ingested. And smoking the drug means its negative effects are transmitted to the brain in less than 10 seconds and may stay in the body up to 36 hours after use.

So just saying no to drugs will be saying yes to stroke prevention.

511. Practice Prudence in the Summertime

As the temperature outside goes up, so does your chance of having a stroke. Studies done in the Negev Desert of Israel and in the Lehigh Valley of Pennsylvania both found that there were more strokes and mini-strokes during the summer months than during the winter months.

The Israel study discovered that the risk of stroke was nearly three times as great on warm days as on cold days. True, the desert is *really* hot in the summer. But researchers in the Lehigh Valley, which experiences a moderate climate, discovered that the peak months for TIAs were June through August, and that higher outdoor temperatures showed "a significant positive correlation for TIAs."

Researchers suggest that when heat waves are predicted you should drink plenty of fluids and try to sit out the heat in an air-conditioned place.

512. Ventilate Coal Stoves

In the Xuhui district of Shanghai, China, stroke is responsible for 17 percent of all the male deaths. Researchers set out to find out why stroke was killing so many people there, and they think they found the culprit—coal stoves.

"Coal fumes were found to be an independent risk factor for stroke," reported the Departments of Epidemiology and of Environmental Health, School of Public Health of the Shanghai Medical University.

If you are using a coal stove in your house for additional heat, make sure that the stove has been properly installed and is well ventilated. If you suspect a problem, have a qualified wood/coal stove installation expert check it out.

FACT OF LIFE

South Is the Stroke Belt

People who live in Georgia, North Carolina, South Carolina, Tennessee, and Alabama are twice as likely to have a stroke as someone living in New York or California. In fact, more people die from stroke down south than do people living up north. Because of this dubious distinction, physicians and researchers have dubbed the southeastern part of the United States "The Stroke Belt."

513. Enlist Family Support

Unfortunately, stroke doesn't discriminate. Anyone can have one. And, although they are rare in young people, the bad habits practiced while young can add to increased risk later in life. So don't make diet and lifestyle changes alone. Get the entire family involved. Family support will go a long way in keeping you, and everyone else, on the stroke strike force.

CHAPTER · 8

INFECTION PROTECTION

They're waiting. Under a damp sponge in the kitchen. On the soap dish in the bathroom. Around the holes in the telephone. Down the sides of the milk carton. Across the knob on your door. On the hands of a stranger.

Everywhere you look, they're waiting—for you. Waiting for the moment they can jump on board and bury themselves in a pore, a cut, a crevice, almost any little niche at all.

They're not really fussy. Some don't even wait for you to pick them up. Some can hitch a ride on the breeze. A movement of air tickles over the countertop, along the floor, around the doorknob, over the telephone, through the bathroom, across an aisle, and drops them all, dead or alive, over every inch of your body until you're covered. Layered. Smothered.

With what? With germs. With bacteria. With viruses and other microbes that all have one thing in common: the ability to make you sick, *very* sick.

Germ Warfare

The microbes come in a variety of shapes and sizes. Some are shaped like rods, others like miniature spacecraft. There's even one that looks like a safety pin.

None of them are very big. More than a million bacteria can inhabit one square inch of skin with room to spare. But what they do to your body has little relationship to their size.

Bacteria are responsible for such life-threatening diseases as tetanus, tuberculosis, syphilis, and toxic shock. Bacteria can also contaminate your food, causing severe food poisoning or even deadly botulism. Viruses are responsible for everything from influenza and hepatitis to polio, rabies, AIDS, and some types of cancer. And once they threaten, the only thing that stands between you and them is your immune system.

Your Body's Best Defense

How does your immune system know a marauding microbe has entered your body? "The immune system is like the police force for your body," explains Terry Phillips, Ph.D., associate professor of medicine and director of the Immunogenetics and Immunochemistry Lab at George Washington University Medical Center. It constantly patrols your body, checking the molecular I.D.'s of every cell. So when a cell's basic identity changes—maybe a virus has moved in, for example—the officer examining that cell identifies it as an intruder and radios its I.D. to the nearest SWAT team. Then the SWAT team surrounds the virus-infected cell and shoots it down. End of cell. End of virus. End of risk to body.

But what if there's a bacterial riot going on in some other part of your body at the same time? Like any good defensive force, your

FACT OF LIFE

Deaths from Infections Are Down

Back in the early 1900s, half of the ten leading causes of death were directly traceable to infectious disease: tuberculosis, diarrhea and enteritis, bronchitis, diphtheria. According to the National Center for Health Statistics, death from infection is becoming increasingly rare, thanks to antibiotics. Today, only one such disease—pneumonia—is in the top ten.

immune system can protect more than one front at a time, says Dr. Phillips. But your body's ability to deploy defensive personnel depends largely on whether or not you've kept it in fighting trim.

Ignore your immune system's basic needs, and even its elite troops will be too tired to fight. Then, when a monster microbe attacks, your defensive forces will be asleep in the barracks instead of battling the enemy.

Don't let that happen to you. Here are the best ways known to keep your immune system at full force.

Defensive Eating

514. Avoid These Diet Traps

An army that doesn't eat right doesn't fight right. A good diet can be one of the most important things you can do to protect yourself against infectious disease.

"We're discovering that the undernourished—those who lack one or more nutrients—such as dieters, fast-food fans, and older folks—may also have impaired immune systems," says Brian Morgan, Ph.D., assistant professor of human nutrition at Columbia University College of Physicians and Surgeons.

Notice we're not talking *malnourished* here—we're talking *bad diet.* "Think balance," advises Dr. Morgan. "Choose foods low in fat, high in fiber, and full of vitamins and minerals."

515. Make Sure You're Vitamin A-OK

Germs are persistent. If they're given a chance to get by your first line of defense—your skin—they'll take it.

Vitamin A is the nutrient that keeps your skin nourished and healthy. Without it, your skin can become dry and cracked—an open door to germs. Vitamin A also helps maintain the protective mucus that lines the mouth, lungs, bladder, stomach, intestines, and cervix.

But vitamin A has another all-important role in your immune system's arsenal. It helps activate disease-fighting T-cells. It appears that vitamin A acts as a switch to turn on T-cells, says Susan Smith, Ph.D., research fellow in the Department of Physiology and Biophysics at Harvard Medical School. "With a vitamin A deficiency, this switch doesn't get thrown."

To get an ample dose of vitamin A, eat plenty of yellow, orange, and dark green fruits and vegetables daily, such as squash, carrots, cantaloupe, spinach, and broccoli.

516. Beta-Carotene Beats Bacteria

Beta-carotene, the form of vitamin A found in fruits and vegetables, may be even better at fighting invaders.

"Lab studies show that this nutrient stimulates the macrophages," says Ronald Ross Watson, Ph.D., of the University of Arizona School of Medicine. These are the large cells that search out cancerous tumors, engulf them, and zap them with a lethal chemical.

Beta-carotene may also be effective against certain bacteria. Researchers at Albert Einstein College of Medicine found that beta-carotene increased immune activity against *Candida albicans*, a bacteria that causes yeast infection.

Beta-carotene is abundant in yellow-orange foods, such as carrots, squash, sweet potatoes, apricots, and cantaloupe, and greens, too, such as broccoli, collards, kale, spinach, and mustard greens.

517. B_6 for a Strong Thymus

It appears that certain B vitamins may play an important role in bolstering your immunity.

White blood cells need B_6 to produce antibodies, and the thymus gland needs it to produce T-cells. But it appears that it may also *enhance* these helper T-cells.

Researchers at Loma Linda University School of Medicine fed a group of mice large doses of vitamin B_6. Those on the high dosage had stronger immune reactions than those not given the vitamin therapy. The reason, theorize researchers, was because of stepped-up T-cell action. These are the cells, by the way, that are often destroyed by the AIDS virus.

This doesn't mean, however, that you should take high doses of B_6. Nor does it mean it is the answer to AIDS. B_6 is toxic in high doses and should be taken only under the supervision of your doctor. The point is that most of us barely get a third of the Recommended Dietary Allowance (2 milligrams), says Terry D. Shultz, Ph.D., assistant professor of biochemistry at Loma Linda. The idea is to regularly eat B-rich foods, such as whole grains, kidney beans, bananas, and black-eyed peas.

518. Vitamin C Protects Cells

Vitamin C has been found to stimulate the production of interferon, a chemical that "interferes" with the reproduction of viruses. If viruses can't reproduce, they can't spread, and when they don't spread, you don't get sick.

Interferon has another mission, too. It triggers tumor destruction. When researchers put 250 milligrams of vitamin C daily in the drinking water of mice, they found that the level of interferon in their blood increased and their susceptibility to leukemia decreased.

The interferon triggered the production of natural killer cells, which destroy tumors, explains Benjamin Siegel, Ph.D., the Oregon pathologist who discovered the link between vitamin C and interferon.

Vitamin C can also do battle with bacteria. Vitamin C "helps keep the white cells healthy," says Dr. Morgan, "and white cells produce antibodies needed to kill bacteria."

519. Vitamin E Fights Cellular Aging

Preliminary research indicates that the anti-oxidant vitamin E may play a key role in preventing the age-related decline in our immune systems.

When Jeffrey Blumberg, Ph.D., assistant director of the USDA/

FACT OF LIFE

TB Is Becoming Rare

Tuberculosis was the leading cause of death in the United States during 1900, accounting for 11 percent of all deaths. Advances in public health and medical science have turned that around to the point where tuberculosis now accounts for only 1,700 out of 2 million deaths annually.

Tufts Nutrition Center, fed aged mice high doses of the vitamin, he found it optimized the vigor of the immune response.

Dr. Blumberg explains that vitamin E works by retarding the production of E_2, a hormone that helps regulate the immune system by calling off T-lymphocytes after they've destroyed infectious invaders. "When we age, though, E2 appears to increase, further suppressing the immune response," he says. "That's where vitamin E comes in—it retards E2 production."

520. Keep Your Immune System Iron-Strong

Iron does more than build healthy blood. It plays a major role in the immune system's ability to fight infection.

Iron is the mineral that makes hemoglobin, the protein that carries oxygen to cells. And a healthy oxygen supply enables the phagocytes—the immune system's first defense against infections—to engulf and kill an invading bacteria.

"If you didn't have enough iron, you could fall prey to a host of bacterial infections, especially in the gastrointestinal tract," says Adria Rothman Sherman, Ph.D., chairperson of the Department of Home Economics at Rutgers University.

Low iron levels can also reduce your resistance to certain viruses. When Dr. Sherman compared iron-deficient rats to those with normal iron intake, she found that the iron-deficient rats had a reduced level of natural killer T-cells.

But don't overdo iron, especially if you already have an infection. It seems that bacteria thrive on iron overload.

Your best bet is to make sure you eat enough iron-rich foods, such as soybeans, spinach, lean beef, potatoes, scallops, broccoli, cashews, turkey (dark meat), and lima beans.

521. Copper—A Lucky Penny for Immunity?

People with a rare hereditary disease called Menkes' syndrome (characterized by low blood levels of copper) often die of pneumonia and other serious infections.

In areas where forage crops are low in copper, cattle and sheep have decreased protection against viral and bacterial diseases.

These are clues to the possible importance of this trace mineral in fighting infections. At Oregon State University, researchers found that when copper-deficient animals were given a copper-enriched diet, their immune systems perked up.

The body needs only small amounts of copper—2 to 3 milligrams should be sufficient, says Tim Cramer, Ph.D., a research professor in nutrition and immunity at the USDA's Grand Forks Human Nutrition Center. You can get that by eating such things as chicken, crabmeat, liver, cashews, dried apricots, mushrooms, and whole-grain foods.

522. Zinc Builds Resistance

"We're finding that zinc is crucial to so many parts of the immune system and that a lack of it may cause damage," says Susanna Cunningham-Rundles, Ph.D., associate professor of immunology at New York Hospital/Cornell Medical Center.

Consider these findings:

- A study conducted at the New Jersey Medical School recently discovered that people with the greatest zinc deficiencies also had the poorest immune responses to various germs. The data suggests that "zinc supplementation may enhance immune functions."
- At the University of California in San Diego, 17 elderly people who took zinc supplements had an increased level of antibodies after three months.
- In a Florida study, elderly people with low-functioning immune systems were given zinc, and their resistance to infection increased.

These studies indicate that zinc may play a protective role, especially in aging immune systems which show a drop-off in T-cell activity. Zinc can be found in foods such as seafood, low-fat beef, pumpkin seeds, calves' and beef liver, dark meat turkey and chicken, Swiss and cheddar cheese, and cashews.

523. Put Salmon on Your Menu

It's the research catch of the day. A school of scientific studies show that eating fish loaded with omega–3 fatty acids—salmon, mackerel, and tuna, for example—can keep your immune system happy as a clam.

In a study lead by Michael Bennett, M.D., professor of pathology at the University of Texas Southwestern Medical Center, a team of researchers investigated the effect of three types of fat on animal immune systems.

Mice were fed diets consisting of either vegetable oil, monounsaturated fatty acids (found in peanut and olive oil), or fish oil. The results: The vegetable oil group responded the worst to infections, followed by the monos. The fish oil group responded the best.

"What it means," says Dr. Bennett, "is that if you are getting all of your fatty acids from vegetable oils and you run into, say, an influenza virus or even a carcinogen, your body may be less able to fight it."

This doesn't mean, however, that you should scratch vegetable oils from your diet. Simply *adding* fish oil to your diet may be all the protection you'll need, he says.

The High-Immunity Lifestyle

524. Make Friends with the Sandman

A good night's rest is a germ's nightmare.

"Sleep is like the mechanic's shop for the immune system," says Dr. Phillips. "During sleep, all your other body functions tend to shut down. Then your food can be used by your immune system."

525. Be a Mellow Fellow

Did you ever notice how you sometimes seem to get sick after extremely stressful times in your life? It's not surprising. Stress tends to shut down your immune system, which in turn opens the door to a host of possible infections.

"We do know that if you're sitting in your office under pressure, and you get upset about it, your immune function will go down," says Katherine Baker, Ph.D., a biologist and researcher at Millersville University of Pennsylvania. Relax, and your immune function goes back up.

Elsewhere in Pennsylvania, researchers at Albright College in Reading found that 20 minutes of deep relaxation can substantially boost your body's output of immunoglobulin A, a soldier of major importance in the body's defense against disease.

If stress has your number, take the necessary measures to get rid of it. (Stress-reducing tips can be found in chapter 11.)

526. A Fit Body Is the Best Antibody

At least that's the way it appears.

"The evidence simply isn't conclusive. But I'd have to say that, based on research and clinical experience, it's clear that *something* happens in the immune system in people who exercise. And I'd have to say that, within certain limits, the effects appear to be positive," says Robert Jones, Ph.D., director of the Prevention and Health Promotion Program of the Department of Family Medicine at Pennsylvania State University's College of Medicine.

How *much* exercise? Boosting your immunity seems to require moderate to medium exercise sustained over a period of time—years, for example, instead of months, says Dr. Jones.

And, he says, "moderate to medium" means that "you ought to feel more energetic when you're through, not less. Your mood should be buoyed, not down. You should have the feeling that you're enjoying yourself. If you're not, chances are you're working too hard."

527. Stop Smoking and Reverse the Harm

No butts about it! Every puff you take puts your immune system in peril. Researchers have found that cigarette smokers have an impaired ability to produce antibodies that fight infections in their upper respiratory tract.

They've also found that disease-fighting T-cells in smokers are less active than the same cells in people who don't smoke.

As you might have guessed, smoking is bad for your lungs. Bronchial cilia, the microscopic hairlike structures in your lungs that defend against infectious invaders, are immobilized by cigarette smoking.

The cilia sweep away the thin layer of mucus in healthy lungs, but in a smoker's lungs, the cilia are weak and can't do the job. The result is a buildup of mucus which brings about the familiar smoker's cough.

Luckily, the harm smoking has done to your immune system goes away once you stop smoking. So for your immune system's sake, don't smoke.

528. Here's Mud in Your Immune System

If you find yourself tipsy too often, you may be tipping the scales in favor of infection.

People who drink a lot have low levels of granulocytes, important fighter cells that converge on infected areas in the body and destroy the invaders.

Alcohol also interferes with your body's ability to produce antibodies against any new infections.

Admittedly, all the studies that show a breakdown of the immune system as a result of alcohol have been done on alcoholics. But, researchers say, there's so much evidence that alcohol has damaging effects at high levels that there's reason to believe it can occur at lower levels.

The message? If you drink, drink in moderation.

529. Listen to Your Mother

Washing your hands before meals and after using the bathroom is a good habit, especially if you want to prevent infections since germs on your hands tend to end up in your mouth. A quick rinse with only water is okay, but if you have soap available, use it.

530. High-Risk Groups Need Flu Shots

The Centers for Disease Control (CDC) recommend yearly flu shots for those it considers at high risk: those over age 65, any adult or child with a chronic pulmonary or cardiovascular disorder, all residents of nursing homes or other chronic care facilities, and those with diabetes or other chronic metabolic disease.

"Vaccination of high-risk people each year before the influenza season is the most important measure for reducing the impact of influenza," states the CDC.

The best time to get your shot is in November, before the active flu season begins, says the CDC. And you should do it every year.

Flu Facts

About half a million deaths have been attributed to the flu in the past 20 years, with roughly 20,000 people dying flu-related deaths every time there is an average epidemic year. But it's not nearly as threatening as it used to be. A 1918 influenza epidemic took more lives than were lost in World War I.

Each new season brings with it a new strain of influenza, and the shots are adjusted to fight the current infection.

Flu shots, however, should be avoided by those known to have an anaphylactic reaction to eggs. Current flu vaccines contain a small quantity of egg protein, which could cause an allergic reaction. If you are hypersensitive to eggs, make sure your doctor knows about the allergy.

531. Good Diet Boosts the Vaccine

Researchers in Canada gave a flu vaccine to 30 malnourished elderly patients and then divided them into two groups. One group ate more nutritiously while the other group did not. Four weeks after the flu shot was given, the people who ate a balanced diet had significantly more antibodies to flu virus than those who were poor eaters.

Eating properly, say the researchers, may help the vaccine provide better protective immunity.

532. Protect against Tick-Borne Diseases

Rocky Mountain spotted fever is a potentially deadly disease (fatal in 15 to 20 percent of untreated cases) caused by a rickettsia, a microscopic organism that lives inside ticks.

The rickettsia are found all over the United States, with the disease occurring mostly in the southeast, from Maryland to Georgia, during the spring and summer months.

Lyme disease (a type of arthritis) is caused by bacteria carried by the deer tick, and it normally is a minor disorder. "But if unde-

tected for a long period of time it may result in ear, joint, or neuro-
logical problems, and in some cases, even chronic arthritis or heart
problems," says Stephan Lynn, M.D., director of emergency medicine at St. Luke's-Roosevelt Hospital in New York City.

Deer ticks live in parklike settings, underbrush, high grass, and
even mowed grass. They are eight-legged creatures that are usually
no larger than a sesame seed.

Take these precautions to help prevent coming into contact with
these disease-carrying ticks.

- Whenever possible, avoid known infested areas.
- When outside in a suspected area, pull socks over your pant
  bottoms and tuck your shirt into your pants.
- Wear light-colored clothing. This will make the ticks easier to
  see and remove before they can travel to the skin.
- Wear long sleeves.
- Wear closed shoes.
- Use insect repellent on pants, socks, and shoes.
- Stay near the center of trails and paths.
- Check yourself and your pets for ticks frequently.
- When you return inside, shower and check your hairlines for
  ticks.

Do not use a match to remove a tick, advises Dr. Lynn. Instead,
remove the tick with fine-tip tweezers, taking care to grasp it as close
to the skin as possible. Pull firmly and steadily to avoid twisting off
its head or mouthparts, which will leave the infection behind. Apply
antiseptic to the bite immediately to prevent further infection.

533. Keep Your Tetanus Shots Current

It's not time to think about a tetanus shot when a rusty nail is
sticking into your foot. Try to stay a step ahead of the problem by
having a tetanus shot every ten years. If your work or leisure activity
puts you at risk for cuts, scrapes, or puncture wounds, then consider
getting a tetanus booster every five years.

534. Protect against Toxic Shock

Toxic shock syndrome is a rare but life-threatening bacterial infection that has been linked to the use of high-absorbency tampons.

FACT OF LIFE

How Clean Is Clean?

One square inch of freshly washed skin may contain a million bacteria. Remember that the next time you give your hands a quick rinse.

A study completed by the Centers for Disease Control found that the risk of toxic shock increased 37 percent for each gram of increase in tampon absorbency.

Use only low-absorbency tampons (read the label before buying), and if you develop a high fever, a sunburn-like rash, severe vomiting, or diarrhea during the course of your menstrual period, remove your tampon and see your doctor.

535. Apply Heat to Minor Wounds

Applying a hot pack to minor wounds may help prevent an infection from occurring. A study published in the *Archives of Surgery* found that localized heat benefits wounds by increasing blood flow and oxygenation.

Oxygen plays a vital role in the clearing of bacteria from wounds, which lead the study's authors to say "the simple expedient of warmth may have value in the prevention of infection."

If you have had a cut that doesn't heal in a couple of days, "put a hot pack, heating pad, or warm towel on it for a couple of hours," suggests John Rabkin, M.D., one of the authors of the study. "Put it on two or three times, and it's likely to help."

536. Practice Safe Sex

Condoms aren't foolproof, but they can lower your risk of contracting syphilis and many other sexually transmitted diseases.

For the most protection, choose latex condoms over ones made from animal skins. Make sure the condom has a reservoir tip so it won't break during ejaculation. Also, never use petroleum-based lubricants like Vaseline with a condom because they can cause it to disintegrate.

And be aware that latex deteriorates over time. Never use a condom that's past its expiration date.

How to Prepare Infection-Proof Food

537. Keep It Hot or Keep It Cold

"There is one very simple rule," says Edmund Zottola, Ph.D., professor of food microbiology, Department of Food Science and Nutrition at the University of Minnesota, St. Paul. "Either keep it hot, or keep it cold."

Don't let a hot dish cool on the counter before putting it in the refrigerator. As it cools, it spends lots of time in the temperature that bacteria love. "The aim is to cool food to 40°F within 4 hours," says Tom Schwarz, assistant director for program development in the retail food protection branch of the Food and Drug Administration. Put the food in the refrigerator right away.

Thaw foods in the refrigerator, not out in the kitchen. If you must take the food out, thaw it in a sealed package under cold water.

538. Have a Nonsmoking Kitchen

If you must smoke, save the cigarettes for after dinner, not while you're preparing it.

"The reason has nothing to do with cigarettes," says Schwarz. "It has to do with putting your hand in your mouth. When you smoke, you touch the end of the cigarette. You get saliva on your fingers, and you transmit it to the food."

539. Don't Taste Too Soon

If you can't resist a taste before the cooking timer rings, you may be biting off more than you expected: a case of "Jewish Mother Disease."

Researchers named it that because women who cooked gefilte fish had the habit of tasting the fish before it was finished cooking. It seems they also had this habit of coming down with an infection.

After much study, they found that when tasting the delicacy, the women were also eating a parasite that was still alive in the partially cooked fish.

Give your food adequate time to cook before you spoon out just a little taste.

FACT OF LIFE

Potent Poultry

One out of every 25,000 servings of chicken will cause someone to become sick, report the Centers for Disease Control. That compares to one illness out of every 250,000 servings of all seafood, including raw or partially cooked shellfish.

540. Cook Chicken Thoroughly

Chicken that is not adequately cooked can harbor salmonella. In its raw form, chicken has been found to be highly contaminated with the bacteria. One Iowa State University study found salmonella in 40 percent of packaged cut-up chicken.

Salmonella, though, can't take the heat. Make sure you cook poultry to an internal temperature of 165°F, which should kill any bacteria lurking inside. That doesn't just apply to freshly prepared poultry. Leftovers should be reheated to 165°, not just warmed up.

541. Keep Infections Out of the Kitchen

"If you're sick, you probably shouldn't be handling food," cautions Dr. Zottola. "The same is true if you have an infected cut, skin irritation, boils, or acne." You're only setting up a risk of spreading infection.

542. Handle Raw Foods with Care

Many food-borne infections have been traced to contaminated equipment. Don't cut up raw chicken and then use the same knife to chop vegetables. Wash it first. If the chicken had salmonella on it, you've just passed it on to your salad greens.

After preparing raw meat or poultry, always scrub your hands, utensils, and cutting board thoroughly with soap and hot water.

Better yet, have two cutting boards, one for meat, one for vegetables, and make sure the meat board gets sanitized. And while we're on that thought, one of the best ways to sanitize your cooking equipment is to run it through your dishwasher.

543. Be a Dine-Out Detective

Most cases of infection by food don't happen at home. In restaurants, be on the lookout for unfriendly invaders.

Here are some restaurant self-defense tips.

- Hot foods should be hot, cold foods should be cold. A hot food that's cooled to below 140° or a cold food that's warmed up past 45° can get you in big trouble. A warm shrimp salad or cool lobster Newburg should be sent back.
- Make sure that the salad bar has tongs available and that they are being used. Notice how big the tongs are. Some restaurants believe small tongs equate with small portions, but finger-sized tongs tend to get dropped a lot. When the tongs land back in the food, so do the germs that are on them.

544. Pass on the Tartare, Please

"Eating raw meat or seafood is not completely safe," says Patricia Griffin, M.D., an epidemiologist at the CDC. "You're taking a risk—there could be bacteria in it.

"We strongly advise against drinking raw milk, too," she says. Make sure the milk you drink is pasteurized.

Dirty or cracked eggs should also not be eaten. The dirt might be chicken manure teeming with bacteria.

545. Be a Smart Turkey

When making a holiday meal, stuff the turkey right before you're ready to put it in the oven. If you pack a bird tightly with warm stuffing and let it sit, the salmonella bacteria inside the cavity will use the time to multiply, even if the turkey is refrigerated.

When cooking the turkey, be sure that the inside temperature reaches 165°F to kill the salmonella. Anything less may make you ill.

546. There's Safety Down Below

When you're trying to determine the pecking order of what goes where in your refrigerator, experts advise keeping the raw poultry on the bottom shelf in the refrigerator.

No matter how tight you may think the chicken's package is, it can still leak. But if it's on the bottom shelf, it won't drip salmonella onto other food.

547. Scrub Away Bacteria

Scrub clean all your fruits and vegetables, especially if you're going to eat them raw. The Food and Drug Administration (FDA) says washing your vegetables is a good way to remove the bacteria that might have gotten onto them in the field or supermarket.

548. Guard against Mold

As your food grows old, it tends to grow mold. Molds can hasten food spoilage and can cause allergic reactions. Under the right conditions, some molds can produce mycotoxins or poisons.

When you discover moldy food, don't sniff it; molds can cause serious respiratory problems. If the food is heavily covered with mold, wrap it carefully and discard it immediately.

Make sure you clean the refrigerator where the food was sitting, and, just to be safe, check out nearby items. Should the food only have a tiny spot of mold, here are some tips on what to do.

- In hard block cheeses, cut off at least an inch around and below the mold spot. Rewrap in fresh wrap and put back in the refrigerator. The same procedure can be followed for hard salami and smoked turkey.
- With jams and jellies, the tiny spot of mold can be scooped out. Next, take a clean spoon and scoop out more jam around the spot. If what's left looks and smells normal, it's okay to eat it. If it tastes fermented, throw it out.
- Firm vegetables like cabbage and carrots can have the spot of mold cut away. You should discard any soft vegetables like tomatoes, cucumbers, and lettuce if they show mold.
- Immediately throw away any moldy soft cheese, cottage cheese, cream, sour cream, yogurt, individual cheese slices, bacon, hot dogs, sliced lunch meats, meat pies, opened canned ham, baked chicken, bread, cake, buns, pastry, corn, nuts, flour, whole grains, rice, dried peas and beans, and peanut butter.

549. Is This Shellfish Warning for You?

Almost 50 percent of raw shellfish, such as oysters and clams, may carry a newly discovered and highly poisonous bacteria that, in rare instances, can cause death in people who have liver disease or whose immune system is weakened or impaired. (For the same reason, these people should avoid swimming in open water if they have a wound that has not healed.)

According to an article in the *Annals of Internal Medicine*, exposure to raw shellfish should be ardently avoided. Cooked shellfish are safe, although you should make sure they are *thoroughly* cooked.

550. Check Canned Goods Carefully

Botulism is a deadly (but rare) disease caused by ingesting contaminated canned or processed food. Some of the 10 to 15 cases reported each year can be traced to commercially prepared food, but 75 percent are usually caused by home-prepared food that's been improperly canned.

To safeguard against this disease, you should inspect all canned and jarred goods for the following signs of contamination: swelling or bulging; foamy or moldy food; or a bad odor coming from the jar.

If you suspect botulism, dispose of the food immediately in a place where you're sure no human or animal can get at it. You should also report it to your state or local health department.

551. Use Caution When Canning

Use extreme caution when doing home canning. Serious, even life-threatening mistakes can be made if proper guidelines are not

FACT OF LIFE

A Deadly Disease

If this cup runneth over, you'd better get out of the way. One normal cupful of botulism carries with it enough bacteria-produced toxin to kill every person on earth. In reality, though, only 700 deaths from this disease have been reported in the last 50 years.

followed. Remember that different foods require different canning methods. For example, greatest care must be taken when pressure-canning all vegetables, seafood, meats, poultry, and freshwater fish. These low-acid foods are the environment in which botulism thrives. Make sure you read and follow all canning instructions carefully.

Also, you should not use a microwave for canning. Canning jars don't get hot enough long enough to kill bacteria when cooked in a microwave.

How Not to Get AIDS

552. Avoid Sex with High-Risk Partners

One way you can contract AIDS is by having sex with someone who is infected with the virus.

Those at greatest risk for having AIDS include homosexual and bisexual men, intravenous drug users, hemophiliacs, female prostitutes, and heterosexuals from Haiti and central Africa.

Obviously it's important to know your mate. Monogamy and condom use will also reduce your risk. But rest assured, you can't get AIDS by having sex with someone who isn't infected.

553. Casual Contact Isn't a Risk

Saliva appears to inactivate the AIDS virus. In studies of households and families with an infected member, AIDS patients shared food and drink, plates, glasses, cutlery, and toothbrushes with uninfected people and no one else got AIDS. In one study of 83 AIDS patients, the virus turned up in the saliva of only 1.

Also, the AIDS virus has not been found in the phlegm or nasal mucus of infected people. All the experts, including former Surgeon General C. Everett Koop, M.D., agree that there's no evidence the virus can be spread through this kind of casual contact.

554. A Kiss on the Cheek Won't Do It

Kissing seems to be safe, too, but Dr. Koop advises against French-kissing someone who might be infected, although transmission through French-kissing has never been documented.

"Even in more intimate settings, there have been no cases of transmission by saliva," says Alan Lifson, M.D., of the San Francisco Department of Public Health's AIDS department. Therefore, the risk of infection from a dry kiss on the cheek or lips is negligible.

555. Hugging Is Harmless

You can't get AIDS from hugging someone with the disease. The virus isn't found in sweat or on the skin. In the household studies mentioned above, people hugged and had lots of close, nonsexual contact. Not one case of AIDS was spread this way.

"The virus has to get into the bloodstream to infect cells," says AIDS expert Margaret Fischl, M.D., of the University of Miami Medical School. "That doesn't happen when you shake someone's hand or hug them."

556. Giving Blood Is Safe

You cannot get AIDS by giving blood. Period. This myth started when people twisted around the concept that it was risky to *get* blood. There's no risk whatsoever when needles are used only once, as they are for blood donation in the United States.

557. Sterilized Needles Are Safe

The AIDS virus may spread on unsterilized needles used for acupuncture, tattooing, or ear piercing. Sterilization, however, eliminates all risks.

A way to make sure the needle is safe to use is to dip it into a 1:10 dilution of bleach, alcohol, hydrogen peroxide, or Lysol to kill the virus. Heating the needle to 140°F for 10 minutes also destroys the virus.

558. Insects Are Not Carriers

The myth that insects spread AIDS got started when researchers theorized that mosquitoes might have spread the virus in Belle Glade, Florida, where an outbreak occurred from 1982 to 1987 among people with no known risk factors.

Evidence taken from the area pointed in other directions, though. First, most people infected with AIDS are between the ages of 20 and 49. Second, after close examination, scientists found that sex and intravenous drug abuse were the actual routes of infection in Belle Glade. And third, there's no evidence of the AIDS virus in insects.

559. Toilets Are Safe to Sit On

Even if the person who used the toilet before you had AIDS, you can't catch the disease off the toilet seat. "The virus can't live on a toilet seat," says Charles Fallis of the Centers for Disease Control. "It dies immediately in the open air."

The virus has sometimes been found in urine, but in quantities so small scientists think the virus isn't transmitted this way.

The AIDS virus has also been isolated in feces, but in 11 studies of more than 700 AIDS patients who lived and shared toilets with uninfected people, the virus has never spread this way.

In no known case has contact with urine or feces, on a toilet seat or anyplace else, led to infection.

560. It's Safe to Eat in Restaurants Where Gay People Work

Your sushi chef has AIDS and his fingers are covered with bandages. Should you be worried that he may bleed into your sauce and you'll catch the disease? No.

Experts say the risks to you are negligible because the amount of virus that might be present in a few drops of blood is scant. Also, the likelihood that the virus could survive passage through the digestive tract is extremely small.

C H A P T E R · 9

STRONG
BONES
FOR
LIFE

She bumps against a table—and her hip fractures. She coughs hard—and a vertebra in her spine collapses.

This isn't a scene out of some horror film. It's the reality of what can happen to a person with *osteoporosis*—the bone-weakening disease that erodes the skeletons of millions of American women. And in many cases, broken bones only set the stage for a bigger tragedy.

"Among women 70 years old who suffer fractured hips, 12 to 20 percent of them die within a year," writes Kenneth Cooper, M.D., in *Preventing Osteoporosis*. The disease itself doesn't kill—what's potentially fatal are the complications (like blood clots and pneumonia) from being hospitalized with a broken hip. But you don't have to be haunted by your own skeleton. Osteoporosis can be prevented—even reversed. The first step is knowing what you're up against.

The Story of Bone

To understand osteoporosis you need to understand that a bone is *alive*—a complex, living tissue that is constantly replacing and repairing itself. When you're young, more bone cells are added than removed. But about the time you're 35, this process reverses itself—more bone is lost than replaced, and your total bone mass gradually decreases. And the bones that are left are porous—full of little holes that weaken the structure.

Osteoporosis isn't easy to spot, however, so most bones are "diagnosed" as osteoporotic when they arrive at a hospital emergency room as fractures of the spine, hip, pelvis, wrist, or shoulder area, says C. Conrad Johnston, Jr., M.D., professor in the Department of Medicine at Indiana University. And these fractures aren't a rarity.

"It is estimated that approximately 33 percent of women over age 65 will suffer at least one vertebral [spinal] fracture," says John Bilezikian, M.D., of the Department of Medicine at Columbia University's College of Physicians and Surgeons.

That's quite a hit list. Here's how you can keep your name off it.

Prevention—at Any Age

561. Check the Strength of Your Family Tree

Scientists believe that the peak bone mass a person can reach is probably genetically determined. You can measure your risk factors by looking into your family history. Or even by just looking at your mother.

Small frames, for example, run in families. So if a mother has osteoporosis, chances are her daughter is at risk for developing the disease also. Whites more than blacks, the underweight more than the overweight, and those who smoke and are sedentary are also at risk. (For a complete profile of someone at risk, see "Weigh Your Risk" on page 238.)

"We conclude that daughters of women with osteoporosis have reduced bone mass in their spine," write researchers in the *New England Journal of Medicine.* "This reduction in bone mass may put them at increased risk for fractures."

562. Start a Bone-Building Program Now

Stronger bones last longer. The best time to build bone mass seems to be from the beginning of adolescence on up to around age 30, says the National Osteoporosis Foundation.

"Young women can increase their bone mass by as much as 20 percent, a critical factor in protecting against osteoporosis," states the foundation.

But preventive measures can be effective at any age—even if you're already showing signs of bone loss.

563. Get Acquainted with Calcium

One of the best ways to build stronger bones is to make sure you have an adequate supply of calcium in your diet.

What makes calcium so important? Bone is roughly two-thirds mineral by weight, and "calcium makes up roughly 40 percent of that mineral," according to Robert Heaney, M.D., professor of medicine at Creighton University and a fellow of the American College of Physicians.

Lack of calcium means lack of bone. In a 14-year study, researchers at the University of California, San Diego, found evidence that "strongly supports the hypothesis that increased dietary calcium intake protects against hip fracture."

The researchers followed 957 older men and women ranging in age from 50 to 79 and found that those who consumed the most calcium had the fewest fractures. "The only factor consistently and significantly associated with risk of hip fracture was dietary calcium," researchers concluded.

Studies have shown that 85 percent of women today over the age of 65 do not meet their daily requirements for calcium. It's not just the elderly missing out either; 70 to 80 percent of women aged 22 to 64 also don't get the minimum requirements.

How much is enough? The Recommended Dietary Allowance

FACT OF LIFE

Milk Is Number One

How important is milk in maintaining bone health? In one Yugoslavian study, researchers found that those who lived in a district where milk consumption was very high had 60 percent fewer hip fractures than those who lived in a community where consumption was low.

Weigh Your Risk

What are your chances of developing osteoporosis? The following are known risk factors. The more descriptive they are of you, the greater your risk.

Some, you will notice, are beyond your control. Others are not. But keep in mind that just knowing your risk and taking preventive measures can greatly reduce your chance of ever getting the disease. The risk factors include:

- Being a woman.
- Your age—the older you are, the greater the risk.
- Early menopause.
- Being Caucasian.
- Eating a low-calcium diet.
- Having a sedentary lifestyle.
- Being underweight.
- Having a family history of osteoporosis.
- Smoking.
- Heavy drinking.

(RDA) is 800 milligrams a day. Some experts, however, say taking 1,000 to 1,500 milligrams a day beginning well before menopause will reduce the incidence of osteoporosis in postmenopausal women. Most experts recommend an average daily intake of 1,200 milligrams, says Mark Zilkowski, M.D., assistant professor in the Department of Family Medicine at the Medical College of Ohio in Toledo.

564. Be Like the Dairy Rich

A good daily dose of dairy products may be all you need to get your essential amount of calcium. Dairy products are the main dietary source of calcium. Since dairy products are taste-pleasing to most, that makes increasing your intake easy. All you have to do is remember that every serving of a dairy product contains about 300 milligrams of calcium. Of course, you'll want to stick to low-fat dairy foods.

The following, for example, provide the recommended 1,200 milligrams of calcium without adding excess fat to your diet.

- One 8-ounce glass of skim milk (300 milligrams)
- One 8-ounce container of low-fat yogurt (350 to 450 milligrams)
- 1½ ounces of low-fat cheese (300 milligrams)
- A daily multiple vitamin containing 300 milligrams of calcium

565. Eat Your Vegetables

Dairy foods are not the only source of calcium. Other calcium-rich foods include green leafy vegetables (except spinach), shellfish, almonds, Brazil nuts, tofu, and sardines. Here's a partial list of non-dairy foods rich in calcium.

Sardines, Atlantic, drained solids, 3 ounces (322 milligrams)
Salmon, sockeye with bones, 3 ounces (203 milligrams)
Soybeans, cooked, 1 cup (198 milligrams)
Broccoli, cooked, 1 cup (178 milligrams)
Tofu, 3 ounces (174 milligrams)
Bok choy, 1 cup (158 milligrams)
Collards, cooked, 1 cup (148 milligrams)
Dandelion greens, cooked, 1 cup (146 milligrams)
Blackstrap molasses, 1 tablespoon (137 milligrams)
Navy beans, cooked, 1 cup (128 milligrams)
Soy flour, defatted, 1/2 cup (120 milligrams)
Mustard greens, cooked, 1 cup (104 milligrams)
Almonds, unblanched, 1/4 cup (94 milligrams)
Kale, cooked, 1 cup (94 milligrams)
Chick-peas, cooked, 1 cup (80 milligrams)
Shrimp, steamed, 3 ounces (33 milligrams)
Scallops, raw, 3 ounces (21 milligrams)

566. Take Supplements for Added Protection

The good news about calcium has been spreading quickly. The *Wall Street Journal* reported that sales of calcium supplements in one recent year were estimated to be $131 million.

Calcium supplements come in a variety of forms, and each kind of supplement contains a different percentage of calcium. If you're unsure that you're getting enough calcium from your diet (and most women don't), you might want to consider taking calcium supplements. Discuss a supplement program with your doctor, who can also advise you as to the type of supplement that's best for you.

Some calcium supplements can carry mild gastrointestinal side effects (constipation and nausea, for example). Calcium carbonate is by far the most common type of supplement and is the most concentrated—40 percent calcium. Other forms include calcium phosphate (31 to 40 percent calcium, depending on the brand), calcium lactate (13 percent), and calcium gluconate (9 percent).

567. Take Tums for the Tummy and Your Bones

If you depend on antacids for indigestion, your best bet is to reach for Tums, because they'll also help your bones. Tums is almost 100 percent calcium carbonate, and it is formulated specifically to break up in your stomach, making the calcium readily available for absorption.

The Calcium Quotient

Increasing your calcium intake can decrease your chances of developing osteoporosis. But many experts, including the National Institutes of Health, consider the Recommended Daily Allowance for calcium too low for women at risk for osteoporosis. Here's what the majority of nutritionists and experts feel the lifelong daily requirement of calcium should be.

- Birth to 6 months: 400 milligrams
- 6 months to 1 year: 600 milligrams
- 1 to 10: 800 milligrams
- 11 to 18: 1,200 milligrams
- Premenopausal women: 1,200 milligrams
- Pregnant and nursing women: 1,400 milligrams
- Estrogen-treated women: 1,000 milligrams
- Postmenopausal women: 1,500 milligrams
- Men: 1,000 milligrams

FACT OF LIFE

Calcium Deficiency Is a Common Problem

If you assume you're getting enough calcium in your diet, you may be wrong. When scientists screen people for nutrient deficiency, they usually find calcium among the top three nutrients that most people are lacking. The other two? Iron and vitamin E.

Doctors, however, do not recommend that you depend on antacids as your sole source of calcium or take them in lieu of a supplement. For one thing, not all antacids are 100 percent calcium carbonate. Some don't contain it at all, and most are aluminum-based.

Also, remember that antacids are a medicine, and like any medicine, should not be abused. And don't take antacids within an hour or two of taking other medication because it could block the absorption of the medicine.

568. Take Your Supplement at Mealtime

A recent study discovered that absorption of calcium from calcium carbonate is impaired in people with little or no stomach acid, a common condition in people over age 60. Doctors, however, feel that everybody could improve their calcium absorption by taking their supplement with meals. So take your supplements with your meals. Or talk to your doctor about taking another type of calcium supplement.

569. Guard against Kidney Stones

When taking a calcium supplement, you should down it with a full glass of water. Why?

Taking daily supplements in the 1,000- to 1,500-milligram range could cause kidney stones in people susceptible to them. If you have a family history of kidney stones, it's a good idea to take calcium supplements only with your doctor's consent.

Once you get the go-ahead, make sure you drink plenty of water. Pebbles don't stay put in fast-moving streams.

FACT OF LIFE

Women Get Too Little Calcium

Experts now claim the Recommended Dietary Allowance (RDA) of 800 milligrams of calcium a day for women is too low to guard against osteoporosis—and most women don't get even that. The Department of Health and Human Services estimates that 75 percent of all adult women get less than the RDA; and a full 25 percent get less than 300 milligrams daily, a figure, they say, insufficent to maintain calcium balance. And the news gets worse: Young women and girls get even less, a fact, notes one doctor, that "must be viewed with considerable alarm."

570. Soak Up the Sunshine Vitamin

Vitamin D is essential for optimal absorption of calcium in the intestine, and doctors say you should get around 400 international units of the vitamin every day. You can do that by spending 15 minutes to an hour outdoors and by including good sources of vitamin D in your diet: saltwater fish, liver, and vitamin D-fortified milk and cereals.

Most doctors do not recommend vitamin D supplements because the vitamin is toxic in high dosages, although a multivitamin with D in it is usually fine.

571. Go Easy on the Soft Drinks

Too many soft drinks could make your bones go soft.

Phosphates, a common ingredient in many carbonated soft drinks, can speed the depletion of calcium from your bones, notes George L. Blackburn, M.D., Ph.D., associate professor of surgery at Harvard Medical School and chief of the Nutrition/Metabolism Laboratory with the Cancer Research Institute at New England Deaconess Hospital in Boston. He suggests you limit yourself to one or two servings of phosphate-containing sodas a day.

Or, better yet, check the labels and choose carbonated beverages that don't contain phosphates. Carbonated mineral waters do not contain any phosphate.

572. Boron: Another Reason to Eat Your Vegetables

Boron is used to make water soft, but it may also make your bones strong. In a study conducted by the U.S. Department of Agriculture, women who took 3 milligrams of the mineral boron lost one-third less calcium than when they were on a diet low in boron.

"The findings suggest that supplementation of a low-boron diet with an amount of boron commonly found in diets high in fruits and vegetables induces changes in postmenopausal women consistent with the prevention of calcium loss and bone demineralization," noted the researchers.

"The boron helped to create a balance of hormones . . . that probably slowed the demineralization of the bone," explains Forrest Nielsen, Ph.D., a USDA nutritionist and one of the researchers on the study.

Boron as yet has no recommended dietary allowance, but a normal balanced diet yields about 1.5 milligrams a day. The best food sources of boron are fruits (especially apples, plums, pears, and grapes), vegetables, nuts, leafy greens, and legumes.

Warning: Boron can be lethal in excessive doses, so don't take supplements without approval from your doctor. The best advice: Get a good daily dose of fruits and vegetables.

573. Manganese Is Important, Too

Laboratory studies in animals indicate that the trace mineral manganese may be as important as calcium in building bones. Fortunately, the average adult diet contains ample amounts of manganese.

The best food sources of manganese are pecans, peanuts, pineapple, oatmeal, shredded wheat, raisin bran, beans (pinto, lima, navy), rice, spinach, sweet potatoes, whole-wheat bread, beef, eggs, tuna, and yogurt.

Milk, by the way, is the best source of both calcium and manganese.

574. Just a Little Spinach, Please

Spinach contains oxalate, a chemical substance that interferes with calcium absorption. Oxalate is also found in rhubarb, and there are traces in soybeans and cocoa. This doesn't mean you should avoid eating these foods. Just do so in moderation if you are at risk for osteoporosis.

575. Know Your Fiber Facts

Yes, it's true that a high-fiber diet, important in regulating the bowels and reducing cholesterol, can also interfere with calcium absorption, says Dr. Blackburn.

But, he says, the health benefits of a high-fiber diet are so significant that you shouldn't cut back for calcium's sake. As long as you're getting the daily amount of calcium suggested on page 240, you needn't worry about the small effect of fiber. Just be aware that too much fiber and not enough calcium could be bad for those at risk of osteoporosis.

576. Watch Those Steaks and Chops

Excess protein binds with calcium in the digestive tract and increases calcium loss in the urine, says Dr. Heaney of Creighton University. He suggests you limit your daily meat intake to 3 to 6 ounces a day. This amount, he says, will have little effect on your calcium status.

577. Hard Drinking Is Hard on the Bones

Heavy drinking has been found to put both men and women at risk for bone fractures, reports the Arthritis Foundation. Men and women who drink heavily have been found to have less bone mass, and they lose bone more rapidly than teetotalers.

Other side effects of heavy drinking—namely, bad eating habits, weight loss, and liver troubles—may also affect bone strength, multiplying the risks of developing osteoporosis.

Experts recommend that if you do drink alcohol, do so in moderation. Limit your intake to two drinks a day.

578. Get Hip to This

Here's just one more good reason to give up smoking. A study conducted at the Brookhaven National Laboratory showed that cigarette smokers had a higher rate of osteoporosis than nonsmokers.

Another study found that women who smoke increase their risk of hip fracture 1.7 times and that 10 to 20 percent of hip fractures can be attributed to smoking.

579. Stay Out of Smoke-Filled Rooms

Even if *you* don't smoke, you could be at risk for osteoporosis if people *around* you smoke.

A study conducted at the Argonne National Laboratory discovered that exposure to cadmium (an element found in cigarette smoke) may speed bone loss in postmenopausal women.

Try to get the people around you to stop smoking, if not for their health, at least for yours.

580. Consider Estrogen Replacement Therapy

Estrogen helps lock calcium inside bones. But menopause shuts down the estrogen factory, and bone health is put on back-order. But there's a medical solution to this supply problem: estrogen pills.

The National Osteoporosis Foundation reports that "estrogen replacement therapy is the most effective method of reducing postmenopausal bone loss." Studies have shown that women who begin taking estrogen within a few years after the onset of menopause have fewer hip and wrist fractures.

"Estrogen would prevent at least 90 percent of the vertebral fractures among postmenopausal women," according to Robert Lindsay, Ph.D., professor of clinical medicine at Columbia University and director of research at Helen Hayes Hospital, New York City.

FACT OF LIFE

There's Benefit in Being Fat

Heavy women are at a much lower risk of developing osteoporosis than thin women. Researchers believe overweight has two benefits: The stress the added weight puts on the bones may help to strengthen them, and the excess fat may help to manufacture additional estrogen, the hormone important to bone building.

If you are at risk for osteoporosis—and 25 percent of *all* postmenopausal women develop osteoporosis—talk to your doctor about estrogen replacement therapy as soon after menopause as possible. "While the introduction of estrogen at any point slows the rate of bone loss in the estrogen-deficient women," says Dr. Lindsay, "the earlier the therapy is introduced, the more effective it will be."

Estrogen replacement therapy, however, is not without risk. It is thought to increase the risk of a type of uterine cancer known as endometrial cancer from 1 per 1,000 women to about 4 per 1,000 women. Many experts feel, however, that in terms of osteoporosis, the benefits far outweigh its risks.

581. Avoid Prescriptions for Bad Bones

Some medications that you may be taking may be the worst medicine for your bones. If you are taking either heparin, a blood thinner, or furosemide, used to treat edema (excess fluid in the tissue) and high blood pressure, check with your doctor about whether it will put you at increased risk for osteoporosis.

582. Move Those Bones

Active bones are healthy bones. A study found that patients restricted to bed rest for 11 to 61 days lost an average of 1 percent of the bone mineral from the lumbar spine. Once out of bed, the bones got back to pre–bed-rest level in approximately 200 days.

Another study of very sedentary 90-year-old nursing home residents found that on the average they experienced "an increase of 4.2 percent in their bone density after performing mild exercises for 30 minutes three times a week."

FACT OF LIFE

Estrogen Saves Bones

Research shows that estrogen replacement therapy would prevent 90 percent of the vertebral fractures suffered by women after menopause and that it can reduce the incidence of hip fractures by as much as 50 percent.

Yet another study showed that "performing aerobic exercise for one hour twice weekly significantly retarded bone loss from the lumbar spine over an eight-month period in healthy women aged 50 to 73."

The mere fact that you are active helps prevent bone loss. A study of 300 elderly men and women in Britain showed that: "In both sexes increased daily activity, including standing, walking, stair climbing, housework, and gardening, protected against fracture."

583. Weight-Bearing Exercise Is Best

Astronauts are active folks, but studies have shown that weightlessness causes a monthly loss of as high as 2 percent of their bone mineral content. Bones need to support weight in order to remain strong.

In fact, studies show that weight-bearing exercise, such as running, cycling, and lifting weights, is the best sort of exercise for your bones.

In a study published in the *Annals of Internal Medicine,* researchers say that "weight-bearing exercise led to significant increases in bone mineral content which were maintained with continued training in older postmenopausal women."

584. Amenorrhea: Too Much of a Good Thing

Exercise is great for osteoporosis, but young women who exercise to the point of missing their periods (a condition called amenorrhea) are actually increasing their risk for the disease. Amenorrhea most commonly occurs in women with low body fat who exercise strenuously, buit it can occur in *any* woman with low body fat.

"Women have to be alerted that, if in the process of exercising they lose their periods, they may lose bone density," says Barbara Drinkwater, Ph.D., an exercise physiologist at Pacific Medical Center, Seattle.

Amenorrhea results when the production of estrogen, an important hormone for building bones, is suppressed.

"The good news is that the loss isn't irreversible," says Dr. Drinkwater. When the women exercisers cut back on the amount they worked out, researchers found that they regained their periods and that their bone mass also increased significantly.

By all means keep exercising; just don't overdo it. Normal amounts of exercise can only help your bones.

585. Fit Walking into Your Life

A brisk 45-minute walk once a day may be all you need to keep on the right path for avoiding osteoporosis. Researchers at Tufts University had nine postmenopausal women take such a walk daily for one year.

At the end of that time the women showed about a 3 percent increase in bone density. An inactive group of women of similar age had a 10 percent bone loss during the year.

So play it safe and take a brisk 45-minute daily walk. "It may not be the minimum required for bone benefits," says William Evans, Ph.D., chief of the USDA-Tufts Physiology Laboratory, "but it's the amount we know works."

586. Garden and Grow Strong

Researchers in the Netherlands found that gardeners had a lower incidence of heart disease than those who preferred just to watch their weeds grow. But they noticed something else: The physical exertion of gardening can help the bones remain strong.

587. Stand Tall

Doctors at the Mayo Clinic found a correlation between strong back-straightening muscles and bone density. They found that the stronger the back muscles, the greater the bone density of the vertebrae.

The next step was to find out if strengthening the back muscles could stop or reverse the loss of calcium from the back.

"We are finding that specific exercises seem to have the greatest effect," says Mehrsheed Sinaki, M.D., one of the study's doctors. "The extension exercises—like arching the back and straightening it—help the most."

Women who did these exercises had less than one-third the spinal fractures of those doing bending or no exercise at all.

If you suspect you already have osteoporosis, check with your doctor before doing this or any other type of exercise—there's a risk of breaking already-brittle bones.

Dealing with the Disease

588. Get in the Swim of Things

Even though swimming isn't exactly a weight-bearing exercise, researchers are still finding that daily dips may help fight osteoporosis.

"Swimming can serve as a gentle way for elderly osteoporotic people to add bone density," says Eric Orwoll, M.D., chief of Endocrinology, Portland, Oregon Veterans Administration Medical Center.

589. Make Your Body Breakproof

Most osteoporotic bone breaks are caused when people fall. Take these measures to cut down on your chances of this happening.

- Have your vision checked and corrected.
- Rise slowly and don't rush to answer the phone or door.
- Know which medications may make you drowsy and use extra caution when you take them.
- Use adaptive devices like canes, crutches, or walkers properly.
- Look out for hidden steps or newly waxed floors.
- Wear low, broad heels and nonskid footwear.

FACT OF LIFE

Bone-Breaking Figures

There are almost 2 million bone fractures a year in women over age 45. Some 200,000 of them are hip fractures. Seventy percent of these fractures can be linked to osteoporosis. It's estimated that 33 percent of all women after age 65 will suffer at least one fracture.

Life-Extension Tool

Personal Emergency Response System

Help is just a phone call away—if you can make it to the telephone. But if you're lying on the floor with a fractured hip, that phone might as well be on Mars.

In an emergency, especially if you live alone, you need someone or something to call for help. That something could be on a chain dangling from your neck.

The device (known by various names that are usually derived from the words "medical alert") is designed so that, in an emergency, it will make the life-saving call for you. It's hooked up to the Emergency Response System, which is available in most areas across the country. Elderly women with osteoporosis are the system's major customers.

"If someone has an accident or other medical emergency, they can push the button on a pendant, sending a signal to a device connected to their phone. This in turn alerts a central monitoring station that help is needed," says Harry Williamson, president of Cross Care Limited, a Pennsylvania distributor of a medical alert system.

All of these systems function 24 hours a day, seven days a week, and work in much the same fashion. "Once the emergency signal comes in, we try to get back to you to see if you are okay," says Williamson. "If we don't get a response, we call your family or a neighbor to go and check on you. We will then notify the police or an ambulance."

To purchase one of these products, you may have to spend between $500 to $1,200 or more, plus a monthly monitoring fee. In some areas, you can get them more cheaply through the American Red Cross or your local county's department of aging. If you can't find them there, look in the Yellow Pages under "Medical Alarms."

In some instances, Williamson says, your medical coverage may cover the cost. "If you're a veteran, the VA (Veterans Administration) will pay for it. One insurance company so far, Mutual of Omaha, will also reimburse you. Otherwise, ask your doctor to prescribe it for you; then you'll be able to claim it on your taxes."

The alarm pendant itself is only about 2 inches long and weighs less than 2 ounces. If you don't fancy wearing something around your neck, there is a style that can be worn on your belt like a pager.

FACT OF LIFE

The Weaker They Are, the Harder They Fall

Three things determine whether or not you'll break a bone in a fall: how hard you fall, how well your tendons and muscles cushion the blow, and, finally, how strong your bones are. The last item—weak bones—is the reason that the majority of broken bones occur in the elderly.

590. Shatterproof Your House

There are plenty of hazards around your home that could cause you trouble if you have osteoporosis. Here's a safety list specially devised for protecting brittle bones.

- Have all the areas of your home lit with fluorescent or glazed bulbs. Don't use bare bulbs because they send a glare which could throw off your eyesight and your step.
- Make sure stairwells and bathrooms are always well lit.
- Use nightlights, especially in the area between bedroom and bathroom.
- Have handrails installed on both sides of all stairways.
- Install a handrail near your tub and toilet.
- Install safety treads in your bathtub.
- Use liquid soaps to avoid slipping on a soap bar.
- Do not wax linoleum floors; use waxless cleansers.
- Get rid of all loose carpets and scatter rugs.
- If young children frequent the house, make sure they put all toys away.
- Keep a sturdy step stool handy for reaching high places.
- Don't leave shoes lying around on the floor.
- Put a nonskid mat near the kitchen sink to avoid slippery spills.
- Make sure the kitchen table and chairs are well balanced.
- Place all electrical cords next to the wall or behind furniture.
- Make sure there is ample walk-through space and that no pathways are blocked by furniture.

Discovery Comes Too Late

Standard x-rays won't detect osteoporosis until 30 percent of your bone has already disappeared. In fact, osteoporosis isn't usually detected at all until the first bone is broken.

591. Learn to Lift Properly

Don't lift objects using your back; use your legs instead. A weak back could snap if you bend over and try to pick up a heavy object, caution experts. So keep your back straight, squat to grasp the object, then lift straight up, using your legs to bear the weight.

Better yet, get someone else to do the lifting for you.

592. Establish a Help Network

No matter how safe your house is, there is always the chance that you may fall and injure yourself. If you live alone, a bone-breaking fall could prevent you from calling for help.

Try to be in at least daily contact with your family or a neighbor, just in case you fall and can't move. That way, help is never far away.

Another thing you can do is to buy an emergency beeper that you can wear around your neck. If an accident happens, you need only press a button, and emergency personnel will be notified. (See Life Extension Tool on page 250 for more information on the device.)

C H A P T E R · 10

■■■■

DIABETES: A LIFE-EXTENSION PROGRAM

Diabetes can short-circuit even the best-laid plans for a long life. As the sixth leading cause of death, it can obviously kill. And it has enough ammunition in its arsenal to send other assassins hot on your trail: 75 percent of deaths among people with diabetes, for example, are blamed on heart disease.

How does diabetes manage to load the gun but get another disease to pull the trigger? By making you an easy target. Simply put, diabetes means you have high levels of sugar in your blood. High blood sugar can actually damage the tiny capillaries that carry oxygen- and nutrient-rich blood from your arteries to the rest of your body. And when neither oxygen nor nutrients can get through to your cells, the resulting injuries set you up for a variety of problems such as heart disease, stroke, and circulatory problems in your arms and legs. Poor circulation is the reason that someone with diabetes has twice the risk of heart disease, twice the risk of stroke, and five times the risk of arterial disease in the limbs as someone without the disease.

And the problem doesn't end there. The impaired circulation in people with diabetes can lead to nerve damage that is itself ultimately responsible for 20,000 amputations a year—one out of every

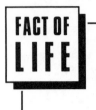

ten diabetics undergoes foot amputation, experts estimate. Others go blind: 25 percent of all new cases of blindness are blamed on diabetes. Moreover, 25 percent of all kidney failure is also blamed on diabetes—as are untold cases of impotence.

That's a lot of threats stemming from a disease that, for the most part, may not ever make you *feel* bad. But all they ever have to be is *threats*. If you have diabetes, there is plenty you can do to make sure you never come face-to-face with the enemy.

A Two-Faced Disease

Diabetes is the result of a body that does not properly secrete insulin, the hormone responsible for processing food efficiently. Insulin acts as a kind of molecular bridge that allows the sugar found in digested food to cross from your bloodstream into your body's cells, where it is broken down into the energy that fuels your body. If there's not enough insulin to build enough bridges to accommodate all the sugar roaming your bloodstream—or if the bridges are too weak for safe passage—the sugar simply accumulates until it reaches such high levels that it begins to bottleneck.

If your high blood sugar is a result of your body not making enough insulin, doctors say you have Type I, or juvenile-onset diabetes, and you'll probably have to depend on insulin by injection to get your blood sugar levels down to normal. This type of diabetes, which usually strikes at puberty (hence, "juvenile"), affects 10 percent of all people with diabetes—about 1 million people.

If high blood sugar is a result of your body not being able to use the insulin that it produces, however, you have Type II, or adult-onset diabetes. And it's by far the most common: 90 percent of all people with diabetes—about 10 million—have Type II. It's also by far the easiest to control.

The Fat Factor

Scientists don't really know what causes diabetes, but they do know that Type II frequently develops in people over the age of 40 who have a family history of diabetes, or had diabetes during pregnancy. And it develops most frequently in those who are overweight.

Between 70 and 90 percent of all those who develop Type II diabetes are obese, and scientists do not think it's a coincidence. Many of them believe that fat plays a pivotal role in the disease's development because fat apparently prevents the insulin your body produces from helping sugar enter your cells. Fortunately, once the fat is gone, your insulin functions better and will help clear the blood of excess sugar. It's such a miraculous and immediate effect that weight loss has become the cornerstone of treatment for Type II diabetes.

Scientists are also looking very closely at the connection between diabetes and a family history of the disease. Given the ten-

Know the Warning Signs of Type II Diabetes

Type II diabetes tends to develop slowly over the years. Fully 50 percent of the people who have it don't suspect a thing. Yet not knowing you have the disease doesn't prevent diabetes from doing its life-threatening damage inside your body.

If you have any of the following symptoms, contact your physician for a diabetes test as soon as possible.

- Frequent urination
- Excessive thirst
- Extreme hunger
- Dramatic weight loss
- Irritability
- Weakness and fatigue
- Nausea and vomiting
- Recurring or hard-to-heal skin sores
- Gum or bladder infections
- Blurred vision
- Tingling or numbness in hands or feet
- Itching

The Risk of Gangrene

People with diabetes are 50 times more likely to develop gangrene than those without the disease. The reason? The impaired circulation caused by diabetes can cut off the blood supply to any given area of the body.

dency of diabetes to run in one particular family or another, it's clear that genetic factors are at work. But in exactly what way is still something of a mystery.

Classic studies of twins, for example, have shown that a twin who develops Type II diabetes after the age of 40 can almost guarantee that the other twin will get the disease. The "concordance rate," as scientists call it, is almost 100 percent. A twin who develops Type I diabetes, however, can promise nothing. If one twin develops Type I diabetes, the other twin develops the disease only 50 percent of the time. In a purely genetic disease, the concordance rate should be 100 percent—50 percent just isn't good enough to prove or disprove a genetic basis.

While the factors that cause diabetes are still uncertain, the factors that can control the condition are not. Fortunately, there is a way to prevent the damage diabetes can cause—and block all the assassins that can rob you of a longer life. The key, doctors say, is to find a way to keep your blood sugar at the same level as that of someone who doesn't have the disease. Here's the way to do it.

The Lifelong, Long-Life Eating Plan

593. Pare the Pudge

Your chance of developing diabetes as an adult literally *doubles* with every 20 percent of excess weight you carry. If you're 60 pounds over your ideal weight of 150 pounds, for example, your risk of diabetes quadruples. So reducing your weight clearly reduces your risk of getting the disease.

As weight drops, doctors have found, so do high insulin levels. Also, the liver, which has been pouring two to three times more sugar than normal into your blood, begins to produce less, and peripheral muscle tissue, previously resistant to the effects of insulin on sugar uptake, begins to use the insulin more easily.

594. Avoid Diet Pills

Weight-loss aids will add to the problems of people with diabetes—not solve them. Over-the-counter appetite suppressants that contain phenylpropanolamine (PPA) can exacerbate the kidney and eye problems that diabetes frequently creates.

595. Make Your Carbohydrates Complex

Manipulating your blood sugar level also means manipulating the level of carbohydrate in your diet. Most people with Type II diabetes should keep their consumption of carbohydrates to less than 55 percent of their total calories, doctors advise, because carbohydrates raise the level of sugar in their blood.

Carbohydrates come in two forms: simple carbohydrates, such as the sugars found in cakes, pastries, and candy; and complex carbohydrates, such as the starches found in vegetables, dried beans, breads, and cereals. Researchers are investigating the idea that simple carbohydrates raise blood sugar more than complex carbohydrates, so it may be a good idea to choose complex carbohydrates more often than simple ones. Complex carbohydrates also frequently contain more fiber, which delays absorption of sugar from the gastrointestinal tract.

596. Eat Fiber at Every Meal

Studies indicate that fiber can help control Type II diabetes if you eat 10 to 15 grams at every meal. That sounds like a lot of chewing until you realize that a couple of dried figs and a bowl of 100 percent bran cereal contain about 15 grams of fiber. One-half cup of baked beans and two slices of whole-wheat bread weigh in at around 13 grams.

Other rich sources of fiber include all varieties of dried beans, peas, lentils, barley, and apples.

597. Cut Down on White Rice

White rice eaten frequently over a long period of time may produce Type II diabetes in some people, concludes a study in *Human Nutrition: Food Sciences and Nutrition.* Scientists aren't sure why, although they do know that diets high in fiber-depleted starchy foods are associated with an increased risk of diabetes. It might be wise to keep white rice as a once-in-a-while side dish and not as a regular part of your diet.

598. Coarse Grains Are Better Than Fine

In a study conducted at the Bristol Royal Infirmary in Great Britain, ten volunteers ate wheat, corn, and oats in the form of whole grains, cracked grains, and coarsely and finely ground flour. The idea was to see how food processing techniques affected the ability of various foods to raise blood sugar levels.

Processing techniques did not alter the way oats affected blood sugar. But the finer both wheat and corn were ground, the quicker the grain was digested and—for wheat flour at least—the higher blood sugar rose.

"Our finding raises the possibility that in susceptible people, regular consumption of finely milled flour increases the risk of diseases . . . like diabetes," say the researchers.

The study suggests that people with diabetes may benefit from replacing finely ground flour with whole or cracked grains, or by using coarsely milled flour. All of these are digested more slowly and are less likely to increase blood sugar levels than finely milled flour.

FACT OF LIFE

Diabetes Hard on Adolescents

The body's ability to use the hormone insulin is impaired during puberty, possibly by high levels of growth hormone. Unfortunately, the result is that adolescents with diabetes frequently have a hard time controlling their blood sugar— just at a time in their lives when they don't want to be concerned with anything that makes them "different" from their peer group.

599. Dream of an Empty Beach after Meals

Sit back, close your eyes, and visualize yourself on an empty beach. Look at the palm trees silhouetted against an orange sunset and listen to the sea gulls. Then dig your toes into the warm sand and let your mind wander along the beach for the next 15 minutes.

If you have Type II diabetes, this simple visualization exercise may have just lowered your blood sugar. In a study conducted at Duke Unversity, 20 people with diabetes were divided into two groups to study the effects of relaxation on diabetes. One group practiced a variety of relaxation techniques, while the other group did not.

The result? People who practiced relaxation techniques after meals could handle 30 percent more sugar than they usually could before their blood sugar levels shot up.

600. Eat Low-Fat Protein

Since you can't live on carbohydrates alone—not if you want your blood sugar to stay around normal, anyway—the American Diabetes Association (ADA) suggests that you eat 12 to 20 percent of your calories in the form of low-fat protein. If that means cutting back on your consumption of meat and cheese, so be it.

601. Eat a Heart-Healthy Diet

Because people with diabetes are predisposed to heart disease, doctors recommend that they eat less than 30 percent of their calories in the form of fat. In fact, many doctors recommend that people with diabetes follow a heart-healthy diet all around. Eating lots of whole-grain breads and cereals, lots of fruits and vegetables, a minimum of even low-fat cheeses and meats, and no egg yolks are ways to keep your heart beating into a healthy and vigorous old age.

602. Substitute Olive Oil for Your Regular Oil

In a four-week study of 10 people with Type II diabetes at the University of Texas Southwestern Medical Center in Dallas, scientists compared the traditional low-fat, high-carbohydrate diabetic diet to a low-carbohydrate diet in which olive oil, a monounsaturated fat, was substituted wherever possible for other fats.

The result? "Glucose levels were actually lower on the mono diet," says Abhimanyu Garg, M.D., who conducted the study. An added benefit was the fact that the diet also lowered two heart-damaging substances—triglycerides and very-low-density lipoprotein (VLDL, a very bad form of cholesterol)—while it raised high-density lipoprotein (HDL), a form of cholesterol that seems to exert a protective effect on your heart.

603. Deep-Six the Fish Oil Supplements

A study at the University of California, San Diego, found that a one-month regimen of fish oil supplements dramatically reduced insulin secretion, while it increased blood sugar levels. Eating fresh fish is good for you, experts say, but if you have diabetes you'd better skip fish oil supplements.

604. Do Your Liver a Favor

Alcohol can affect your blood sugar level so severely that experts recommend you drink no more than the equivalent of 2 ounces of alcohol twice a week.

Keep in mind alcohol's potentially damaging effect on the liver and the fact that it's the liver that is in charge of storing and releasing sugar to your body. The last thing someone trying to control their blood sugar wants is a liver that is screwing it up.

605. Eat before You Drink

Eating before you drink is a piece of advice that has been handed down from father to son and mother to daughter for centuries. But for people with diabetes, it's a matter of life and death, reports the National Institute of Diabetes and Digestive and Kidney Diseases. Alcohol on an empty stomach can lead to such low blood sugar in someone with diabetes that it triggers shaking, dizziness, and collapse.

Unfortunately, people who don't know you have the disease may simply assume you're drunk and not summon emergency medical attention. So eat before you even get near an alcoholic beverage.

606. Think Small Six Times a Day

Along with what you eat, when you eat is one of the cornerstones of keeping your blood sugar levels consistently normal. That's because your body can actually handle a larger number of small meals better than it can handle a few big meals. The reason? The smaller the meal, the less insulin is needed to handle the sugar from each meal. The result is that you end up with a more constant blood sugar level.

What's the best schedule? Plan your three major meals—breakfast, lunch, and dinner—evenly throughout the day and then add three in-between snacks, suggests Karl Sussman, M.D., associate chief of staff for research and development at the Denver Veterans Hospital and past president of the American Diabetes Association.

How Sweet It Is

607. A Sweet Strategy to Sneak Sugar Past Your Body

In the past, people with diabetes were told that they couldn't eat sugar because it would send their blood sugar level soaring.

Today, however, doctors have found a way to sneak sugar into your body without sending your blood sugar level through the roof. You can have a food containing sugar, doctors say, if it's a carbohydrate and contains only a small percentage of sugar; if it's spaced evenly throughout the day and not gulped down in one mind-bending binge; and if it's eaten in the context of a mixed meal, not as a single food.

608. Fructose Is Better Than Sucrose

Fructose is a sugar that manufacturers sometimes use as a substitute for sucrose (table sugar) in sweets and baked goods.

Fructose, doctors explain, is handled a little differently by your body than sucrose. Fructose passes more slowly than sucrose into your blood from the gastrointestinal tract, for example, and, unlike sucrose, it is metabolized in the liver rather than left to wander your bloodstream. As a result, there is little increase in blood sugar as long as your diabetes is under control to begin with. If you eat too much fructose, however, it will raise your blood sugar.

609. Soft Drinks Are Hard on Diabetes

You wonder how they managed to fit the liquid into the can when you realize that one 12-ounce can of pop has *9* teaspoons of sugar in it. Guess what that does to the blood sugar levels of someone with diabetes?

When choosing a soft drink, says the ADA, look for one that's labeled "sugar-free" or "diet." Better yet, pass on the fizz and choose fruit juice instead.

610. Take Advantage of Sugar Substitutes

Use sugar substitutes to sweeten food whenever possible. "All the sugar substitutes on the market—saccharin, aspartame, and others—are useful in helping a diabetic person tolerate their diet better," says Dr. Sussman.

Using sugar substitutes in tomato sauce can make the difference between an exciting plate of pasta that keeps you on a healthy diet and a boring plate of pasta that makes you blow the diet to smithereens.

611. Learn How to Spot False Friends

It's true that foods labeled "dietetic" or "diabetic" contain no sugar. But they frequently do contain fat and lots of calories—both of which can sabotage your efforts to keep blood sugar down by encouraging you to gain weight.

Some of these products are actually higher in fat and calories than their nondiatetic counterparts. So next time you pick up something "dietetic," check the ingredient label for hidden time-bombs—before you put it in your cart. Read the labels carefully!

FACT OF LIFE

The Dollars and Cents of Diabetes

The cost of treating diabetes is staggering. Direct and indirect costs amount to over $20 billion dollars annually. That's nearly 5 percent of the total U.S. health-care costs.

The Active Life

612. Exercise Can Bring Blood Sugar Down to Normal

When combined with the proper diet, exercise can actually bring blood sugar levels down to normal in people with Type II diabetes.

"Exercise appears to help muscle cells take up and use sugar, even when there are lower levels of insulin in the blood," says Gerald Reaven, M.D., an endocrinologist at Stanford University. That effect helps people with Type I diabetes use their insulin more effectively, and in people with Type II diabetes—where the body's inability to use insulin is the major problem—it practically cancels out the disease.

Experts in diabetes say that aerobic exercises like swimming or cycling are good, but everybody's favorite seems to be walking.

"Brisk walking is an excellent exercise for diabetics in good shape," says Henry Dolger, M.D., former chief of the Diabetes Department at Mount Sinai Medical Center in New York City. It's easy on your body, and there is very little risk of serious injury.

613. Don't Do Double-Time

If you happen to miss a workout or two, don't try to make it up by doing the next workout faster or twice as long. A brisk workout lowers blood sugar perfectly, but warrior aerobics can cause a life-threatening drop in some people—particularly those who are taking oral diabetes drugs or insulin.

614. Be Prepared for Low Blood Sugar

Occasionally exercise can lower your blood sugar so far that you get nervous, shaky, and weak. You may also be sweating, have a headache and blurred vision, or become very hungry. These are the symptoms of hypoglycemia, a low blood sugar condition that can cause life-threatening problems.

Fortunately it's easy to stave off. Just stick some food or fruit juice in your gym bag where you can get it if you experience any of these symptoms. A couple of bites or a few sips, and you should be right as rain. If you're a walker, you can tuck a snack or a box of juice in your pocket. Food and beverage packagers have become quite creative in making their products more portable, so stroll through the supermarket and figure out what might be easiest to keep at hand.

615. Build Your Exercise Program around Your Meals

People who are taking insulin should exercise an hour after meals to avoid exercising on an empty stomach. This will help them avoid lowering their blood sugar to hypoglycemic levels.

On the other hand, people with diabetes who do not take insulin should try to exercise *before* meals. This practice will help regulate their appetite and promote weight loss.

Foot Care

616. Wear Running Shoes

Given the problems people with diabetes have with their feet, the type of shoe you wear is of major importance. But what's the best type?

After studying the feet and shoes of 100 people with diabetes, podiatrist Scott Soulier, D.P.M., a consultant to the Utah diabetes control program in Salt Lake City, concluded that regular shoes do not pad or cushion the foot sufficiently to prevent the types of calluses to which people with diabetes are prone. But running shoes do. Moreover, they serve as a convenient and inexpensive alternative for custom-made therapeutic shoes.

617. Size Up New Shoes Carefully

Break in new shoes by walking around on a carpeted surface for an hour or so to find out if they're likely to cause any irritation. If they do, have that spot checked by your doctor within 24 hours and follow his advice as to how you should protect it in the future. You may have to junk the shoes, but chances are your doctor will be able to figure out how you can make them work.

Once your shoes have passed the carpet test, however, you can start wearing them on a regular basis. The ADA recommends that you wear them for 30 minutes the first day, then add another 30 minutes each day until you can comfortably wear them all the time.

618. Keep Your Feet Fit

Because of the impaired circulation and related nerve damage caused by diabetes, people who have the disease must pay particular attention to their feet. A small blister or callus may be insignificant to most people, but even a simple irritation may be life- or limb-threatening to someone with diabetes. And complicating the problem is the fact that many people with diabetes have a hard time feeling irritations on their feet in the first place.

For that reason, here are some tips from the American Diabetes Association that will go a long way toward keeping your feet fit.

- Check your feet before and after exercise. Look for any breaks in the skin, redness, blisters, or unusual swelling. Also have someone else inspect your feet, particularly if your vision is impaired. If any of these occur, or if you feel any pain in your feet, see your doctor.
- Never "shave down" calluses yourself. Have them treated by a professional.
- Wash your feet daily, making especially sure to dry between your toes.
- Keep your feet well moisturized, but don't put the moisturizer between your toes.
- Never walk barefoot.
- Avoid over-the-counter remedies such as wart removers for foot problems unless you've talked with your doctor first.

Medical Care

619. Wear a Medical Alert Bracelet

In an emergency, it's vitally important that medical personnel know you have diabetes. If you're unconscious and can't talk, they'll have no way of knowing you have diabetes. That's why you need to wear something—a medical alert bracelet or necklace, for example—that will tell people your problem when you can't.

Many of these medical alert bracelets and necklaces can be opened and a scaled-down version of your medical history inserted. At the very least, the bracelet should include your name and address, your physician's name, address, and phone number, a clear description of your medical condition, and a list of any medications you're taking.

620. Use OTCs with Care

When you reach for an over-the-counter (OTC) remedy, don't read just the dosage. Check out the ingredients as well. "Many over-the-counter products contain sugar and other ingredients, like alcohol, that can elevate your blood sugar," says Robert Silverman, M.D., Ph.D., chief of the diabetes program branch of the National Institutes of Health. "Mostly it's the cold-related products that you should be careful with, but it's important to read all OTC labels. And always check the label for any warning directed to people with diabetes." If you're not sure about some ingredients, ask your pharmacist for more information.

621. Talk to Your Doctor about Aspirin

Aspirin taken in normal doses—one or two 325-milligram tablets every 4 to 6 hours—is not likely to have much of an effect on your blood sugar levels.

However, the ADA cautions that the large doses—three to four tablets every 4 to 6 hours, for example—sometimes taken by people with arthritis can lower blood sugar levels. And, although people with diabetes generally *do* want to lower their blood sugar levels, aspirin can foul up the efforts of someone who is controlling blood sugar levels so tightly that there is little margin for error. The result of even a slight miscalculation can be that blood sugar gets knocked down to hypoglycemic levels.

So talk to your doctor before you start taking large amounts of aspirin. You may need to alter the dose of any diabetic medication you're taking, or you may want to consider using an aspirin substitute such as acetaminophen (Tylenol and Panadol contain acetaminophen), since it has no effect on blood sugar.

Life-Extension Tool

NovoPen

More and more doctors are recommending that people taking insulin for their diabetes are better off giving themselves several shots a day instead of just one or two. But how do you carry around a vial of insulin (which needs refrigeration) and a handful of syringes discreetly?

NovoPen, a kind of preloaded syringe that looks like a sleek fountain pen and can be carried in a lapel pocket, may provide the answer. It holds 150 units of insulin—about a week's worth for many people with diabetes—and needs no refrigeration. You might want to ask your physician whether or not he thinks it's for you. It's available through your local pharmacy from the Squibb-Novo Company.

---

622. Check Your Blood Sugar Levels Yourself

People who have diabetes should check their own blood sugar levels, advises the Juvenile Diabetes Foundation. This is because someone who periodically checks their levels can immediately correct them—by eating a carbohydrate to bring them up, for example, or taking a brisk walk to bring them down—when there's a problem.

It also has an added benefit, a somewhat psychological one. "It's kind of a motivating force," says Dr. Sussman. "When you check your blood sugar level you are making yourself aware of your diabetes. And the evidence is strong that the more people test themselves, the more likely they are to achieve diabetic control."

623. Check Your Blood, Not Your Urine

Although most people with diabetes are accustomed to monitoring their blood sugar levels themselves by dipping a chemically treated piece of paper into their urine and watching for a particular color change, the Juvenile Diabetes Foundation points out that it takes anywhere from 20 minutes to 2 hours for changes in blood sugar levels to show up in urine. As a result, a urine test can show "normal" levels when your blood sugar is actually reaching dangerously high levels.

The foundation recommends that anyone with diabetes use a self-administered blood testing kit to check blood sugar. The discomfort of pricking your own finger is minimal, given that the result is tight control over the disease.

624. Check Your Tester Every Three Months

If your blood sugar testing involves placing a drop of blood on a plastic strip that is then chemically analyzed and read by a mechanical device, you need to have the device checked every three months for accuracy.

"Every three months, do two tests," advises Dr. Sussman. "Do one on your machine and send one to the laboratory to see if yours is giving accurate results. If not, contact the manufacturer to find out how it can be fixed.

"It's also a good idea to check your technique in performing the blood glucose test, not just the device. Often, wrong results come from poor technique rather than from the metering device not functioning properly," he says.

LIFE
WITHOUT
STRESS

Pliny the Elder, a famous Roman scholar, escaped the eruption of Mt. Vesuvius in A.D. 79, only to die of a sudden heart attack soon after. Medical historians speculate that the stress of fleeing a volcanic eruption triggered what's called ventricular fibrillation—that is, his heart started to beat wildly and erratically until it just gave out.

Over the centuries, doctors have recognized that emotional stress—especially extreme fear, anxiety, anger, or grief—can trigger sudden and unexpected death. More recently, medical journals have reported a link between frequent or persistent stress and potentially life-threatening conditions such as asthma, high blood pressure, heart disease, stroke, diabetes, cancer, and alcoholism. The *British Medical Journal*, for example, reports a study indicating that women who'd been successfully treated for breast cancer were more likely to suffer a recurrence if they'd undergone severe stress than cancer victims experiencing less pressure. And stress has even been linked to speeding the deaths of AIDS victims.

A Vicious Cycle

Stress invites disease by assaulting the defenses of your immune system. Disease-fighting cells are wiped out, leaving you more susceptible to disease. "The argument is not that stress produces an infection," say John B. Jemmott III, Ph.D., of Princeton University, and Steven E. Locke, M.D., of the Harvard Medical School, in *Psychological Bulletin*. "But it impairs immunologic functioning and makes the person, if exposed to an infectious agent, more likely to develop the disease than he or she would have been if not under stress."

Stress can get you in an indirect way, too. People often smoke, overeat, or drink too much alcohol when they're under stress, and those habits can shorten life by causing cancer, heart disease, stroke, emphysema, or liver disease, according to the U.S. Department of Health and Human Services. An average 40-year-old man who smokes more than 40 cigarettes a day, for example, snuffs about 8 years off his life.

So, what makes life so stressful? Researchers have come up with a list of stressful situations that include both positive and negative "life events," like getting married or divorced, getting promoted or losing your job, experiencing the birth of a child or death of a family member, buying a house or defaulting on your mortgage, and going on vacation or spending a week in the hospital. Yes, even the good things in life can be potentially bad for us—if we don't know how to deal with them properly. And for those who don't, says Australian cardiologist Zelman Freeman, "life is a terminal illness."

Beating the Odds

But *you* needn't be a victim of disease by stress. In fact, if you put yourself in the right frame of mind, you'll go a long way in avoiding its repercussions altogether.

Scientists investigating the mind/body relationship have discovered that stress per se doesn't make you sick. Rather, your *interpretation* of the stressful event and how you react to it determines how well you handle it. For example, a summons from the boss to one person could draw feelings of anticipation: "Oh, good. He wants to praise me." But another person will view it with dread: "Oh, God. What did I do now?"

Such differences in how two people can interpret the same stressful situation is why one will thrive on stress, using it to nourish his spirit and increase the quality and length of his life. The other may just cave in.

Make Friends, Live Longer

Attitude, too, influences "stress hardiness." Take hostility, for example. Studies have found that people who are cynical and easily irritated have difficulty making and keeping friends. (No surprise there.) Yet research shows that having a network of trusted friends, relatives, and co-workers protects against the lethal effects of stress.

Evidently, say researchers, combining a lot of stress with little social support can dangerously increase your risk for developing life-threatening illnesses like heart disease.

What's more, people who are hostile tend to attract trouble like magnets. The University of Utah researchers found that hostile

---

When It's Time to Talk to a Therapist

If stress becomes unbearable, don't hesitate to seek professional help. Private counseling or a stress-management program tailored to your specific problem will help.

If you can't identify the exact source of your stress, make a list of the problems at home and the physical symptoms that accompany them. As with any problem the first rule is to recognize that you are suffering. From there, the cure can be as easy as a walk in the park as you breathe deeply—smiling all the way!

In search of a new direction? Try contacting one of the following organizations.

The American Institute of Stress
124 Park Avenue
Yonkers, NY 10703

Stresscare Systems, Inc.
272–30 Grand Central Parkway
Floral Park, NY 11005

Stress Vector Analysis
Medicomp, Inc.
1805 Line Avenue
Shreveport, LA 71101

FACT OF LIFE

Fights Can Lead to the Bitter End

Arguments are the leading precipitators of homicide and accounted for nearly 4 out of 10 murders during one recent year for which statistics were gathered.

people experienced far more daily hassles than friendly, agreeable people—and, in general, they experienced more personal blows. In contrast, a friendly and agreeable attitude actually helps reduce conflict in life and invites support from others—sort of a "Nudge not, lest ye be nudged" state of mind toward everyday sources of stress.

The following tips will help you achieve the mental and physical state of well-being so important to living a stress-free, disease-free longer life. The first few tips that follow will help you handle stress in general. You will also learn strategies on how to handle everyday hassles, cope with conflicts, and relieve pressures you may be feeling at home, at work, or in your personal relationships.

Building a Stress-Resistant Attitude

625. Find a Friendly Shoulder

"The feeling of being loved and cared for by friends and family goes a long way in protecting you from the negative effects of stress," says Nelson Hendler, M.D., a psychiatrist at Johns Hopkins Hospital in Baltimore. Surround yourself with people who will be there when the going gets tough. And give them the feeling that you will do the same for them.

626. Slip into Someone Else's Shoes

Try to see a conflict from another person's point of view, advises Redford Williams, M.D., an expert on heart health and author of *The Trusting Heart: Great News about Type A Behavior*. "By trying to understand another's behavior from his viewpoint, you might gain the same sense of perspective. In most cases, you'll find your anger slipping away."

627. To Forgive Is Divine

Wrongs and retributions can be a tiresome burden to carry, says Dr. Williams. "By letting go of the resentment and relinquishing the goal of retribution, you may find that the weight of anger lifts from your shoulders, easing your pain, and also helping you to forget the wrong."

628. Learn to Weather Disappointment

Whether it's a minor letdown, like friends who cancel dinner plans, or a major defeat, like being denied an anticipated promotion, disappointments are always stressful. The big problem isn't the practical repercussions—two empty place settings at the table or loss of anticipated income—but the blow to the ego.

The secrets to weathering disappointment with your ego intact include the following:

- Don't blame yourself. Work by several researchers has shown that people who tend to blame themselves for misfortune are more susceptible to disease.
- Don't make a catastrophe out of something that doesn't have to be a catastrophe. Remind yourself that the sad event doesn't mean you'll never be happy again.
- Substitute other goals or activities. Instead of focusing on a letdown, concentrate on alternatives, or make new plans.

629. Don't Blame Yourself

Accepting responsibility for your actions is good; blaming yourself for every misfortune is not. Based on his pioneering work with hundreds of prisoners of war, hostages, Holocaust survivors, and other victims of severe stress, psychologist Julius Segal says that always assuming that your own behavior or character led to misfortune leads to hopelessness and depression.

630. Find the Right in Your Wrong

When faced with difficulty or defeat, redefine the situation. "How can you see a situation differently so that it becomes a learning experience rather than an exercise in blame or guilt?" says Joan Borysenko, Ph.D., in her book *Minding the Body, Mending the Mind.*

631. Speak in Positives, Not Negatives

While occasional swearing might help you vent anger, other words and phrases can be highly debilitating. Here are some examples.

- Take the word "problem" out of your vocabulary, and replace it with the word "challenge."
- Beware of thoughts that start with "I should," "I ought to," "I have to," "I feel obligated to," "I owe it to him," "I deserve." People often think they "must" do something, when in fact they don't.
- Instead of saying, "I can't stand your clutter all over the place," say, "I don't like it." Whenever you promote "I don't like it" to "I can't stand it," you're confusing your wants with your needs and generating an incredible amount of stress. Most of the events we think we can't stand are easily endured.

632. Just Say No

"No" is the most lifesaving word in the English language, says cardiologist Robert Elliot, M.D., especially for heart attack candidates, who tend to try to do more than is realistically possible.

633. Call Time-Out

Give yourself mini time-outs, says Joel Elkes, M.D., director of the behavioral medicine program at the University of Louisville. Don't let yourself become overwhelmed by tasks and obligations, but see them in perspective. Accept what you can do and don't waste time worrying about what you can't do.

634. Take a Second Look at Your Values

The high life isn't everything if your lifestyle is bringing you hassles instead of happiness. Take inventory of your work and living habits. Ask yourself if more family time wouldn't make you happier than a larger home that means more upkeep, more commuting time to work, and more bills. Maybe simplifying your life and cutting your obligations would make you happier.

FACT OF LIFE

Nice People Live Longer

Death rates from heart disease are four to seven times higher among people with hostile attitudes, according to studies by Redford Williams, M.D., an internist with the psychiatry department of Duke University Medical Center in Durham, North Carolina.

635. Grin, Giggle, Smile, Laugh

Evidence indicates laughter protects against the effects of negative stress by triggering the brain's release of endorphins, the body's natural painkillers.

Here are some ways to build more laughter into your life.

- Keep a "silly scrapbook." Collect funny cartoons, humorous anecdotes, remarks you overhear and other items that leave you chuckling. Then, when you need a humor fix, leaf through the book or pin a "laugh scrap" on your bulletin board.
- Make a "silliness check" at 4:30 in the afternoon. "At that point, if you haven't laughed yet, you should," says Steve Allen, Jr., M.D., son of comedian Steve Allen.
- Spend time with people who enjoy a good laugh. "Get together regularly with friends to share funny stories about daily disasters—with an eye towards constructive solutions," says Marjorie J. Ingram, director of the Creative Response to Stress Project at the Saratoga Institute.

636. Accept Life's Fizzles

Coming to terms with your frustration can greatly relieve the stressful feelings it generates.

"Accept frustration as part of the price for getting things done," says William Knaus, Ed.D., author of *How to Conquer Your Frustrations*. "There's no getting around it: You simply have to accept that things aren't going to be the way you want them to be all of the time. You can't always win."

The Power of Positive Thinking

637. Make a Peace Pact

When you're feeling hostile, cynical, irritable, or impatient, repeat a word that evokes enough emotion to suppress your stress—peace, love, trust, or patience, for example—suggests Dr. Williams.

638. Start Thought Stopping

A study published in the *Journal of Personality and Social Psychology* suggests that a major cause of depression is the inability to distract yourself from the negative thoughts everyone has from time to time.

For people who dwell on one all-consuming negative thought all day long, Dr. Williams recommends a technique known as thought stopping. As soon as you realize you're having these thoughts, yell "Stop!" as loudly as you can (in your mind). "Surprisingly, those thoughts will often stop," says Dr. Williams.

639. Memories Are Good Medicine

Relive happy memories. In times of stress, train yourself to look back and remember a pleasant experience or satisfying moment. "You might choose your wedding, or the birth of your child, or being recognized for an achievement by someone whose opinion mattered a great deal to you," says Anees A. Sheikh, Ph.D., professor and chairman of the department of psychology at Marquette University in Milwaukee, Wisconsin. "Any scenes of events when you felt secure, elated, or successful will do. And don't merely recall these events to mind—relive them."

640. Give In to Gravity

During the day, you spend a great deal of time fighting the force of gravity. Dr. Sheikh designed the followed imagery technique to help let gravity take over and reduce stress.

Let every muscle, every fiber, every cell in your body be pulled down and down, farther and farther. Feel your body and mind slowing down. There is no rush, nowhere you have to go, nothing you have to do. Tensions and frustrations gradually seep out of your system. You feel at ease and at peace, with yourself and with the universe.

641. Consult Your "Inner Adviser"

This ancient technique, also described by Dr. Sheikh, can connect you with an inner source of wisdom, to help counteract stress, anxiety, or depression that seems to come out of nowhere.

Close your eyes and visualize a wise and compassionate being who knows you completely. Perhaps this inner adviser is someone you respect and admire or feel deep affection for, or who understands you in a special way. Or perhaps the figure is a divine being or religious figure. In your mind's eye, move toward this inner adviser until you are face-to-face. Then talk with this guide about things that are bothering you. Ask questions about anything that's on your mind. Wait patiently for the answer.

642. White Out Worry

Caught up in a swirling cloud of worry? Try this imagery exercise, also offered by Dr. Sheikh:

Relax and imagine you're sitting in a great meadow on a perfect day. The sky is filled with rainbow lights, and one shaft of white light has found you. It's brighter than one hundred suns. You feel it warming the top of your head. Now it penetrates the top of your head and flows into your body, into your chest, your arms, your hands, right down to your fingertips, your abdomen, your legs, feet, and toes. The light cleanses you, dissolving all negative emotions and thoughts, which leave you in the form of dark smoke blown away by a gentle breeze. You're left feeling free and joyful.

643. Write to Yourself

"Journal writing provides a soothing, relaxing way to get in touch with feelings and sort out stressful conflicts in your life," according to Martin G. Groder, Ph.D., a psychiatrist in Chapel Hill, North Carolina. Left unexpressed, certain negative feelings can lead to illnesses—some of them life-threatening.

"In a hectic lifestyle, journal writing is like meditation or taking long walks, one of the few sources of solitude," says Dr. Groder. "It's safe, available, and you can do it on a rainy day."

Some journal writing hints:

- Pick a comfortable, private, safe place to write.
- Don't just list events. Express concerns, opinions, and reflections.
- Write about different kinds of feelings in different kinds of ink, like red ink for adventurous solutions, black ink for conservative, practical solutions, or purple ink for romantic fantasies (like escaping to a tropical island).
- Take measures to ensure that what you write will stay private.

Instant Stress Relievers

644. Go Chase a Butterfly

Take a stroll in the park. Along the way, collect leaves or watch the squirrels. Weather's bad? Watch the drama of building thunderheads. Stuck indoors? Buy yourself a bunch of flowers. Experts say nature breaks for the spirit can diffuse a lot of stress.

"When we're overloaded with everyday concerns, nature takes us away from our problems," says David C. Glass, Ph.D., a professor of psychology at State University of New York at Stony Brook. "The break allows us to restore our energy and could have tremendous benefits in alleviating negative feelings."

645. Let There Be Music

Whether you prefer serenades by Mantovani or Blue Öyster Cult, music can be a powerful stress reduction tool.

"The right music can take you from a highly tense state to a relaxed yet alert state in as little as 30 seconds," says Steven Halpern, Ph.D., a pioneering music composer, performer, and producer. Calming music has been used to reduce distress and pain among people in dentists' offices, childbirth centers, coronary care units, and migraine headache clinics.

Of course, the wrong tunes can *give* you a migraine. Your best bet is sedative music—music with a slow, easy rhythm of approximately 60 beats per minute—as regular as your heartbeat at rest. Also, instrumental pieces—notably performed by flute, harp, piano, and string ensembles—tend to be more soothing than vocal numbers.

Life-Extension Tool

Relaxation Tapes

The sounds of nature or musical harmonies can dissolve tension in minutes, helping you to stay calm in the wake of trying circumstances or control tension before it builds to an unhealthy level. Since uncontrolled stress is a risk factor for cardiovascular disease and other life-threatening medical conditions, listening to relaxation-inducing tapes can be an enjoyable way to keep a lid on anxiety and its life-shortening effects.

Here are some relaxation audiotapes to choose from. Ask for them wherever audiocassettes are sold, or contact the supplier, if listed.

- *Music and Nature.* Three-cassette set includes: Peaceful Evening, Misty Forest Morning, and Radiant Sea. From Vital Body Marketing, Manhasset, New York.
- *Interludes.* Four-cassette series includes: Fireplace, Tropical Beach, Babbling Brook, Thunderstorm. From Great American Studio, New Rochelle, New York.
- *Sounds of Nature.* Series includes: Ocean Waves, Forest Sounds, Gentle Rain, Creek in the Forest, Reflections of Reflections. Order from Valley of the Sun Publishing, Malibu, California 90265. In California, phone 1–800–225–4717. Outside California: 1–800–421–6603. Or order from the Center for Marine Conservation, Catalog Order Department, P.O. Box 810, Old Saybrook, Connecticut 06475–0810. Phone 1–800–227–1929.
- *Songs and Sounds of the Humpback Whale.* From the Center for Marine Conservation, P.O. Box 810, Old Saybrook, Connecticut 06475–0810. Phone 1–800–227–1929.
- *Rainy Day Meditation.* From Valley of the Sun Publishing, Malibu, California 90265. In California, phone 1–800–225–4717. Outside California: 1–800–421–6603.

(continued)

Life-Extension Tool—*Continued*

- *Island Sunrise.* Valley of the Sun Publishing, Malibu, California 90265. In California, phone 1–800–225–4717. Outside California: 1–800–421–6603.
- *Deep Relaxation.* By Sirah Bettesse, Ph.D. From TDM/McGraw Hill.
- *The Rush-Hour Refresher.* From Enhanced Audio Systems, Emeryville, California.

If a visual sojourn appeals to you, you might consider an underwater odyssey, courtesy of the following videocassettes: *The Worlds Below,* with narration and music, or *Ocean Symphony,* music only. Both cassettes in VHS format only, from the Center for Marine Conservation, on page 279.

---

646. Take a Deep Breath

If you find yourself waiting for an important phone call or sweating out other delays, take a few deep breaths. Expand the abdomen first, then the chest. When you exhale, collapse the chest first, then the abdomen. Learn to accept that waiting is no big deal. Realize that trying to be in control is not helpful here, says psychologist Dr. Greenspan.

647. The Feel-Better Phenomenon

A massage or hot bath may do wonders to relax you. But don't overlook the benefits of a brisk walk or some other type of physical activity that you enjoy. Exercise burns off excess adrenaline, the by-product of your body's response to stress.

"Exercise may also induce a kind of 'relaxation response' by flooding your body with endorphins, natural opiatelike painkillers released by the brain and other organs," says Daniel M. Landers, Ph.D., of the Exercise and Sports Research Institute, at Arizona State University in Tempe.

Other research suggests that exercise directly reduces anxiety and tensions. And people who take part in vigorous physical activity consistently report a dramatic increase in psychological well-being. In short, fit people handle stress better.

Generally, the best kinds of exercise for counteracting stress are continuous, rhythmic aerobic activities such as running, walking, cycling, swimming, and cross-country skiing. Stop-and-go activities such as tennis, racquetball, and basketball are less potent stress aids but are still worthwhile if you enjoy then.

Bettering Your Relationships

648. Angry? Think Things Through

When you disagree with someone, do you attack them, snub them, or talk things out calmly? If you take the third tactic, you're doing your blood pressure a favor. From 1971 to 1972, researchers at the University of Michigan examined the relationship among stressful marital situations, blood pressure, mortality rates, and the way people cope with anger. In a follow-up study done 12 years later, they found that people with high blood pressure who suppressed their anger when they were unjustifiably attacked by their spouse were more than twice as likely to have died during the ensuing 12 years as those who said they would express their anger or protest.

"The key issue is not the amount or degree of your anger, but how you cope with it," says Ernest Harburg, M.D., researcher for the study. He explains that both suppressing your angry feelings or venting your anger can lead to greater stress. Reflective coping—that is, waiting until tempers have cooled to rationally discuss the situation—is the best choice, because it restores a sense of control over the situation and helps solve the problem.

649. Walk Away from Tension

If you and your mate are having problems with your relationship, walking together may be a way to alleviate stress. "The tension can be dispersed through the exercise, rather than channeled into an outburst of emotion," says Cynthia Strowbridge, a psychotherapist in New York City.

Walking together can often ease communication. Away from sedentary settings, silent pauses occur more naturally. We tend to think of communicating strictly in terms of talking, but walking in silence with someone close to you brings a strong feeling of connection. "We forget how intimate it is to be wholeheartedly with another person in silence. Being in step together, out-of-doors, can be amazingly healing to body and spirit," says Strowbridge.

Away from the distractions of television, telephones, and household demands, you have the time and opportunity to enhance your sense of commitment to each other.

650. Friction? Talk on Neutral Territory

When problems get in the way, get away—to dinner, a weekend in the mountains—anywhere away from home. But don't think you can immediately discuss your problems. Unwind a bit first.

When you do finally talk, first talk about what's right in the relationship, then discuss what would be helpful to change. Defensive people are rarely, if ever, willing to talk. And if you try to make the other person guilty, forget it. You'll never solve any problems; in fact, you'll only create new ones.

651. Double Life? Double Trouble

Two doctors in New Rochelle, New York, observed firsthand what too much love can do to a man's heart and health. "Two cases we have seen in our coronary-care unit exhibited a striking similarity that we feel singles out a particular source of stress as a contributing factor to myocardial infarction," the doctors report.

The source of this stress? Being involved with two women at once. "We were struck by the youth of the patients, the severity of their disease, and the singular nature of their emotional predicament," the doctors commented.

"We propose that multiple spouses or fiancés may present such severe psychological stress as to accelerate the course of coronary artery disease, thereby qualifying as a new risk factor not previously identified in the literature," they conclude.

The moral of the story? Stick to one romantic commitment at a time.

652. Kids' Feelings Count, Too

Children may bring joy to a home, but raising them also creates a significant amount of stress. For starters, to avoid contributing to their stress and ultimately yours, don't lump them together as "the kids." Also:

- Respect a child's privacy. As long as they keep their own rooms clean, you won't have to clean up after them and inadvertently misplace important belongings.
- Let children participate in household decisions. Being authoritarian and dogmatic doesn't work, says one psychologist and father of four. Teamwork is the key. Hang up a family calendar. Hold meetings to juggle schedules. Block out time in advance for family activities.
- Establish clear rules. To prevent misunderstanding, write them down and post the list for all to see. (And be prepared to explain your reasons for each rule.)

653. Make a Play Date with Your Kids

If work is coming between you and your children, set aside time or make an appointment to spend some time together. If you can't make it right away, set a date and keep it, says Kenneth Greenspan, M.D., of the Center for Stress and Pain Related Disorders at Columbia-Presbyterian Medical Center in New York City. "Say that on Saturday afternoon, you will take one of your children to lunch or shopping. That goes a long way even though that child doesn't see much of you during the week. It's important for the child to know beforehand and not just have these events come up sporadically."

654. Don't Bring Office Problems Home

"I'm convinced that the pattern of unloading daily stresses on friends and family bears an enormous risk," says Barbara Mackoff, Ph.D., author of *Leaving the Office Behind*. It's possible to use up their patience and concern. And the consequences may be anger, problems with your marriage, your children, or your love life—all from taking out your stress on your family. Leaving your cares at the office, on the other hand, may help you return to work refreshed and able to work better.

Home Sweet Home

655. Garden for Inner Tranquillity

Imagine for a moment the fresh, earthy aroma of sun-warmed soil, seedlings standing on parade as they're bathed in the soft mist of an early morning spray . . .

A garden can yield more than fresh fruits and vegetables. Roger Ulrich, Ph.D., associate professor of geography at the University of Delaware, and an expert in the field of plant/people relationships, has conducted studies which show fairly substantial physiological and emotional changes occurring when people are exposed to plants. Their blood pressure falls, their muscles loosen, and their heart rate slows.

Researchers in the Netherlands have found that people who lovingly tend their plants have significantly fewer heart attacks than those who don't. Gardening lowers blood pressure and increases the body's resistance to stress, the researchers conclude.

656. Settle for "Good Enough"

Don't expect to have the cleanest house, the whitest clothes, the most well-behaved children. Trying to be perfect can lead to stress.

The answer: Decide what you can be flexible about and where you won't compromise.

657. Plan the Great Escape

Create an atmosphere in at least one place in your home where you'll find it especially easy to relax: new furnishings for the bedroom, a shower massage in the bath, soft lighting in the den—a setting where you can let your imagination take you away from it all.

658. Organization Is Essential

Ever laugh at closet organizers, space savers, and filing cabinets for the home? Think again. Were you laughing the last time it took you an hour to find your car keys?

Designate a special place for all those items you lose often and get in the habit of putting things where they belong. (And that goes for the office, too.)

659. Conquer Clutter

The best anyone can say about housework is that it feels good when you're done. And if you think about it, the most stressful part of housekeeping isn't finding fingerprints on the toaster or dustballs under the couch—it's dealing with encroaching clutter: mountains of cups and glasses in the kitchen sink, newspapers and magazines strewn over the coffee table, and kids' toys everywhere you step. Conquer clutter and you go a long way to reducing the "visual stress" it creates. Here's how, according to Don Aslett, author of several books on housekeeping.

- Insist that each family member—children and adults—pick up his or her own mess.
- Create a control center in each room for communal clutter—like mail. In the bathroom, stow hairbrushes, combs, hairdryers, and other grooming paraphernalia out of sight in a drawer or bin, or out of the way on shelves or hooks, so it's not strewn all over the vanity.
- Keep your decor simple. Lots of vases, knickknacks and ornaments have to be straightened, dusted around, worried about, or picked up after they topple.
- Declare an Assault-on-Junk Day. Mobilize your spouse and kids to help you clean out the backlog of clutter in the attic, garage, basement, or other clutter-prone area of the house.

660. Delegate Housework

Meals, shopping, laundry, and lawn care take time, even if you have a microwave oven, a power mower, and other helpful appliances. Don't tackle housework alone. If all adults in the household are working outside the home, hire all the help you can afford. (A trustworthy and reliable neighborhood teenager is a good substitute for professional—and more expensive—help.)

661. Family Ties Need Time to Bind

"Don't work 20 hours a day and still expect to spend quality time with your family," says Nelson Hendler, M.D. "Cut back. And if your hours still don't permit enough time, flextime (going to work earlier and leaving earlier) might be a lifesaving and sanity-saving option."

What's Your Stress Quotient?

Scientists say that the amount of stress in our lives is not as important as how we react to that stress. To find out where you stand in your own vulnerability to stress, give some honest thought to the following questions and circle the number in the appropriate column.

	Usually	Sometimes	Rarely
1. You are easily annoyed or frustrated.	3	2	1
2. You hate to lose.	3	2	1
3. You get angry but don't show your feelings if someone crosses or criticizes you.	3	2	1
4. You get very impatient if made to wait in a line.	3	2	1
5. You have a way of taking on more responsibility than you feel comfortable with.	3	2	1
6. You have trouble asking for help when you think you need it.	3	2	1
7. You resort to alcohol, tranquilizers, or other drugs to help you cope.	3	2	1
8. You discuss problems with other people you feel you can trust.	1	2	3
9. You have trouble apologizing when you make a mistake.	3	2	1
10. You blame yourself and worry when you make a mistake.	3	2	1
11. You let people know if they've hurt your feelings.	1	2	3
12. You feel you give more to family and friends than you receive.	3	2	1
13. You take time to relax or enjoy recreational activities and entertainment.	1	2	3
14. You find time for daily or almost daily exercise.	1	2	3
15. You smile and laugh a lot.	1	2	3

(continued)

What's Your Stress Quotient—*Continued*

Scoring

Now add up your answers and see where you stand.

15–25: Low risk. Congratulations on being a cucumber. The cool way in which you handle life's daily hassles should help you live happily and long.

26–35: Moderate risk. You're a cucumber with splashes of Tabasco sauce. Your personality and methods of handling stress put you in moderate danger of developing a stress-related illness.

36–45: High risk. You're a Mexican red pepper. Your coping strategies put you at high risk of a stress-related illness, and you should make efforts to chill out. Try being easier on yourself and less critical of others. Get better at sharing problems rather than keeping them bottled up. Try, too, to release tension through enjoyable exercise, recreational activities, and relaxation.

SOURCE: Adapted from a more extensive questionnaire appearing in *Health Risks* (The Body Press, 1986, A Price Stern Sloan, Inc. Company, Los Angeles, California) by internist and cardiologist Elliot J. Howard, M.D., of the Lenox Hill Hospital in New York. .

662. Get a Handle on Home Finances

Make a budget and plan to stick to it. A big source of family stress is not how much money you have, but how you're going to spend it. A well-thought-out, written budget can relieve the stress of wondering why you always seem broke no matter how hard you work. Also:

- Decide on a goal, then work toward it. Do you want to buy a house? A new car? Start a retirement plan? Write down what you want to do, when, and how you will arrange to finance it.
- Keep an emergency fund for surprise expenses like new tires, a broken water heater—or even an economic recession.
- Consider automatic payroll deduction. To force yourself to save, authorize your bank to automatically deposit your check and transfer a specified amount to your savings account.

663. Do As the Islanders Do

Researchers who studied family life on the tranquil island of St. Lucia in the Caribbean uncovered a secret: Giving children responsibility in the operation of the household—tending gardens, running errands, looking after younger brothers and sisters—encouraged an active, self-reliant coping style that endured for life.

Work Happy

664. Get Some Satisfaction

Monotonous work has been associated with coronary heart disease. The stress of conflicting job demands has been linked to increased heart rate and blood pressure. Some ways to deal with job dissatisfaction include:

- Ask for more guidance, more freedom, more money—whatever it is you need. To help ensure success, present your case calmly and rationally.
- Recognize what's not your fault. If you're a waiter where the kitchen is slow and a diner's impatiently waiting for his food order, explain the situation. Same goes for an auto service salesperson dealing with a client who brings his or her car in for repairs which take longer than expected.
- Consult a career counselor if you feel trapped in an intolerable situation.

665. Overwhelmed? Find Out Why

Sometimes people think they hate their jobs, when, in reality, they just lack the skills to do the job properly. If that's the case, go to your boss or personnel administrator and ask for training in how to manage, delegate, or do the job properly.

666. Lists Work Wonders

Whether you work at home or in an office, write "Things to Do" lists daily. On each, rank four to six items in order of importance. Do them in that order, but don't worry if you don't finish everything.

If you're really into making lists, think about all the things you do that waste time and write them down. Concentrate on avoiding all items on this list. You'll find yourself with extra time, and that "To Do" list will get done before the alarm sounds.

667. Deadlines? No Problem!

Reducing the stress of deadlines is a matter of setting up priorities, scheduling your time accordingly, and then making an effort to stick to both priorities and schedule. Time management experts recommend this step-by-step strategy.

- Decide which deadlines are rigid and which ones are flexible. Getting a new job by the first of the year is flexible, for example. Registering your car by the due date is not.
- Figure out how long a task will take and how much time you can spend on it. Be realistic.
- Think of the project in very specific steps. Then assess the time required for each.
- Take steps to ensure that you'll be able to do what you have to do. Set aside time to work uninterrupted and gather all the information or materials you'll need.
- Finally, *do* the job. Waiting until the last minute and then having to work in a panic is stressful.

668. Take Time to Unwind

De-stress before you go home at night. Spend time alone, exercise, or identify and connect your feelings with the people and events in your day rather than pouncing on the first person you see when you walk through your front door.

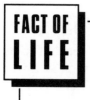

FACT OF LIFE

Money Breeds Misery

In one survey, people earning more than $30,000 per year cited financial and work-related problems as the most frequent causes of stress in their lives.

More Practical Tips

669. Don't Try to Read People's Minds

Don't assume you know what another person is thinking and feeling. Your reactions are likely to be off base since they are based on assumptions, not facts.

670. Keep a Stress Log

Take notice of the activities you're involved in throughout the day to discover what might be behind your stressed-out outlook.

Do you drink too much coffee every morning? People insist they can't get started without it, but one study shows that men who drank nine or more cups of coffee each day were more than twice as likely to have irregular heartbeats.

Is your workday full of stress with no chance to relax? Emotional stress boosts adrenaline while it increases your likelihood of arrhythmias. Slow down and relax as often as possible. Researchers at the Harvard School of Public Health say that "psychological stress profoundly lowers the cardiac threshold for ventricular fibrillation"—the dangerous kind of arrhythmia that makes your heart beat randomly and recklessly, resulting in sudden death.

Have you just had a shouting match with a co-worker? Acute anger seems to wreck your heart's rhythm the most, since the emotion releases chemicals in your body that restrict arteries leading to your heart.

671. Easy Does It

Eating, playing, and working in moderation rather than in excess are often overlooked ways to avoid undue stress.

672. Fret Not

In other words, "Don't sweat the small stuff and remember it's *all* small stuff," says Robert Elliot, M.D., a University of Nebraska cardiologist.

EXERCISE—
FEEL GOOD
FOR A
LIFETIME

Imagine yourself sprinting along a forest trail, soaking in the scent of pine with every breath without ever getting winded. Imagine yourself cycling on a winding rural road, past cows and farmhouses, feeling invigorated and rejuvenated as you zoom to the crest of each rise. Imagine yourself swimming through a pool so effortlessly that the sun sparkling off your wake seems to generate the power of each thrashing stroke. Best of all, imagine doing it all and feeling this great until you're 60, 70, or even beyond.

An impossible dream? Not at all.

Regular exercise is the single most important thing you can do for yourself if you want to live a long and healthy life. Not only that, research has shown it can actually help you *extend* your life. Level of fitness, they found, is directly related to the rate of mortality. And you don't have to be a marathon man or woman to extend your lifespan, either. Moderate levels of physical fitness, the type "attainable by most adults," appear to be protective against early death, claim the researchers.

Exercise will not only help you live longer, it will help you feel *younger,* too. "Regular exercise can give you the equivalent of ten

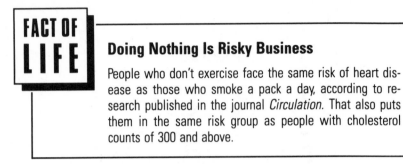

FACT OF LIFE

Doing Nothing Is Risky Business

People who don't exercise face the same risk of heart disease as those who smoke a pack a day, according to research published in the journal *Circulation*. That also puts them in the same risk group as people with cholesterol counts of 300 and above.

years' rejuvenation," says exercise researcher Roy Shephard, Ph.D., of the University of Toronto. One of the ways it helps us retain our vitality is by helping us avoid the debilitating effects of many age-related diseases. In fact, many of the problems we experience as we age are caused not by disease at all but by deconditioning.

Exercise, in a nutshell, keeps us in shape and extends our youth.

Recline and Decline

Without exercise, however, life becomes a different chain of events. Research has come up with a whole list of negative repercussions as a result of living a life of sloth.

You shorten your life. A study of 10,224 men and 3,120 women conducted at the Institute for Aerobic Research in Dallas over an eight-year span found that death rates from all causes were highest among the unfit and lowest among the most fit. Death rate, they found, declined according to the increased level of a person's fitness. What's the common demominator? "Higher levels of physical fitness appear to delay all-cause mortality," they say, "primarily due to lowered rates of cardiovascular disease and cancer."

In another study, Ralph S. Paffenbarger, Jr., M.D., headed a research team that studied the relationship between lifestyle and longevity among 16,936 Harvard alumni. He found that the more active you are, the longer you are likely to live.

In his study, men who burned 2,000 or more calories per week in activities like walking, stair climbing, and playing sports lived longer than men who burned less than 2,000 calories a week with physical activity. And the men who burned at least 3,500 calories a week by staying active lived the longest.

You risk heart disease. The Harvard study also found that men who were physically active were 31 percent less likely to die of a heart attack, stroke, or other cardiovascular disease than fellow alumni who were sedentary. And, said the study, men who engaged in little or no exercise tended to have higher blood pressure—a key risk factor for heart disease—than those who were active.

In another study at Ball State University, researchers collected data on a group of men over four years to find out if a correlation exists between the incidence of coronary heart disease and an individual's fitness level. They found that those with a low aerobic capacity have a higher risk of developing premature coronary artery disease than those who are more fit.

You gain weight. The Harvard study also showed that men who never or rarely exercised weighed more than more active graduates. The reason: Basal metabolic rate (the rate at which calories are burned to fuel the body's basic biological functions) slows down with age—about 2 to 3 percent every ten years after age 20.

As the decades roll by, we tend to eat more and exercise less, explains Elizabeth Applegate, Ph.D., nutrition director of the adult fitness and cardiac rehabilitation program at the University of California, Davis. As a result, we gain fat and lose muscle, the body's most metabolically active tissue. The result? Metabolism slows more in overweight nonexercisers.

You replace muscle with fat. As you grow older, your body's proportions of fat and muscle change: Muscle tissues gives way to fat. After age 30, the average individual loses muscle fibers at a rate of 3 to 5 percent every ten years. By age 60 you may lose up to 30 percent of your muscle power.

You run out of steam. In general, as we get older our bodies become less efficient at performing physical activities. We tire more quickly. In the laboratory, scientists measure this change by the decrease in vital lung capacity, better known as VO_2 max. Among sedentary folks, this decline occurs at a rate of about 1 percent every year after age 25. Loss of muscle and decreases in the efficiencies of the heart and lungs all contribute to this overall loss of stamina.

You lose flexibility. As we grow older, we stiffen. This loss of flexibility makes movement more difficult and ages our appearance. The reason? Disuse causes connective tissue—ligaments, joint capsules, and tendons—to lose their flexibility. A fact, say researchers, due more to a sedentary lifestyle than the aging process.

A Long Life for the Active

Aging, however, is a different process for those who are active. Regular exercise bestows a special kind of vitality—to the body *and* mind—that transcends aging. Study after study has proven it: Active people feel better, look younger, and live longer. Put exercise in your life, and you'll enjoy countless benefits, including the following:

You protect your heart. Being unfit in itself is enough to cause a heart attack or stroke, according to research published in the *New England Journal of Medicine*. But exercise helps lower cholesterol, triglycerides, and blood pressure, all leading causes of heart disease.

Not exercising is like tacking many years of wear and tear on your heart, according to Lars G. Ekelund, M.D., Ph.D., an associate professor of medicine at the University of North Carolina at Chapel Hill.

But a simple program of aerobic-type exercise—such as walking for about 30 minutes three times a week—can reclaim those "lost" years. Regular exercise may raise HDL (high-density lipoprotein), the "good" kind of cholesterol, and lower LDL (low-density lipoproteins), the "bad" cholesterol.

You slow the aging process. Regular aerobic exercise throughout life will not only protect you from heart disease but also hold off aging. That's the conclusion of a ten-year study conducted by Michael L. Pollack, Ph.D., at the University of Florida's Center of Exercise Science.

Dr. Pollack studied 25 runners and competitive walkers who

FACT OF LIFE

Exercise Improves the Mind

Early research indicates that exercise may not only prevent the brain from fading as we get older, but may actually sharpen the mind. One study compared men and women who exercised vigorously for at least 75 minutes a week with those who exercised less than 10 minutes a week. When tested, the high exercise group had better memories, quicker reactions, and more accurate reasoning—even after age and education were taken into account.

Are You Getting Enough Exercise?

You're not exercising enough if:

- You buy a new pair of tennis shoes every two years because the old ones are dirty, not worn out.
- You have so much power equipment that you don't work up even a mild sweat when doing yard work.
- You take the elevator to go up one floor.
- You ride around a parking lot looking for a parking space close to the store entrance.

You're probably getting enough if:

- You can climb to the third floor without stopping to catch your breath.
- Your most heavily used shoes have neither wing tips nor high heels.
- Your muscles aren't sore the day after washing both cars.
- Bowling or playing golf once a week isn't your sole means of exercise.

You're getting too much exercise if:

- You feel you could use a nap after working out.
- You feel tired the rest of the day.
- Your muscles ache most of the time.
- You need orthopedic devices, ice bags, and massage to keep up your exercise routine.
- Your spouse comments that it's nice to have you around the house for a change.

averaged 62 years of age at the study's end. "Treadmill tests showed that their aerobic capacity, a reliable measure of aging, was better than that usually found in lean, unathletic 25-year-olds," according to Dr. Pollack.

"Earlier studies have shown that people of all ages, if they begin a proper exercise program, can improve their aerobic capacity by 15 to 20 percent," says Dr. Pollack. "Our research proves that you can start a regular exercise program as late as your forties and your loss of aerobic capacity will be less than 5 percent per decade—instead of the usual 10 percent—as long as you maintain your level of training."

You stay firm and trim. It's a proven fact: Aerobic (oxygen-

FACT OF LIFE

Women Flex, Men Fish

When it comes to leisure-time activities, men most enjoy fishing, while women prefer to get out there and swim, according to a poll of 2,019 adults conducted by the Gallup organization. Next to fishing, men liked swimming, with playing pool and weight-lifting tied for third. As for women, bicycling came in second, with aerobic dance taking third.

burning) exercise can help you burn fat, build muscle, and stoke your calorie-burning furnace all at the same time. And exercise revs up your metabolism so you burn more calories. That translates into a body that's firm and trim.

One study which compared men in their fifties with men in their twenties found that the more a man exercised, the lower his percentage of body fat—regardless of age.

You help guard against cancer. In 1985, the American Cancer Society began recommending exercise to protect against cancer. Although the supporting evidence is mixed, studies suggest that exercise reduces the risk of cancer, according to Edward R. Eichner, M.D., professor of medicine at the University of Oklahoma. Dr. Eichner says that exercise may prevent cancer in three different ways— by reducing obesity, by augmenting the body's immune defenses, and by prompting people who start to work out to make other healthful changes in their behavior, like quitting smoking or eating more nutritious food.

You build stronger bones. You'd think that with all the abuse your body takes during exercise you'd put wear and tear on your bones. But that's just not the case.

"There's no doubt that exercise is beneficial to the bones," says Barbara L. Drinkwater, Ph.D., of the Pacific Medical Center in Seattle, Washington. "The more bone you can store in the bank, the better. Even more important is slowing down bone loss. Active people maintain bone better. We lose it less rapidly."

Peter Jacobson, M.D., an orthopedic surgeon at the University of North Carolina Chapel Hill School of Medicine, agrees. Any exercise that involves some pounding—running, playing tennis— seems to slow the rate of bone loss, he says.

You handle stress better. Unrelenting stress contributes to a number of disorders, many of them life-threatening. But exercise may be an effective antidote. Exercising for 40 minutes can result in reduced stress levels for up to three hours, says John Ragland, Ph.D., of the sports psychology laboratory at the University of Wisconsin. In comparison, an equal period of rest and relaxation reduces stress for only 20 minutes.

Studies also indicate that exercise can lift your spirits by stimulating the release of natural mood-elevating chemicals called endorphins.

You build endurance and agility. People who remain physically active throughout their later years can gain as much as a 25-year advantage in performance over people who retire to their easy chairs, reports Vincent Mor, Ph.D., of Brown University. A study of 4,500 people between the ages of 40 and 85 found that physically active 70-year-olds could perform physical tests as well as 50-year-old couch potatoes. Better yet, only moderate activities such as walking and gardening appear necessary to keep the aging body more agile.

Get into Gear

Of course, the best way to reap all these wonderful life-preserving benefits is to "get aerobic." Aerobic exercise is the kind that gets your heart pumping fast. The kind that makes you feel good about yourself when it's all over. The kind of exercise that gives you the extra energy to soar through any day—at any age.

The American College of Sports Medicine recommends that, to benefit the heart, you need to exercise 30 minutes a day for a minimum of three times a week. And it's never to late to start (though if you're over 40 and starting an exercise program for the first time, you should get your doctor's okay).

But aerobics is only part of the exercise prescription. Doctors who specialize in longevity can't stress enough the importance of *keeping active.*

The following tips can be helpful to anyone in pursuit of a longer life through exercise, whether you're taking your first step into a walking shoe or aiming to break a 4-minute mile.

Rx for Exercise

673. If You Like It, Try It

Many people wonder if there's one perfect exercise, one that delivers aerobic benefits, flexibility, and strength all in one. Top picks include swimming, jogging, aerobic dance, cross-country skiing, and stationary bicycling—but only if they appeal to you.

"A perfect exercise is one that you stay with," says D. W. Edington, Ph.D., director of the University of Michigan Fitness Research Center. "You have to ask yourself what you like to do. After all, in order to get the full aerobic benefit from exercise, you've got to do it for at least 30 minutes three times a week. If you can't stand swimming or skiing, no matter how 'perfect' it may be [from a physiological standpoint], it'll do you about as much aerobic good as tic-tac-toe."

"If you try one exercise and you don't like it, don't give up on all exercise," says Gail Johnston, the director of the Aerobics and Fitness Association of America's specialty certification program, Fitness for the Overweight. "Shop around."

674. Take Personal Limitations into Account

You'll be more likely to stick with a workout that accommodates (not ignores) your body's individual foibles. If you're overweight, try swimming or pool exercise classes; fat floats, lifting weight off stressed joints. If stiff muscles or arthritis slows you down, take up yoga or join a stretching class. If you have stamina to spare but feel flabby, try a light weight-lifting program.

675. Any Time, Just the Same Time

People often ask experts, "What is the best time to exercise— morning, noon, or night?" The best time is any time that it's convenient for you.

If a morning workout gets your pulse hopping and your energy popping, fine. But if the very thought of an A.M. workout makes you groan and hide under the covers, schedule it later. But don't put off exercise until you've finished everything else you have to do. If exercise is last on your list, you may never find the time.

An added hint for success: Exercise at the same time every day. "If you get used to exercising at a particular time, it becomes part of your life," says Howard Flaks, M.D., public relations chairman for the American Society of Bariatric Physicians.

676. Swim to Your Heart's Content

If you're looking for a form of exercise that's easy on the joints but will also give you an aerobic workout, try swimming.

As for which stroke is the best to use, it's always a good idea to alternate between a variety of them. Moving in order from most to least strenuous, you'll find the crawl, backstroke, breaststroke, and finally, the least strenuous of them all, the sidestroke. The doggy paddle doesn't count.

677. Approach Aerobic Dance a Step at a Time

Aerobic dancing can be a great form of exercise—if you approach it sensibly. If aerobics is new to you, and you start out too quickly, you could injure yourself. So begin gradually. Start by doing it easily—"low-impact" classes are best for beginners—and then work up the difficulty level if a more running-oriented dance approach appeals to you.

Where you dance is as important as how you dance. According to Edward Percy, M.D., an orthopedic surgeon who specializes in sports medicine, look for a dance floor that's cushioned, but not too soft. "The surface should be cushioned enough so that there is some give, but it shouldn't be so soft that the foot sinks into it."

When looking for an aerobic dance shoe, Dr. Percy advises choosing one that is soft and flexible with a softly cushioned sole, a slightly built-up heel, and a flexible toe area that will bend when you do.

678. Row, Row, Row Your Imaginary Boat

For a great whole-body workout, climb aboard a rowing machine. Researchers at the Work Physiology Laboratory at Ohio University tested 60 men and 47 women on rowing and cycling machines on four separate occasions, and the rowing machine consistently proved to be more taxing.

For all workloads tested, heart rates, oxygen consumption, and calorie burning were greater on the rower. Rowing involves not just the muscles of the legs (quadriceps), but muscles of the chest, back, trunk, and arms as well.

And of course, if you get an opportunity to row a *real* boat, you'll be up to the task.

679. Frequency Wins over Endurance

Small, frequent exercise sessions are better than occasional, prolonged sessions. According to physiologists at the University of Nebraska, three 30-minute exercise routines burn twice as much fat as two 45-minute sets. Why? Every exercise session speeds up your body's metabolism and decreases hunger. The three-time-a-weekers gained the advantage of increased metabolism and decreased hunger for an extra day.

680. Double Your Pleasure

You can avoid boredom, develop a wider range of fitness, and avoid overuse injuries by cross-training—participating in more than one fitness activity. Many joggers, for example, also bicycle. Many people who take aerobic dance also run, walk, and weight-train.

681. Be Prepared for Rainy Days

A well-designed exercise regimen should contain a contingency plan for bad weather. Buy a new or used stationary bicycle. Thirty minutes at 15 mph will give you a good workout. Or invest in a rowing machine, or even a treadmill.

At the very least, invest in a good rain suit, so that you can hit the road at any time.

682. Chart Your Progress

Small, interim goals are easier to achieve than one single ultimate goal. Set up some small markers of success and keep a written record of your improvement.

For example, you may set goals that lead up to 3 miles of walking by the end of the first month. Your next goal could be to decrease

FACT OF LIFE

A.M. **Ambition**

A Phoenix doctor who prescribes exercise for his patients says that 75 percent of his patients who exercise in the morning stick with it. Afternoon exercisers have about a 50 percent compliance rate, and only about 25 percent of those who say they'll work out in the evening actually get around to it.

the amount of time it takes to make those 3 miles. Then you may aim again for distance.

You can also keep a log of your vital statistics—weight, resting pulse, and blood pressure, for instance. If one of your goals is weight loss, you may want to take before and after photos for your diary.

Charting your progress is crucial because the feedback is encouraging, and you can proudly show your results to others.

683. Be Patient

Don't expect too much too fast. In exercise studies, researchers typically follow participants six to eight weeks before significant drops in heart rate, blood pressure, and weight are noted. So don't quit before you've given your program a chance to take effect. After all, you didn't get *out* of shape overnight. One consolation: The more unfit you are, the sooner you'll see results.

684. Psych Yourself Up

If you know you should get out and exercise but have trouble establishing momentum, try this: About an hour before you lace up your walking or running shoes, start thinking about the course. Imagine how good it will feel to get outside in the fresh air and how invigorated you'll feel afterward. Reflect on the physical and emotional benefits that come with a good workout.

Granted, you're not about to play the Super Bowl or World Series, but the stakes, in terms of your health and well-being, can be just as high.

Stay on Target with Your Heart Rate

One of the life-lengthening benefits of exercise is a stronger heart. And to strengthen your heart, you have to work it hard enough to increase its muscle mass and aerobic capacity. The way to do that is to push your heart to beat to its "training heart rate"—at least 60 percent of its maximum capacity.

To calculate your training heart rate, subtract your age in years from 220. Now calculate 60 percent of this figure. This is your minimum training heart rate.

If you are age 40, for example, you would subtract 40 from 220, giving you a base of 180. A training rate would be 60 percent of that number, or 180 times 0.60, which equals 108 beats per minute. If you want to train more vigorously, increase the 60 percent to 70 percent. You should never exceed 80 percent.

The simplest way to measure your heart rate is to count your pulse for 10 seconds, then multiply by 6. The easiest way to do this is to place a finger—not your thumb (which has its own pulse)—on the pulse at your wrist. The accompanying chart shows the 10-second pulse rate at 60, 70, and 80 percent capacity for various age groups. Are you within your target heart rate zone?

Age	Heart Rate (bpm) 60%	70%	80%	Age	Heart Rate (bpm) 60%	70%	80%
20–21	20	23	27	54–55	17	19	22
22–25	19	23	26	56–59	16	19	22
26–27	19	23	26	60–62	16	19	21
28–29	19	23	26	63–65	16	18	21
30–35	19	22	25	66	15	18	21
36	18	22	25	67–70	15	18	20
37–44	18	21	24	71–74	15	17	20
45	18	21	23	75	15	17	19
46–51	17	20	23	76–78	14	17	19
52–53	17	20	22				

685. Half a Workout Is Better Than None

If you must, cut workouts short occasionally, but don't scrap them entirely, says Art Mollen, D.O., director of the Southwest Health Institute in Phoenix, Arizona. Even if you aren't gung-ho 100 percent of the time, keep in the swing of your workout schedule by doing *something*. The idea is to maintain momentum; it'll keep you from getting completely derailed.

686. Become an Exercise Scout: Be Prepared

If your sweatsuit and shoes are ready and waiting for you when you wake up, you'll be less likely to skip your morning workout. If you routinely work out on your lunch hour or after work, pack all your gear the night before. Or keep a week's worth of clean socks and togs in your car at a time.

687. Or Sleep in Your Sweatsuit

If the temptation of the warmth under the covers tends to win you over on cool, dark mornings, try this unusual but effective alternative: Sleep in your sweatsuit. That way, leaving a warm bed to go out into the cold air won't be so much of an adjustment.

688. Plan to Succeed

Surveys show that most people drop out of regular exercise programs within the first six months. Don't be one of them.

There are certain factors essential to sticking with an exercise program, according to James E. Rippe, M.D., director of exercise physiology and nutrition at University of Massachusetts Medical School. For an exercise program to maintain the stick-to-itiveness that it requires, he says you must:

- Develop a specific plan.
- Establish realistic expectations.
- Use reliable equipment.
- Establish a specific time and place to work out.
- Vary activities (to reduce boredom).
- Enlist the support of friends and family.

Taking these steps can help you beat the dropout odds.

The Power of Walking

689. Fit Walking into Your Life

Don't underestimate the power of walking. New scientific research—and a lot of it—focuses on walking's benefits as an aerobic exercise. In fact, researchers are finding that walking can hold its own when pitted against more vigorous forms of exercise, such as jogging and aerobic dance.

According to studies performed at Stanford University School of Medicine, brisk walking can reduce your risk of cardiovascular disease about 80 percent as effectively as jogging.

690. Deck the Malls

Some malls open their corridors to walkers before they open the stores for shopping, so you can get in a couple hours of exercise before the crowds arrive. In winter, the greenery and controlled climate are a welcome change if you live in a snowy region of the country.

691. Learn to Be a Fitness Walker

But don't try to walk across America your first time out. Take it easy and build up to greater distances. According to Robert Brown, M.D., Ph.D., professor of behavioral medicine and psychiatry, University of Virginia, Charlottesville, take one mile at a time.

Measure out a 1-mile course using your car's odometer, says Dr. Brown, then walk the course at a pace you can easily tolerate. Every day walk the same course while keeping track of your time. The day

FACT OF LIFE

Exercisers Make Better Workers

A recent Gallup poll found that 62 percent of regular exercisers said that working out makes them feel more energetic on the job; 43 percent said they felt more creative; and 45 percent said they felt more self-assured.

you walk it in under 15 minutes, you will have broken the magic mark.

Next goal: walk 2 miles in 30 minutes. Then 3 miles in 45 minutes, and, finally, 4 miles in one hour. If you can keep up this pace every other day, you can consider yourself a real fitness walker.

692. Walk a Dog, Any Dog

Have you ever considered getting a dog for a walking companion, but realized that your lifestyle just wouldn't accommodate the commitment involved? Maybe you and your local humane society can work something out: They have dogs, and you have walking time!

At the Humane Society of New York, Sarah C. Haywood oversees a volunteer cadre of dog walkers. Encouraged by a sign in the window saying, "Volunteer! Walk a dog!" people with time, energy, and compassion for animals sign out a pooch and ramble around the city. Everybody benefits!

693. Get To Know Them There Hills

Need to cram a 4-mile walk into a 30-minute time slot? Do a 2-mile stint uphill. If you walk up a hill with a 5 percent grade—a hill that rises about 5 feet for every 100 feet—you'll get a great aerobic workout. And you'll burn about 45 percent more calories than you would walking on a flat surface.

694. Put on a Little Weight

If you want to burn a few more calories and increase your aerobic fitness, try carrying hand weights when you walk. Start with 1-pound weights. Carry them with your arms bent and swinging. Then gradually work up to 2- or 3-pound weights.

"Use hand weights during walking, and you can burn more calories per mile than you would while running," says Bryant Stamford, Ph.D., director of the exercise physiology laboratory at the University of Louisville School of Medicine in Kentucky.

Hand weights are not recommended for those with high blood pressure.

695. Plan a Walking Vacation

A walking tour makes the perfect spring, summer, or fall vacation. In the United States and Canada, some chambers of commerce have put together walking tours, especially in cities with historic or restored areas. If you're venturing abroad, your travel agent may be able to provide information about walks in foreign countries.

696. Put the Right Shoe Forward

Any walking program should start off on the right foot, so you'll want to get a pair of comfortable sneakers or walking shoes.

Look for a shoe that has a well-cushioned, even springy heel. The shoe should also be sturdily constructed and have a comfortable fit. Also, buying a shoe that controls the tendency of your foot to roll inward will take a lot of stress off your ankle and leg.

Extra Ideas for Extra Energy

697. Two Succeed Better Than One

Women who exercise with their husbands are twice as likely to maintain a regular fitness program than if they work out alone, say researchers from St. Francis Medical Center in Peoria. Earlier, those researchers found that men were 66 percent more likely to continue a regular exercise program when their wives joined them.

698. Climb the Stairs to Fitness

Include stair climbing in your repertoire of workout activities. Stairs are the equivalent of a 50 percent incline, so you'll want to go slowly, though. Caution: Don't attempt stair climbing if you're overweight. It could dangerously stress the heart, according to a lung specialist at the University of Texas Medical Branch at Galveston.

699. Learn to Cross-Country Ski

If you live in snow country, take a class in cross-country skiing. It's a superb way to get a great workout while enjoying the wonders of nature.

Cross-country skiing is a whole-body workout: You use your arms *and* your legs, and you travel a considerable distance at a steady pace, making cross-country skiing one of the best aerobic conditioners there is—better than jogging, according to many sports medicine doctors. Sustained effort, using all major muscles in the upper and lower body to vigorously push the legs back and pole your way along the terrain, builds overall fitness superbly.

Beginners will also find that their strength increases with their initial efforts, but that effect wears off as you gain experience—you *are* strong, rather than becoming strong.

And here's an added bonus for the calorie-conscious. Two hours' worth of cross-country skiing burns up more than 1,000 calories and tends to raise your metabolism for hours afterward, burning up still more calories.

700. Make Like a Kid and Play Outdoors

For most adults, winter means slippery sidewalks, spinning car tires, and grimy slush. But when you were a kid, snow meant *fun*, and playing in the snow for hours was a blast: You spent hours building snowmen, sledding, and skating. So get out there and enjoy the fun. Borrow a neighbor's kid or a nearby niece or nephew, if you need an excuse to play.

701. Shape Up at the Seashore

Next time you take a trip to the beach, make it a fitness trip. Get up extra early while the air is still cool and crisp and rent a bike. Or ask a companion to join you and rent a bicycle built for two and ride along the boardwalk.

Instead of lying on the beach all afternoon, take a long stroll along the beach. Challenge yourself to see just how far you can go.

FACT OF LIFE

The Generation Gap

Middle age just ain't what it used to be. A nationwide survey found that in the 1980s, people 45 and older did more bicycling, camping, hiking, tennis, and skiing than the same age group did 20 years ago.

702. Dance, Dance, Dance

Psst! Wanna get some exercise without calling it exercise? Learn ballroom dancing. Or tap dancing. Or square dancing, Irish jigs, bellydancing, flamenco, or the Texas two-step, for that matter.

Dancing is an enjoyable way to keep active and get plenty of exercise. And fast dancing, if sustained, can give you an aerobic workout. Check out classes at your local Y or adult education at your area high school.

703. Garden and Grow Fit

If your idea of a good time is tugging at obstinate dandelions, lugging bags of manure around the yard, or waltzing a wheelbarrow across bumpy rows of raised soil, you're in luck. It's also good exercise.

Gardening, in fact, can even give you an aerobic workout, says Peter Jacobson, M.D., an orthopedic surgeon in Virginia Beach, Virginia, "Gardening gives you the same exercise as going for a steady walk, although it's not as aerobic as running," says Dr. Jacobson. "It can be part of setting reasonable, achievable goals to exercise."

704. Work around the House

Putting a new roof on the garage, remodeling the family room, and waxing the car may not qualify as aerobic in the clinical sense of the word, but they can contribute to overall health and fitness.

"Work around the house can be a great form of exercise," says Ronald LaPorte, Ph.D., associate professor in the department of epidemiology at the University of Pittsburgh. "But too often it's erratic or seasonal. If activities around the house and yard are going to be a form of exercise, be as consistent as possible," he says.

705. Make Entertaining Exercise

A fun way to incorporate more exercise into your schedule is to combine home entertainment with exercise. Instead of just listening to records, dance to them. Addicted to television sitcoms? Try pedaling a stationary bike while you watch. Or run in place or do push-ups during commercials.

FACT OF LIFE

A Reason to Start—And Stop

Looking for a way to give up cigarettes—forever? Take up exercise. Statistics show that people who exercise are twice as successful at quitting than those who don't exercise.

706. Go out of Your Way to Exercise

Walk to the newsstand instead of getting home delivery. Use fewer wastebaskets, so you have to walk more to toss refuse. Park half a mile from work and walk the rest of the way. Get off the bus two stops too soon.

You get the idea. Cut out the shortcuts and soon a little extra exercise will be as natural to your daily activity as eating, sleeping, and brushing your teeth.

707. Become a Globe Plotter

Keep track of your mileage and use pins or a bright marking pen to plot an imaginary course on a map of your state, the nation, or even the continent. You may be intrigued to see how far your fanciful trek takes you.

Think of the bragging rights: You'll be able to say, "I walked across four states this past winter."

708. Form an Exercise-for-Lunch Bunch

Chances are, your co-workers are in the same boat you are— they mean to exercise but can't seem to fit it in. So get together at lunchtime for a brisk hour-long walk.

709. Music Makes Exercise Easier

If you haven't already done so, add music to your workouts. Music lowers perceptions of fatigue and pain, allowing you to push harder with less apparent effort. That in turn encourages you to stick with an exercise program—and increases your pleasure in the bargain.

Certain musical rhythms also improve muscular coordination. A Stanford University study suggests that people can perform physical activities—from household chores to weight lifting—better with a catchy beat in the background.

In short, music "enhances your rapport with your body," says Kenneth Bruscia, Ph.D., a music therapy professor at Temple University. "It increases endurance, regulates breathing rates, and establishes a mood for physical activity."

710. Arrange for Away-from-Home Workouts

If you belong to a health club, find out if it offers reciprocal arrangements with other clubs. You may be able to use a facility near your vacation or business travel location.

Or find a hotel that has a pool or exercise room. More and more hotels that cater to business travelers are opening health clubs on the premises.

Life-Extension Tool

The Performance "BioScan" Heart Monitor

Here's a device that can warn you instantly if you're overtaxing (or undertaxing) your heart during exercise.

The Performance BioScan is a wireless unit that features an elastic chest belt/transmitter and a water-resistant receiver that can be strapped to your wrist or handlebar. The liquid-crystal display shows a pulse range of 10 to 240 beats per minute (bpm) and features upper and lower limit alarms that can be set in 10-bpm increments. (This is a key feature, because the most effective training occurs at 70 to 85 percent of your maximum heart rate). Once set, an alarm sounds when you are exercising too lightly or too vigorously.

The device, which is made in Japan, is designed primarily for serious athletes who want to train at peak performance, but it also serves as an effective safety instrument because it can warn you immediately when you are overstressing your heart.

The BioScan costs approximately $130 and can be purchased in Performance bike shops or by calling its mail-order number, 1–800–727–2453.

Fitness Smarts

711. Invest in a Good Pair of Shoes

After you've chosen your sport, invest in a good pair of shoes to go with it. Lots of time and money have been poured into improving shoe design, and yesterday's all-purpose sneakers have given way to specialized shoes for walking, running, tennis, aerobics, and more. And what's good for one exercise isn't necessarily good for the other.

Aerobic shoes, for example, are designed for the impact of an indoor floor, not the pounding of muscle and bone against the open road. The result could be injury.

The new activewear shoes are engineered for comfort and performance of a given activity and to ease stress on feet and joints, so you'll be less likely to be sidelined by pain or injury.

There are, however, what are called cross-training shoes, suitable for more than one activity.

712. Attention Beginners: Start Out Slowly

While your goal may be to exercise for 20 or 30 minutes at a clip, that may be too much if you've never exercised, says Gail Johnston, of the Aerobics and Fitness Association. So start exercising for as long as you feel comfortable.

If 5 minutes a day is the most you can bear, then so be it. When you become comfortable with that much, maybe a week or so later, increase it by another 5 minutes, and so on.

713. Warm Up First

Sudden starts and stops tax your heart and muscles. For safety's sake, spend at least 5 to 10 minutes before your workout getting your circulation going. If you exercise outdoors in the winter, do some warm-up exercises in the house before you go out.

Don't confuse warming up with stretching, cautions Peter Lemon, Ph.D., professor of exercise physiology at Kent State University in Ohio. "Warming up is rehearsing the exercise slowly. If you walk, for instance, walk slowly for the first few minutes. *Then* stretch your muscles slowly—don't bounce."

714. Cool Down

Don't just stop your workout and head for the showers. Wind down slowly by doing a less strenuous version of the exercise you just performed.

Swimmers can swim slowly around the pool. Walkers can slow down to a stroll. When you exercise, blood collects in your arms and legs. Cooling down allows it to flow back to your brain, bringing with it the added oxygen it picked up from exercising.

Gradually decrease your activity until your heart returns to close to its resting rate. Winding down for 5 minutes or so is easier on your heart.

715. Become a "Three-Percenter"

Don't wear yourself out exercising too hard. Experts will tell you that increasing your exercise pace gradually will help you increase your aerobic capacity better than struggling against too-tired lungs.

Plus, you'll help avoid the soreness and possible injury that often besets an exerciser who leaves the starting gate too fast. You can prevent muscle soreness by increasing your workout speed, weight, or distance no more than 2 or 3 percent weekly.

But if you do get sore muscles, don't stop exercising altogether. Instead, engage in a light aerobic workout emphasizing muscles that are not sore. Aggressive stretching or premature intensive use of sore muscles can further aggravate the problem.

Keep in mind that even something as good as exercise could be harmful in excess: Animals forced to exercise at relatively high intensity on a constantly moving treadmill or in a tub of water actually have increased cancer rates.

716. Give Your Stomach a Break

Wait at least 2 hours after eating before exercising, suggests Clark. Reasons: When you're doing intense exercise, blood flow to the stomach decreases (as more blood goes to muscles) and food sits undigested. Food also makes some people feel sluggish, possibly hampering performance.

Also, wait 4 hours before exercising after a heavy meal, says Clark.

FACT OF LIFE

Executive Success

A survey of executives at 800 corporations found that 80 percent exercise daily. Preferred activities? Golf, racquet sports, jogging, and swimming.

717. Hit the Watering Hole

If a camel can slurp down 30 gallons of water before heading out on a trek, you can surely manage one tall glass. Exercising in warm weather dehydrates your body more than you might realize. Even if you're not a heavy-duty perspirer, you lose lots of water through a process known as insensible perspiration. You can develop muscle cramps and feel drained of energy.

So drink up before you head out and drink another big glass when you get back. And if you can, take a few sips *during* your workout, too.

By the way, sugary drinks are absorbed into the body much more slowly than water. So avoid sugary drinks when you're dry. Alcohol before, during, or after exercise is not a hot idea, either. Alcohol has a diuretic effect, releasing fluids from the body just when it craves fluids the most.

718. Watch Your Weight in Hot Weather

If your 30-minute workout on a hot, humid day drops a remarkable 5 pounds from your body, don't pat yourself on the back. It's not fat you've lost (unfortunately, shedding fat is not that easy), but water. You should drink it right back up.

If you sweat heavily, you can lose a lot of water during a workout and some valuable nutrients along with it.

To make sure you've replenished your water, weigh yourself before and after a workout, advises Nancy Clark, R.D., director of Nutrition Services at Sports Medicine Systems in Brookline, Massachusetts, and author of *Nancy Clark's Sport Nutrition Guide Book*. If you weigh less the second time on the scale, drink enough water to get back to your original, pre-exercise weight.

By the way, 2 cups of water weigh 1 pound.

FACT OF LIFE

Breast Cancer Linked to Inactivity

Researchers at Harvard University found that women who had been active in basketball, swimming, tennis, track, gymnastics, volleyball, or other sports in college later developed significantly less breast cancer than their inactive peers. Their sedentary classmates had twice the risk for breast cancer as well as two and a half times more cancer of the uterus, ovaries, cervix, and vagina.

719. Dress Warmly for the Cold Outdoors

Plunging mercury can test an exerciser's mettle. But if you're outfitted properly, winter walking or jogging can be invigorating. Here are some helpful hints.

- Cover your face and lips with petroleum jelly. (Water-based moisturizers can freeze on your face.)
- Wear mittens, not gloves.
- Layer your clothing. The inner layer should be polypropylene, which wicks away perspiration; the second layer should be wool, which traps body heat; and the outer layers should be water-resistant yet capable of letting water vapor from your body escape.
- Wear a warm hat. You lose as much as 40 percent of your body heat through the top of your head.
- To keep your feet warm and dry, try a pair of wool socks with polypropylene liners. In comparison, two layers of regular socks will make your shoes too tight, and as a result your feet will feel colder.

720. Save Your Knees—Scurry like Groucho Marx

Taking longer strides and running with your knees bent—even just a little—helps reduce the amount of shock to the body, says Thomas McMahon, Ph.D., a Harvard University professor of applied mechanics and biology.

"Bending your knees just 10 degrees when you run reduces by

80 percent the amount of shock transmitted through the body," says Dr. McMahon. "Groucho running" does require more energy, giving you an extra workout for your effort, he adds.

721. Bathe Away Muscle Soreness

Taking a warm bath after your workout will untense your muscles, especially when you're just beginning an exercise program.

"You may feel a little muscle soreness a few days after you start any exercise program," says Steven I. Subotnick, D.P.M., a sports podiatrist from Hayward, California. "But don't worry; it won't last long. Keep exercising, and the pain will soon go away. But if you have pain that interferes with your activities or gets worse, see a doctor."

Note: *Hot* baths don't help; they can cause swelling. A *hot tub*, because of its pulsating action, can actually be beneficial.

722. But Don't Ignore Habitual Pain

If you ache after every workout, you're either exercising too hard or too infrequently. Either way you're setting yourself up for injury. Instead, take a slow, steady approach to exercise.

723. Try a Post-Exercise Rubdown

After a hard workout, a massage can help tired muscles rally. One theory about massage's effectiveness is that it helps eliminate metabolic waste products like lactic acid that form in tired muscles and impede performance. Massage also increases blood flow to an area and helps relax muscles, improve performance, and prevent injury.

724. Carry Your I.D.

Most people carry identification with them when they travel or drive a car, but few exercisers bother to carry any identification when they hit the road. Unfortunately, such an oversight could spell disaster if an accident occurs while you're running, biking, or hiking.

That's why Michael Sivore, M.D., president of Medical Information Systems, Inc. in St. Louis, Missouri, created the Health Access Card, an emergency information card. "The Health Access Card gives people the option of having their medical histories at their disposal, which proves useful in emergencies," says Dr. Sivore. "And to make it easy, we designed a card that can be laced to a runner's shoe."

The basic card ($10, plus postage and handling) stores simple emergency information (contacts, insurance information, allergies, prescriptions, significant past medical histories, doctors' comments, and so on), and options for the card allow space for up to three additional letter-sized sheets of medical information—such as EKG tracings or blood test results. For more information, contact Medical Information Systems, Inc., 714 Gravois Road, P.O. Box 540, Fenton, MO 63026.

725. If You Bike, Wear a Helmet

Compared with cyclists who don't wear helmets, cyclists who do have an 85 percent lower risk of head and brain injury in an accident. That finding was reported in *The New England Journal of Medicine,* and we think it speaks for itself.

CHAPTER · 13

ACCIDENTS AND
EMERGENCIES:
YOUR PERSONAL
PROTECTION
PLAN

If you're like a lot of people, you probably think that accidents are just a matter of bad luck—you happen to be in the wrong place at the wrong time, or you're at the mercy of factors beyond your control. Though chance *is* one factor, you actually have more control over your fate than you might think. Consider:

- Of the 48,700 people killed in auto accidents in one recent year, nearly two-thirds of the victims—32,400 people— would still be alive today if they (or somebody else) had not been driving recklessly. Speeding, not surprisingly, was most responsible, followed by failure to yield the right of way, drifting over the center line, passing improperly, turning illegally, and tailgating.
- Drinking is implicated in half of all fatal motor vehicle deaths. In one recent year, drinking was the cause of approximately 22,000 deaths and 320,000 injuries.
- Nearly 80 percent of all fires happen in the home, killing approximately 6,000 Americans each year. Fire officials say most of these deaths could be avoided if smoke detectors were properly maintained.

- Accidental falls kill more people over age 65 than any other injury. One study of an elderly population in one community found that 44 percent of all falls were caused by hazards in and around the house (tripping over rugs or objects or slipping on ice, for example). And 1 out of 5 people who fell as a result of tripping over something had tripped over the same object before!
- Each year, nearly 1,000 people are killed or paralyzed in diving accidents. Alcohol and drugs are associated with many of them.
- Seventy percent of boating fatalities are caused by falling overboard. Many of these deaths could be prevented if boaters would wear personal flotation devices.

Needless Deaths

All of these deaths—and many, many more—could have been avoided. Yet accidents happen all the time. Every hour, nearly 11 Americans will be killed in some sort of accident, and another 170 will suffer a disabling injury. That's 258 deaths a day, and 1,810 a week.

Accidents are responsible for killing approximately 94,000 people in the United States each year. That makes accidents the fourth leading cause of death in America (behind heart disease, cancer, and stroke) and the number one cause of death in those under age 40.

More than half of these deaths are the result of road accidents. Falls are the second leading cause of accidental death, followed by drownings, fires, poisonings, and choking. And none of these statistics account for crimes of violence—which involve nearly 50,000 people a year—or disasters such as floods, tornadoes, earthquakes, and airplane accidents.

But an accident doesn't have to happen to *you*. As we said, you have a lot more control over your fate than you might think. Do you, for example, always drive defensively? Do you know how to control a skid or avert a head-on collision?

Do you take defensive action against crime? Do you know how to secure your home or avoid confrontation? Do you know how to escape a burning house?

FACT OF LIFE

The Safest Way to Fly

Large airlines are the safest to fly, followed by commuter airlines, air taxis, and private planes. At least that's how it stacks up when you compare the safety records of these four modes of air transport in one recent year. Taken into account were total accidents, fatalities, hours flown, and miles covered.

Do you know how to avoid danger when caught in a vulnerable situation, such as swimming in a strong current? Would you know what to do if you were caught in an earthquake or a tornado?

Remember, accidents don't just happen to other people. Defensive living combined with a little knowledge and quick action can go a long way toward keeping you safe and secure.

Home, Safe Home

726. Fallproof Your House

Are you headed for a fall? Inspect your home for hazards, using this checklist adapted from guidelines developed by Rein Tideiksaar, Ph.D. and Arthur D. Kay, M.D., co-directors of the Falls and Immobility Program, Ritter Department of Geriatrics and Adult Development, Mount Sinai Medical Center, New York. If you spot potential booby traps in your home, correct the situation as soon as possible.

Exterior. Are sidewalks even? Are steps in good repair? Do steps have handrails? Are handrails securely fastened? Is lighting adequate? If not, are step edges clearly marked with colored tape?

Interior. Are stairways adequately lighted? Are adequate night lights in place? Do throw rugs have secure (nonskid) rubber backings? Are rooms uncluttered so you can get around freely and easily? Are linoleum or vinyl floors nonslippery? Are cabinets and shelves easy to reach without stretching?

Bathroom. Are skidproof strips or mats in place on the floor of the tub or shower? Is the toilet seat high enough to enable you to get on and off easily? Is the medicine cabinet well-lit, so you can read labels clearly? Are floors nonslippery (that is, not highly waxed or covered with a fluffy, easy-to-trip-over throw rug)?

Bedroom. Is the bed high enough to easily climb into and out of? Are rugs and carpets nonskid or well-anchored to the floor? Is lighting adequate? Are light switches easy to reach? Do night lights mark the route from the bed to the bathroom?

727. Don't Flirt with Fire

The key to surviving a house fire is to prevent, not put out, a fire. Here are some fire prevention strategies from the American Red Cross.

- If an electric motor or appliance is giving off smoke, immediately pull the plug or turn off the power.
- Have your chimney checked and cleaned regularly to avoid chimney fires.
- Keep portable heaters away from combustible materials like drapes, couches, and stacks of paper. And burn only the type and grade of fuel recommended by the manufacturer.
- Store gasoline and other flammable liquids in tight metal containers, preferably away from the house and never near heating equipment or pilot lights. And don't smoke when using flammable materials.
- Make sure you provide smokers with plenty of good-sized ashtrays.
- Before you go to bed, check for smoking-related fire hazards, especially if you've been entertaining guests who smoke. Look under cushions, couches, and chairs for smoldering cigarette butts. Some furniture fabrics produce toxic gases when burning, increasing the danger of death by asphyxiation, or lack of oxygen.
- Empty ashtrays into a container of water, not a wastebasket.
- Display live Christmas trees for no more than two weeks and don't stand your tree near a fireplace, wood-burning stove, portable heater, radiator, or other heat source. Also, don't decorate the fireplace mantel with boughs or other flammable materials.

911: The Number That Could Save a Life

If you're faced with a life-threatening medical emergency, call the nationwide medical help phone number: 911. If 911 doesn't operate in your area, consult the inside front cover of your phone directory for the phone number of your local Emergency Medical Services, poison control center, or police, fire, or ambulance service.

When you call for help, be prepared to give the following information, so action can be implemented quickly.

- Where the emergency situation is, with cross streets if possible
- What phone number you're calling from
- What happened—heart attack, auto accident, electrical shock, fall
- How many people need help
- What's being done to help the victim or victims

728. What to Do When the Lights Go Out

Keep a flashlight with fresh batteries where you can easily find it if the power goes out for any reason. Don't use candles, which are hazardous because of the high risk of fire.

729. Do Your Hair in the Bedroom

The bathroom is no place to stockpile electrical appliances such as hair dryers, curling irons, electric hair curlers, and electric shavers. At the very least, they should be stored and used as far from the sink and tub as possible. People have been electrocuted attempting to retrieve appliances that have accidentally fallen into the water.

730. Keep Your Kitchen Counter Clear

For the same reason, electrical appliances such as radios, irons, blenders, can openers, and toasters should be stored away from the kitchen sink. For added safety, keep them unplugged when not in use. Also, you should have any appliance repaired if it gets wet, to avoid fire or electrocution.

731. Strategic Planning for Smoke Detectors

Eighty percent of all fire deaths occur where people are sleeping, while they're sleeping, according to the American Red Cross. And the leading cause of fire death is asphyxiation (lack of oxygen), not flames. Fire quickly consumes oxygen, thereby increasing the carbon monoxide concentration in the air. In addition to the threat of smoke and noxious fumes, superheated air, which often reaches 300°F, can knock you out or kill you in minutes.

An early warning system provides occupants of a burning house with a critical commodity—escape time. According to the International Association of Fire Chiefs, smoke detectors can double your chances of surviving a house fire. To protect yourself and your family:

- Install a smoke detector on each level of your home at strategic locations such as the kitchen, basement, stairwells, and hallways near bedrooms.
- Keep a flashlight near the bed and in other convenient locations to facilitate a safe, swift exit in the dark or smoke.
- Check smoke alarm and flashlight batteries once a month.

732. Make Battery Changes Standard Procedure

Have you tested your smoke detector lately? According to the International Association of Fire Chiefs, three out of four homes have smoke detectors, but as many as half the smoke detectors are useless because the batteries are old or missing.

Fire officials advise people to install fresh batteries in their smoke detectors and flashlights once a year—preferably in October, when they change their clocks from daylight saving time to standard time. "Linking the annual battery change with the fall time change is designed to make this important safety 'anniversary' easy to remember and act upon," says Chief Ronald Coleman, association president.

733. Plan a Great Escape

In one minute, a house fire can triple in size. That doesn't leave you much time to figure out the best way out of the house. So every household should formulate an escape plan. Practice evacuating in the dark with your eyes closed, because if fire breaks out at night (as most home fires do), that's exactly how you'll have to exit. If you have to make your way through a smoke-filled room, you'll need to crawl on your hands and knees with your head low to avoid breathing smoke. So practice this, too.

If you live in a two- or three-story building, you should install a safety ladder or other means for reaching the ground safely. Designate a spot for your family to gather outside, so you can account for everyone.

The peak season for house fires is December and January, so you might want to hold a fire drill every fall to refresh your memory.

734. Learn to Stop a Fire Before It Spreads

When used correctly, fire extinguishers can keep small fires from becoming big ones or help clear an escape route through a small fire, says the Red Cross. Fire extinguishers are labeled A, B, and C, depending on which kind of fire they are designed to consume.

- Extinguishers with a green A on the label are appropriate for paper, cloth, wood, rubber, and some plastics.
- Extinguishers with a red B on the label are appropriate for flammable liquids (oils, gasoline, kitchen grease, paints, solvents), the most likely causes of fires that break out in the kitchen, basement, workshop, or garage.
- Extinguishers with a blue C on the label are appropriate for electrical fires (motors, power tools, appliances, wiring, fuse boxes).

You can also buy a multipurpose dry chemical extinguisher labeled A-B-C to put out most types of fires.

To be safe and effective, a fire extinguisher must be easy to get to quickly and must be operated by someone who knows how to use it. So make sure extinguishers are visible and accessible. Read the directions *before* an emergency arises. Your local fire department can show you the best place to keep it and how to mount it properly.

735. Safety Is Your First Priority

If a fire breaks out, don't waste precious time trying to phone the fire department from your burning house. Alert everyone who lives with you about the fire and telephone 911 or the fire department from a neighbor's house.

Car and Driver

736. Everyone Should Have a Belt

Seat belts save lives. It's a proven fact. More than 11,000 people involved in car accidents over a recent four-year period survived because they were wearing seat belts at the time.

Using front-seat safety restraints reduces the risk of death by 40 to 50 percent and the risk of injury by 45 to 55 percent, according to a National Highway Traffic Safety Administration estimate. And since laws requiring the use of seat belts have been enacted in 31 states, death rates from highway accidents have dropped substantially.

Although the law in most states applies only to front-seat passengers, backseat passengers should consider buckling up, too. One British study found that rear-seat passengers are actually more likely to be thrown from a car at impact than the driver or a front-seat passenger.

737. Don't Be a Dope

The last thing you want in a car is a slow foot on the brake or a hand that hesitates on the wheel when the fool up ahead makes a sudden stop or an animal darts across the road.

Yet that's exactly what you'll have if you take any one of dozens of medications. Which ones? Painkillers, antihistamines, antidepressants, sedatives, and high blood pressure medications can affect your ability to drive, pharmacists say. So if you're taking any of them, check with your pharmacist to make sure it won't affect your reflexes. And if it does, ask your doctor to prescribe a similar medication that doesn't.

738. Don't Drive under the Influenza Bug

The next time you come down with a bad cold or a bout of the flu, you might want to use the following bit of news as an added incentive to stay home: British researchers report that driving under the influence of a flu virus may be as hazardous as driving under the influence of alcohol.

The Medical Research Council's Common Cold Unit in Salis-

Life-Extension Tool

Auto Air Bags and Safety Restraints

Beginning with the 1990 model year, all autos sold in the United States were required to have passive restraint systems—automatic safety belts or air bags. Air bags are concealed in the steering wheel or dashboard. On impact, an air bag is activated by a sensor in a car's hood. In a fraction of a second, the air bag inflates to cushion a motorist against the impact of a crash, preventing the driver from being slammed against the steering wheel, dashboard, or windshield.

Air bags are available in many current cars. Air bags have significant advantages over seat belts alone, claims the U.S. Department of Transportation: They are more effective at preventing head injury, a major cause of death and disability from auto collisions, and they reduce the severity of head, face, and torso injuries sustained in front-end collisions, the most deadly kind of collision.

The department estimates that the combination of air bags and mandatory seat belt laws will save almost twice as many lives as mandatory seat belt laws alone.

But remember, air bags are meant to be used along with, not instead of, seat belts. They can't protect you against side, rear, or rollover collisions. So you should still make it a habit to buckle up.

---

bury, England, gave flu victims performance tests. Their reaction time was at 43 percent of capacity—considerably worse than the reaction time of those who were drinking moderately.

Colds, too, reduce driving skill, say the researchers. Cold victims bombed on tests of hand/eye coordination.

739. It's Dangerous to Be Driving Mad

Hot heads are as dangerous as bad brakes or bald tires. In one survey, 1 out of every 5 drivers killed in auto accidents had suffered an emotional upset within 6 hours before they crashed. So keep your cool and try not to drive when you're in a state of emotional turmoil—say, after an argument or when you're under some sort of stress, says Ming T. Tsuang, M.D., Ph.D., professor of psychiatry at the Harvard Medical School and chief of psychiatry at the Brockton–East Roxbury V.A. Medical Center in the Boston area.

FACT OF LIFE

The Accident-Prone Personality

The personality traits most associated with automobile accidents are belligerence, uncontrollable anger, hostility, and immaturity, says a report published in the *American Journal of Psychiatry.* The person who has these traits also has difficulty dealing with authority figures and has a tendency toward risk-taking. Surprised?

740. Avoid Highway Hypnosis

Fatigue is a factor in approximately 1 out of 10 collisions, according to the American Automobile Association (AAA). To keep from getting drowsy, especially on long trips, take these precautions.

- Don't start out on a long drive right after eating a heavy meal. Digestion makes the body sleepy. On the other hand, a light meal or snack will help you concentrate.
- Roll down your window for fresh air. Or turn the dashboard vents toward your face and activate the fan to revive yourself with fresh air. "People tend to make their cars too comfortable," says James Solomon, training administrator for driver improvement programs of the National Safety Council.
- Turn on the radio. A talk show will keep you more alert than music.
- Cool your face. Solomon says long-distance truck drivers often carry an insulated plastic bag (the kind used for lunches and beverages) filled with ice and a damp cloth. Every once in a while, they wipe their faces with the damp cloth. "It helps them stay alert," says Solomon.
- In bright sunshine, wear nonglare sunglasses. Glare strains your eyes and triggers fatigue.

741. Keep Your Stereo Way Down Low

If you're having trouble focusing on traffic while driving, you might want to check the volume on your radio. Psychologists at Clarkson University in Potsdam, New York, found that when car stereos were cranked up, drivers—in this case, volunteer college students—couldn't see as far or as well. They theorize that visual acuity is decreased when decibel levels are high.

742. Plan a Pit Stop

Never drive more than 2 hours without taking a rest break, says Solomon.

Pull off the road at a rest stop, get out of the car, and walk around. Stretch your legs to get your circulation pumping and relieve fatigue. If you feel like it, go ahead and take off your shoes and socks, too. Cooling your heels can clear your head. If it's possible, switch drivers.

Eat a light snack, too. A study conducted in Sweden showed that eating does more to improve driving performance than a rest break without food.

743. Smoke Gets in Your Eyes—And in Your Way

An analysis of 595 car crashes found that people who smoke while driving are 50 percent more likely to have an auto accident than nonsmokers. And in simulated driving tests, smokers were involved in three times as many accidents as nonsmokers.

According to the National Safety Council, the carbon monoxide in cigarette smoke interferes with your eyes' ability to adapt to darkness, making night driving risky. Researchers also theorize that rooting around for cigarettes, matches, lighters, and the ashtray distracts attention from the road. Also, smoke fogs the windshield, irritates your eyes, and triggers coughing fits, all of which interfere with driving.

744. Caution: Car Phone on Board

Car phones may be convenient, but unless you use common sense, they can also be dangerous.

"A car traveling at 55 miles per hour travels 80 feet in a second—plenty of distance for disaster if you've diverted your attention from the road," says the AAA's Frank Kenel.

Statistics show that motorists with car phones mounted on the dashboard are half as likely to have an accident as those with phones on the center console.

"On the dash, a car phone is more in the driver's line of vision," says Susan Cowan-Scott, spokesperson for the California Highway Patrol (CHP). "If it's on the console, you have to look down and keep your eyes off the road more." Even safer, says a CHP study, are speaker-phones with hands-free dialing and one-button autodialing.

745. Improve Your Night Vision

At night, you can see about one-sixth as far as you can see in daylight, which may account for the fact that 57 percent of all collisions happen at night.

To help improve your night vision, you should:

- Regularly clean the soot, salt, and bugs off your headlights and turn-signal lights.
- Regularly wash your windshield, inside and out and keep your windshield wipers in A–1 working order. Studies show that smeared, dirty, or scratched windshields not only reduce vision but also increase glare by scattering light from headlights of oncoming cars.
- Most important, slow down after dark.

746. A Bright Idea for Older Folks

The older you get, the more vulnerable you are to poor night vision, says Burt Skuza, O.D., executive director of the Minnesota Board of Optometric Association's task force on vision concerns

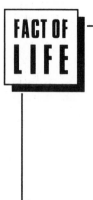

FACT OF LIFE

Roads Are Safer

It appears cars and drivers are safer now than they ever were, even though there are more cars on the road. In the 75-year stretch from 1912 to 1987, road deaths in the United States dropped signficantly: 91 percent, from 33 deaths per 10,000 registered cars to 3 per 10,000. In 1912, there were 3,100 fatalities when the number of vehicles totaled 950,000. In 1987, there were 48,700 fatalities, but registrations soared to 186 million.

among older Americans. As you age, the retina—the "film" in the back of the eye that receives outside images—responds more slowly to changes in light. So older people find headlight glare more troublesome and don't readjust to darkness as easily as they did when they were younger.

If you find this is happening to you, it's best to turn the wheel over to someone else at night.

747. Don't Be a Flasher

If a driver in the opposite lane neglects to dim his or her high beams, don't flick your high beams on and off, says the National Safety Council's James Solomon. All that does is blind the other motorist, making the situation more dangerous. Instead, move a little farther to the right and look as far down the road and off to the right as possible without taking your eyes off the road.

And don't use your high beams at all during fog; they'll cause glare.

748. Sunglasses by Day Improve Vision by Night

Wear sunglasses if you're going to spend a lot of time outdoors on a bright day and plan to drive at night. Sunglasses help to preserve your eyes' store of visual purple, a substance that helps your eyes adapt to the dark, says the National Safety Council. Without daytime protection from sunglasses, your ability to see at night declines markedly.

749. Brighten Up a Rainy Day

Some states now require that all drivers turn on their low beams on dark, rainy days.

Daytime running lights, which turn on automatically when the car is started, are required in some European countries, and studies indicate they can save fenders and lives. In Finland, daytime crash rates dropped 27 percent after drivers began to turn on their headlights during the day in winter. In Sweden, there's been an 11 percent reduction in head-on collisions since the passage of a law that requires day and night use of headlights.

FACT OF LIFE

Death by Drinking Is Down

Anti-drunk-driving campaigns appear to be having an impact: The number of drunks involved in fatal car collisions has gone down. Although the number of drivers involved in fatal car accidents increased 8 percent in a recent four-year span, the number of legally drunk drivers involved in fatal crashes dropped from 30 to 26 percent, according to National Highway Traffic Safety Administration Statistics.

750. The Caution Flag Goes Up at Dusk

Dusk is the most common time for fatal accidents to occur. According to the Pennsylvania Optometric Association, the contrast between the brightness in the sky and the darkness on the road makes it difficult to see. Using your lights should help improve your vision.

751. Keep Pace with Traffic

On highways and freeways, drive at a legal speed that matches the speed of other traffic, recommends the AAA. Driving much faster or slower than the general flow of traffic will increase the risk of a collision. Choosing the speed used by most drivers will also reduce conflict, making driving more relaxed.

752. Green Light: Count to Three

When you're stopped at an intersection, don't assume that all the traffic has cleared when the red light turns green, says Lt. Herbert Grofcsik, commanding officer of the driver training unit at the Philadelphia Police Academy. "Drivers crossing in front of you might try to beat the yellow light. Or the driver across from you might dart out to make a left turn in front of you."

Apparently, this happens a lot. A survey conducted over a 45-hour period on midweek traffic at a major urban intersection found that 7 out of 20 drivers ran a red light.

To be safe, wait 3 seconds and look both ways before you pull out after the light turns green and proceed with caution.

753. You've Got to Be a Block Ahead

Driving in heavy traffic requires a constant series of decisions. At high speeds you have less time to make safe choices.

To anticipate changing conditions, the AAA says you should make a habit of looking ahead and noting traffic and road conditions within the distance you estimate you'll cover in the next 12 seconds. At 30 miles per hour, 12 seconds is the equivalent of ⅒ mile, or 1 city block. At average freeway speeds, a 12-second lead amounts to ⅕ mile, or 2 city blocks.

The 12-second rule will alert you to hazards far enough in advance to slow down, change lanes, or otherwise avoid trouble. Also, it gives you time to pump your brakes, which will flash your brake lights and warn vehicles in your wake, reducing the risk of a rear-end collision.

754. Know When to Back Off

Tailgating is dangerous. At 30 miles per hour, it takes 4 seconds—about 44 feet, or 5 car lengths—to stop. The AAA says that's the distance you should keep between you and the car in front. As your speed increases or decreases, so do the time and distance required to brake to a stop.

Take a Lesson from Jackie Stewart

How does three-time world champion race car driver Jackie Stewart handle the open road?

"I use exactly the same techniques in my road driving as I do in my race driving," Stewart told *Car and Driver* magazine. Good driving, says Stewart, takes "the three C's: concentration, conscientiousness, and consideration." These qualities "are as important on a racetrack as they are on the street," says Stewart.

According to *Car and Driver* editor Rich Ceppos, who accompanied Stewart in an outing in a Ford Taurus, Stewart drives at the speed limit, yet his driving almost seems slow, because he's so smooth, precise, and polite. "It's as though there's an egg between his foot and the gas pedal," comments Ceppos. Maybe that's why Stewart won 27 Grand Prix races—and finished in one piece.

To gauge your potential stopping time, pick a point ahead and count "one thousand one, one thousand two, one thousand three, one thousand four." Do this until you have a fairly good idea of what a 4-second lead looks like, and use that as your safe following distance.

Also, keep in mind that this formula applies to normal traffic volume under good weather conditions. In bad weather, a car needs two to ten times more distance to stop than on dry pavement.

Here's another helpful benchmark: If you can read the nameplate showing the make of the car in front of you, you're following too closely, no matter what the weather. So back off.

755. Know the Rules of the Road in the Rain

When you drive your car in the rain or on wet pavement, the tires push a wave of water ahead of them. At low speeds, this isn't much of a problem. But as you increase your speed—to 30 or 35 miles per hour and higher—that wave can become a slippery film between your tires and the road surface. This phenomenon is called hydroplaning. Light cars are more apt to hydroplane than heavy cars. Hydroplaning is also more likely if you have too much weight concentrated in the rear of your car.

You know you're hydroplaning if you try to turn the wheel but the car keeps going forward. Or you hit the brakes and get no response. Or, in a front-wheel drive car, you try to speed up but can't. The wheels may be turning faster, but they aren't touching anything but water, so they just spin.

FACT OF LIFE

Local Streets Are More Dangerous Than Interstates

More fatal motor vehicle accidents occur on local urban streets than on the interstates of urban and rural areas combined, according to National Safety Council statistics. Still, overall, rural areas are the scenes of most traffic deaths.

If you're hydroplaning, don't slam on the brakes. "Ease off the gas," says Solomon. "As the car slows, that wave starts to dissipate and the wheels start to touch the road again."

A light shower can be just as dangerous as a heavy downpour. Whenever it rains, oil and grease that accumulate on the road mix with dust and rainwater to form a slick and risky combination.

756. Are You Skidding?

If your car goes into a skid, your first impulse may be to brake hard and fast. *Don't.* If you hit the brakes, the wheels will probably lock, causing your tires to slide instead of roll. When that happens, you lose your ability to steer, and you'll continue to skid, either off the road (if it's banked) or in a straight line (if it's not).

The secret to controlling a skid is in steering, not braking. Just a few minor adjustments to the wheel, combined with taking your foot off the pedals, will often do the trick. Here's what to do, according to the National Safety Council:

- If your rear wheels start to skid and the back of the car swings around toward the front, take your foot off the accelerator and turn the steering wheel in the direction you want the front of your car to go. If the rear of your car is sliding to the left, for instance, steer left. Don't oversteer, though, or your wheels will start skidding in the opposite direction. As your wheels regain their grip on the road, accelerate smoothly and gently and counter-steer until you're in the direction you wish to go.
- If your front wheels start to skid—in other words, if your car plows straight ahead regardless of whether you've turned the wheel left or right—take your foot off the accelerator and wait for the front wheels to grip the road again. As your car slows down, you will regain steering ability. Steer the wheels gently in the direction you want to go. Gently accelerate when you have the car back under control.
- To prevent your car from skidding in the first place, make it a habit to drive at a smooth pace and always allow plenty of braking distance, especially in rain, snow, ice, or heavy traffic.

757. Pump Wet Brakes into Action

Total brake failure in cars is rare. But occasionally, poor maintenance or driving through puddles of water can weaken your brakes. If you hit the brakes and they don't respond, pump them a few times, pressing down gently and letting up again. Heat from the friction will dry the brake linings or pads and restore braking power.

758. "Squeeze Brake" on Ice and Snow

Pumping the brakes works on clear or wet pavement. But don't pump the brakes if you find yourself skidding on ice or snow-covered roads. According to the AAA, the most efficient way to brake on a slippery surface is to disengage the clutch (if you have a manual transmission) or shift into neutral (if you have an automatic transmission) and apply a technique known as squeeze braking.

Using steady pressure, apply the brakes firmly, to a point just short of locking, then ease off the brake pedal slightly, but not completely. Reapply the brakes to the point just short of locking and hold. This technique, says the AAA, gives you the best combination of braking effort and steering control.

759. Driving a Three-Wheeler Takes Skill

Coping with a tire blowout is a lot like controlling a skid. Here are some basic instructions.

If your car lurches to one side, you've blown a front tire. If the car sways from side to side, fishtails, or pulls toward one side, you've blown a rear tire. Either way, don't brake. Instead, take your foot off the gas. Grip the steering wheel firmly—it'll wobble like the dickens—and try to steer to correct any change in direction caused by the blowout. Brake only after you have the car under control. Turn on your four-way hazard flasher lights, look for a safe place to pull over, and slowly ease your vehicle off the road.

760. Head Off a Head-On Collision

A head-on collision is the worst kind of collision. If you see another vehicle headed straight for you, don't freeze. If you act quickly, you may be able to avert disaster.

Your first instinct is to look for an escape route. For example, head for the right shoulder or turn off into a side road, if possible. Turn enough so that if you get hit, you get hit at an angle. Don't slam on the brakes: You might lock the wheels, making any maneuver impossible.

The idea is to do whatever is necessary to avoid being hit head-on. A blow at an angle reduces the force of the impact—and your chances of serious injury.

Two Wheels for the Road

761. Sign Up for Motorcycle School

Riding a motorcycle requires a whole new set of driving skills. If you own a motorcycle or plan to buy one, consider attending a motorcycle safe-driving school. Whether you're a novice or an experienced rider, you'll learn how to ride a motorcycle correctly and safely.

To locate motorcycling courses in your state, call the Motorcycle Safety Foundation at 1–800–442–6826.

762. Helmet Law: Listen to the Victims

If you want to feel the breeze rushing through your hair, buy a convertible. Buzzing down the freeway with nothing but thin air between the road and your head is not worth the risk. Most deaths and serious disabilities from motorcycle accidents are due to head

FACT OF LIFE

Helmets Do Save Lives

In 1966, Congress voted to withhold federal highway funds from states without compulsory helmet laws. Forty-seven states eventually complied, and motorcycle fatalities plummeted. Ten years later, Congress repealed the act, and 26 states repealed or weakened their helmet laws. The number of motorcycle fatalities rocketed again—44 percent over the next three years.

injury. Should you crash, a proper helmet can save your life or protect against permanent brain damage and disability.

When the Safety Helmet Council of America interviewed motorcycle accident victims, 86 percent said they were traveling within the speed limit and on dry, clean road when they spilled. More than half were traveling at less than 35 miles per hour. Yet in nearly two-thirds of the accidents, the riders hit their head on the road surface. All were wearing helmets, and most agreed that without protection, they'd be dead. When mentioning their helmet, nearly every survivor commented, "It saved my life."

763. A Helmet Should Fit like a Glove

"The helmet that offers the most protection is the full face helmet. It completely wraps around and protects your head and face," says Doug Fitts, manager of the California Motorcyclist Safety Program, a state-mandated program run by the California Highway Patrol.

Helmets, like hats, come in many sizes, and it's important that you buy one that fits. An ill-fitting helmet could easily come off in an accident.

A correctly fitted full face helmet will not have a gap inside between your head and the helmet. Make sure the cushioning inside it fits right up against your face and chin.

764. Stay Upright When Avoiding Accidents

"There's no such thing as a fender bender on a motorcycle," says Fitts. "Any accident, no matter how minor, could result in a serious injury. In a car, you have steel wrapped around you; on a motorcycle, you're wrapped around the steel."

It used to be that riders were taught to lay their bikes down if they were about to hit something. Research now refutes that advice.

"Laying the bike down would actually increase your total stopping distance," says Fitts. "It's well known that leather slides farther than rubber."

"Normally, it's best to keep the motorcycle up on both wheels and use the powerful brakes that bikes now have. Modern motorcycles can stop far shorter than an automobile can," says Fitts.

765. Sunglasses Don't Offer a Shade of Protection

"Sunglasses are potential safety hazards when worn while riding a motorcycle at freeway speeds," says Fitts. "When the wind blows on your face, debris can fly behind the glasses, and it can get into your eyes. Buy a helmet with a face shield, and you won't have to worry about all that."

766. Shield Yourself from the Wind

A motorcycle windshield works just like your car's windshield: It deflects air and debris around you and keeps bugs out of your teeth.

"A windshield or fairing [the molded plastic piece that covers the handlebars] offers a great amount of protection," says Fitts. "It stops you from being pelted with things, and that gives you the ability to concentrate on riding instead of dodging flying objects."

767. Wear Fall Fashions When You Ride

When you ride a motorcycle, don't dress for the ride, dress for the fall you may have. That means no shorts, no bare feet, and no riding without a shirt.

"Wear protective long-sleeved clothing made of leather or any type of heavy, strong material," says Fitts. "Don't ride with sandals or sneakers on; wear sturdy over-the-ankle footwear. And while you're at it, a good pair of riding gloves will go a long way in protecting your hands."

FACT OF LIFE

Weeknights Are Safer

According to traffic statistics, more than half of all fatal motor-vehicle deaths occur on Friday, Saturday, or Sunday. Peak hours for fatal crack-ups: from 4:00 P.M. Friday to 2:00 A.M. Saturday, and from 6:00 P.M. Saturday to 3:00 A.M. Sunday.

768. Oil Spills Could Cause Your Spill

Cars that burn oil and drip fluids not only spoil the environment, they make a dangerous environment for you to ride in.

"Be careful when driving through areas where vehicles have been stopped," says Fitts. "Oil and grease can drip off cars and trucks, and should you drive through it and try to turn, you could slide and spill. Watch out for accumulations of these drippings at intersections and in parking lots."

Safer Waters

769. Learn the Ropes

The rules of the water are a lot different than the rules of the road. Unfortunately, you don't need a driver's license to take the helm of a private boat. Before you shove off, you should be familiar with motorboat or sailboat handling, marine terminology, navigation and piloting, weather, traffic regulations, navigational lights, what to do in an emergency, and all other aspects of good seamanship.

The U.S. Coast Guard strongly recommends that all boaters take a boating course with a local auxiliary unit. In one recent year, there were 946 boating fatalities in the United States, according to the Coast Guard. Only 100 of the people involved had taken a safe-boating course.

If you don't know of a Coast Guard Auxiliary flotilla in your area, call 1–800–368–5647, or write to the U.S. Coast Guard Auxiliary National Board, Inc., 9449 Watson Industrial Park, St. Louis, MO 63126–1575.

770. Keep Your Head in the Clouds

Don't depend on TV's Action Jackson from last night's weather news to give the "sky's clear" send-off today. Weather can change rapidly. Before getting under way, check the weather report. Be alert to signs of impending bad weather and know the National Weather Service Storm Advisory Signals and where they're flown in your area.

Here are a few ways to predict weather by observing the clouds.

- Crowded, dense, dark, and towering clouds indicate changing or worsening weather.
- The sharper the edge of a thundercloud and the darker its color, the more violence it contains.
- The weather will change if cloud color, shape, and size change.
- When cumulus clouds (puffy and white) become cumulo- nimbus clouds (dark, tightly wrapped, and churning) you can expect a squall within 60 to 90 minutes.

771. Know Your Limit

Three simple rules govern your passenger capacity: Don't over- load, keep the load low, and distribute the load evenly. If your boat carries a label indicating its weight capacity, adhere to it. If not, use the following formula to determine the maximum number of people your boat can safely carry: Length times width of boat divided by 15 equals the maximum number of people on board. The "nautical per- son" is considered to be 150 pounds.

772. Wait Until You Dock to Pop the Cork

Alcohol is a prominent factor in boating deaths and accidents. It's the reason that operating a boat under the influence of alcohol became a federal offense in 1984. Violators can get a year in jail and a $5,000 fine.

773. Don't Stand Up in a Small Boat

A four-year study of accidental drowning deaths in North Car- olina found that men and fishing are not as compatible as you might think: Fishing is second only to swimming when it comes to drown- ings, and 98 percent of the victims are men.

"The story of the fisherman who has been drinking beer, stands up in the boat to urinate overboard, falls out of the boat and drowns is well known among coroners," notes James P. Orlowski, M.D., in *Pediatric Annals*.

774. Jump Ship with the Greatest of Ease

Sudden immersion in cold water can cause rapid, uncontrolled breathing, cardiac arrest, and other life-threatening problems, triggering what the Coast Guard calls sudden disappearance syndrome—someone falls in the water and never comes up again. If for some reason you must enter the water, says the Coast Guard, button up your clothing, don a personal flotation device, and enter the water slowly. Also, stay with the boat and get as much of your body out of the water as possible. This will help prevent loss of body heat.

775. Dress to Float

It's a common belief that someone dressed in long pants and waders will sink immediately should he fall in the water. Not necessarily true; such clothing can be a lifesaver.

Air trapped in the clothing can provide considerable buoyancy, and if you bend your knees, you can also get air trapped in your waders. If you remain calm and stay on your back with your knees bent, you should be able to paddle slowly without exhaustion.

If, however, you find your gear or waders are pulling you down, you should remove them immediately. The idea is to expend as little energy as possible until you can get out of the water.

776. An Ocean Is Not a Big Swimming Pool

Swimming in oceans and rivers is a lot different from swimming in a pool. "Don't assume that a hundred laps in your pool at home means you can swim the Colorado River," says Duncan Morrow, spokesman for the National Park Service. "Your pool isn't equipped with cold water, logs, and riptides." So don't push your limits and save enough energy to swim back to shore safely.

For safe open water swimming, also remember the following:

- Avoid hazardous areas such as dams, boat ramps, or areas with heavy boat traffic.
- At the beach, check to see if a warning flag has been raised and don't swim if the water or weather is rough.
- If you're caught in a current, don't try to swim against it. Swim away from the current at a perpendicular angle and then back to shore.

FACT OF LIFE

Salt Water Is Safest for Swimmers

Drownings occur more often in fresh water than salt water. Even in states bordering the seaboard, far more drownings take place in pools, rivers, and lakes than in the sea. Drownings involving boats also occur more frequently in fresh water.

777. Think Before You Dive

More than 70 percent of diving accidents result from plunging into shallow water of 4 feet or less.

"A swimming hole that was deep enough to dive into last year may be shallow this year, due to lack of rainfall," says John F. Ditunno, M.D., project director of the Regional Spinal Cord Injury Center of the Delaware River at Thomas Jefferson University Hospital in Philadelphia. Don't assume you know the depth, even if you're familiar with the location.

The American Red Cross offers additional safe diving advice.

- The first time you enter the water, slip in or walk in. Jumping into shallow water can be dangerous, too.
- Don't dive from the edge of a pool or low dock or from a springboard 20 inches or less above the water unless the water is at least 8 feet deep.
- If the diving board is 26 inches above the water, the water should be at least 10 feet deep; if 30 inches, water should be at least 12 feet deep, and if 39½ inches (1 meter), at least 16 feet deep.
- Never dive headfirst into an aboveground pool.
- Never dive off the sides of diving boards, ladders, or pool equipment, or off the sides of piers or rock jetties.

778. Party out of the Pool

Statistics shows that one-half of all drowning victims have significant levels of alcohol in their blood. Drinking alcohol before entering the water impairs your judgment, disorients your senses, and impairs your reflexes and swimming ability. Alcohol is also a vaso-dilator—it widens your blood vessels, promoting heat loss. This increases your chances of suffering hypothermia, or dangerously low body temperature.

779. Don't Battle the Mane

Swimming pools and hot tubs with suction-fitted drains pose a special danger to people with long hair: If the grate or cover on a sidewall drain is missing or broken, your hair can get snarled in the outlet, trapping you beneath the water level.

So if your hair is long, securely pin it up on your head or don a bathing cap before you enter a pool or hot tub.

Crime Stoppers

780. Give 'Em What They Want

If you're nose to nose with a robber, don't put up a fight. Crime experts say you should hand over your cash, credit cards, watch, or jewelry—whatever the assailant wants.

"It may run counter to current 'macho' thinking, but it's usually better to accommodate a criminal than to fight him," says Deputy Commissioner Robert F. Armstrong of the Philadelphia Police Force. "In the case of a street robbery, for example, you're best off giving the assailant what he wants. He's happy, and you're still alive."

Make a conscious effort to identify your attacker and report the crime to the police at once.

781. Burglars Hate Surprise Visitors

Burglars want to avoid confrontations—that's why they like to visit when you're not home. If you return home and see signs of a break-in—a door ajar, a screen slit, a window broken—don't enter the house. Back out of the driveway or keep walking to the nearest phone booth or neighbor's house and call the police. The only ones who should stop a burglary in action are those trained to do it: the police.

782. Give Your House That At-Home Look

Don't advertise that you're away by turning out the lights and leaving the garage empty for extended periods of time, says the National Crime Prevention Council. You should:

- Leave lights on and the radio playing, preferably tuned to a talk show.
- Use inexpensive timing devices to turn inside lights, the radio, or television on and off at different times.
- Have a neighbor or friend stop by your home frequently if you're going to be away for an extended period of time.
- Never leave a key "hidden" outside.
- Give your watchdog the run of your home. A penned-up dog is a small threat to a would-be burglar.

783. Make Sure Your Home Is Secure

When it comes to protecting your life and possessions, you're only as safe as your security system. The National Crime Prevention Council says the following is the best way to keep out the unwanted.

- Make sure outside doors, including the door between your house and garage, are constructed of solid, 1¾ inch metal or wood and fit tightly in their frames. Hinges should be on the inside, so an intruder can't unscrew the door from its hinges.
- Secure exterior doors with deadbolt locks.
- To secure a sliding glass door, place a rigid wooden dowel in the track. Or install a commercially available patio door lock.
- Keep windows locked at all times and, if necessary, fit them with metal grilles.

784. Don't Invite Trouble into Your Home

If someone knocks at your door, you should be able to identify the caller before you open the door. The National Crime Prevention Council recommends installing a peephole, wide-angle door viewer, or other device that allows you to see who's at your door without opening it. A short chain between the door and the jamb is not a good substitute because any intruder can easily break it.

785. Play Possum and Play It Safe

If you hear someone breaking into your house, don't confront him—he could be armed. And if you wake up and someone is in the room going through your belongings, pretend to be asleep. Wait until the intruder leaves, then call the police.

786. Don't Dance with Danger

You can cut your chances of being mugged or robbed by following this advice from the National Crime Prevention Council.

- When walking at night, travel the busiest street available (even if it's the longest route) and avoid passing vacant lots, alleyways, and construction sites.
- Stand tall and confident and be alert to what's happening around you.
- Women should carry their handbag crosswise over their shoulders and keep it firmly gripped. Men should carry their wallets in an inside coat or pants pocket, not in a rear pocket.
- When walking to your car, have your keys ready so you can unlock the door quickly. Check the backseat to make sure no one is hiding there, get in, and lock the doors *before* starting your car.
- If a motorist stops to ask you for directions, do not get close to the car; reply from a distance.
- In apartment buildings, hotels, and office buildings, familiarize yourself with emergency buttons on elevators. Stand near the controls, and if you're attacked, hit the alarm and as many floor buttons as possible.

FACT OF LIFE

Full Moon Brings Out the Worst in People

It's not superstition after all! More crimes are committed during a full moon than at other times of the month, according to a report in the *British Medical Journal*. Other studies have linked a full moon with aggressive behavior, injuries, murders, suicides, and admissions to hospitals for psychiatric problems.

Freak Accidents and Flukes of Nature

787. Don't Go Wild in the Wild

"Many of the accidents we see in the national parks are the product of a mind-set that doesn't recognize the parks for what they are—very different from the urban environment," says the National Park Service's Duncan Morrow. "People need to know that in many respects a park—any park, anywhere—is an alien environment and, like any new environment, it has its own set of rules."

Here are some basic tips for surviving in the woods.

- Pay attention. Gawking at gorgeous scenery leads to car wrecks and falls—the two leading killers in national parks.
- Don't feed animals or leave food out near a campsite. Wild animals are too unpredictable.
- Don't approach or get between *any* mother animal and her young. "Get between the gentlest-looking doe and her fawn, and she'll attack," says Morrow, "and when she's through, you'll look like you've been in a knife fight."

788. Get out of Harm's Way

Your chance of winning the million-dollar lottery is probably greater than your chance of being struck by lightning, especially if you know what to do when caught outdoors during an electrical storm.

- Avoid open areas where you're the tallest object. Stay away from hilltops, fields, beaches, bodies of water, tall isolated trees, electrical fences, telephone poles, and flagpoles.
- If you're with a group, have everyone spread out so that if one person is struck, the bolt won't jump to other people.
- Take shelter, if possible, in a closed automobile with a metal roof, or in thick woods.
- If you're in the forest, take refuge under a thick growth of small, not tall, trees.
- If no shelter is available, curl up on the ground, preferably in a ditch, gully, or culvert. Squat down with your hands drawn in and your feet close together to decrease potential contact points for lightning. Avoid wet soil if possible, since water is a

good conductor of electricity. If possible, position yourself on
a rubber raincoat, plastic sheet, or some other nonabsorbent
material to help protect against ground currents. Do not lie
flat.
- Stay away from metal equipment such as bicycles, umbrellas,
golf clubs, fishing rods, tent poles, or tractors.
- Remove your jewelry; it can attract lightning.

789. It's Good to Have Some Funnel Vision

Auntie Em and Toto may have known what to do, but if you're
a westerner who happens to be passing through Kansas at the same
time as a funnel cloud, you're headed for trouble if you don't know
the drill. Here's what you may need to know.
- Head for cover *real* fast if you hear a tornado warning. It
means a twister has been sighted, and you should seek shelter immediately. If you wait until you see or hear the tornado
or flying debris, you're already in serious danger.
- If you're inside a building, find shelter on the lowest floor,
preferably the basement, away from windows. Central areas,
including closets, interior hallways, and central stairwells, are
best. Avoid rooms along the outside of a building.
- If a basement isn't available, choose an inner hallway or some
small area away from windows.
- Protect your head and neck, areas most vulnerable to fatal
injuries during a tornado, by getting under something heavy
and using your arms to protect your head.
- If you live in a mobile home, seek shelter in a permanent
building. A mobile home can become *dangerously* mobile in a
twister.
- A car is the *last* place you want to be, says the National Safety
Council. If you're in your car and you see a tornado, don't try
to outrun it: Tornados are swift and erratic. If possible, leave
the car and find shelter in a building or drive away from the
tornado's path at a right angle. If the tornado is hot on your
heels, abandon your car and lie in the nearest ditch.
- Don't get under a car or next to one: In high wind, the vehicle may roll over onto you.

790. Shake, Rattle, and Roll

Most Californians know what to do in an earthquake. In the San Francisco earthquake of 1989, the residents were credited for knowing how to react, which many believe saved lives and avoided panic. Instructions are even given on the front page of California phone books. But not all earthquakes happen in California.

When an earthquake strikes, actual earth movement causes few deaths. It's the world collapsing around you that's your biggest threat.

Should you feel the earth move under your feet, here's what American Red Cross says you should know.

- If you're in the kitchen, turn off the stove at the first sign of shaking.
- If you're in a building, take cover under a desk or table (hold onto the legs so it won't creep away from you) or in an interior doorway.
- The National Safety Council says that if you're out on the road during an earthquake, it's best to stay in your car. The quake may shake the suspension system of your car until your teeth chatter, but your vehicle is still better than no protection at all. But don't park near buildings, highway overpasses, or utility wires.

Self-Help Emergency Action

791. Do-It-Yourself CPR

If you think you're having a heart attack and begin to lose consciousness, start coughing vigorously—about once every second. This "do-it-yourself" version of cardiopulmonary resuscitation can keep you conscious long enough to summon help. The technique was developed by John Michael Criley, M.D., chief of cardiology at the Harbor UCLA Medical Center in California. (If someone else is having a heart attack and you don't know how to administer CPR, you might be able to save their life by instructing them to keep coughing until help arrives.)

"Coughing causes the muscles of the abdomen and chest to

contract in such a way as to keep blood moving through the heart and to the brain," explains Dr. Criley. "[We've found] that the technique can maintain blood flow to the brain at levels equal to or greater than a normal heartbeat, and that consciousness can be maintained for a minute and a half, possibly longer."

792. You Can Stop Yourself from Choking

Make a fist with one hand and place the thumb side on the middle of your abdomen slightly above the navel and well below the tip of your breastbone. Grasp your fist with your other hand and give a quick upward thrust.

You can also lean forward and press your abdomen over any firm, nonsharp object, such as the back of a chair, a railing, or a sink.

793. Stop, Drop, and Roll

Fire needs oxygen to burn. So if your clothing catches fire, trying to run away or flailing your arms and legs will only fan the flames. Instead, you should follow the Stop, Drop, and Roll rule, endorsed by the American Red Cross.

- Stop wherever you are.
- Drop to the floor.
- Roll over and over to smother the flames.

794. Anaphylactic Shock: Be Prepared

For some people, certain drugs (like antibiotics or anesthetics), insect bites (like wasp stings), foods (like seafood or nuts), or exertion can cause the most serious allergic reaction possible: anaphylactic shock.

If you're one of them, within minutes of exposure to the allergen, your skin will begin to feel warm and start to itch. Your throat will feel as though it's closing, and your breathing will be labored. Hives, swelling, light-headedness, and weakness may also occur. You could even pass out. If untreated, anaphylactic shock can be fatal within 5 minutes to 30 minutes.

If you're at risk for anaphylactic shock, you should carry an emergency treatment kit that contains epinephrine, a synthetic hormone you can inject into your system to stop the reaction.

Lefties: Be Careful Out There

Statistics show that, on the average, people who are left-handed live nine months less than people who are right-handed, seemingly because lefties have more than their share of accidents. Corollary: Left-handed men have more than twice as many motor vehicle accidents as right-handed men.

Researchers attending a conference of the American Academy of Allergy and Immunology reported several cases of fatal allergic reactions to food in which all the victims knew of their allergy and had survived previous reactions. Some even had their treatment kits with them. Yet none of them took their medicine, the one step that could have saved their lives.

The researchers emphasize that sensitized individuals *must* carry and self-administer epinephrine at the first sign of a systemic reaction to avoid possible tragedy.

CHAPTER · 14

GROWING UP HEALTHY

Somewhere, in the early seconds of the year 2000, a child will be born. The event may go largely unnoticed, dimmed by the hoopla of the world greeting the birth of its next millennium.

But in a quiet hospital room away from all the confetti and paper hats, the newborn baby will lie cradled in his parents' arms. Theirs will be a night filled with hopes and dreams—hope for the next generation, dreams about a child growing up in good health and prosperity.

Those born in the year 2000 will have a lot to look forward to, not the least of which will be a very long life. According to figures from the Social Security Administration, boys born during that year will have an average life expectancy of 72.2 years; girls can expect to outlive them by another 8 years.

Now imagine the same scene, only 300 years earlier. The bedroom is dark and humid, the windows and drapes shut to keep out the noise and the dust from the street. Outside, an eighteenth-century celebration is going on as the residents of London usher in the new year of 1700.

Inside, a mother and child meet for the first time. And there are dreams. As the old midwife nods knowingly, the young mother talks not of hope that her new baby will live a long life, but of hope that the child will just survive. Life was much less of a sure thing back then.

The Age of Inopportunity

In the eighteenth century, two-thirds of the children born in the metropolitan area of London died before they were 5 years old. Two-thirds. Today the odds are much better for the 381,101 children born worldwide every day. Now, for every 100 children born, only 1 dies.

Writing in a book called *Domestic Medicine* published in 1784, one English doctor expressed shock at what he faced: "It appears from the annual register of the dead that almost one half of children born in Great Britain die under twelve years of age."

Children were no match for the infectious diseases of the eighteenth century. Smallpox, typhus, typhoid, measles, and diphtheria cut a deadly swath through the turn-of-the-century playgrounds. These epidemics, noted one writer, killed "as rapidly as wildfire can eradicate dry stubble." During one smallpox outbreak in Sweden, of the 300 children affected, 270 died.

Life was so tough for the young back then that even teething was "one of the most fatal affections of infancy." And if you were unlucky enough to catch a childhood disease, odds were against you that you'd ever make it to adulthood.

It wasn't until the end of the century that the fight against these infant killers intensified. That's when, for the first time, children were inoculated against diseases. And the massive dying stopped.

A Genuine Lifesaver

It was Edward Jenner, M.D., an English country doctor, who helped firmly root what appears today to be an ever-growing life span. In 1796, Dr. Jenner noticed that dairy workers never seemed to contract smallpox; instead they came down with a disease called cowpox. He took a perfectly healthy boy, an 8-year-old named James Phipps, and inoculated him with some "lymph from a cowpox sore taken from the hand of a milkmaid." James suffered some minor symptoms but escaped the disease.

Then the real test came. In July of 1796, Dr. Jenner introduced live, and possibly fatal, smallpox virus into James's system. James stayed healthy. A couple of months later, Dr. Jenner did it again. James still remained a healthy little boy. The rest, so to speak, is history.

FACT OF LIFE

Kids Winning over Leukemia

Kids may be winning the fight against leukemia, the disease that's the biggest threat to young lives. According to *Clinical Pediatrics*, acute lymphoblastic leukemia (ALL) is still the cause of more deaths than any other childhood disease after the first year of life—but during the last decade the survival rate has improved to 65 percent.

In time, other vaccinations appeared, and the results were just as dramatic. Polio had always been a serious childhood disease of almost epidemic proportions. In 1952 there were 58,000 reported cases alone. After a vaccine was discovered in 1955, reported cases dropped to 15,000 the following year. By 1986 there were only 8 cases.

Today children are routinely vaccinated. It's the law. In order to go to school, they have to get their shots before they get their books.

Modern Threats

Nowadays accidents have replaced illness as the number one killer of infants and children. The National Safety Council reports that nearly 4,000 children aged 1 to 4 die each year as a result of injuries sustained in an accident. Motor vehicle accidents top the list as the most common cause of death, followed by fires and burns, drownings, falls, and choking on food and other objects.

Disease, however, cannot be downplayed. Although modern medicine has established a safe harbor against childhood diseases, popular practices are setting them up for developing life-threatening conditions and illnesses later in life. The American Academy of Pediatrics says that about 80 percent of obese children go on to become obese adults. Heart disease risk factors—such as high cholesterol and high-fat diets—are being detected in the young. Studies claim America's children are out of shape, and a report from the Public Voice for Food and Health states that poor dietary habits can even be traced right to the school. The average school lunch, states the organization, contains 39 percent of calories from fat—9 percent above what the American Heart Association considers healthful.

But kids today are luckier than ever before. Vaccines have made many former commonplace diseases, such as croup and measles, almost unheard of today. And you can teach your children to eat right and get the right kind of exercise. You can prevent accidents from happening.

The bottom line is, you can take the lead in starting your child off on a long and healthy life. Here's how.

A Head Start on Good Health

795. Immunization Is a Must

Measles, mumps, rubella (German measles), polio, pertussis (whooping cough), diphtheria, tetanus, and hemophilus meningitis (Hib) may be rare today, but they aren't unheard of. Nor are they harmless childhood illnesses. All of them can kill. But they're also easily preventable. The American Academy of Pediatrics has developed a recommended immunization schedule (see the chart on page 354) that tells you just when the inoculations are needed.

If you don't happen to have a pediatrician or family physician, call your local public health department. The department usually has supplies of vaccine on hand and may even give the shots free.

796. Be Cautious with Hib

When your child nears his scheduled appointment for his Hib shot (usually in his eighteenth month), pay close attention so that he doesn't come into contact with a child who already has hemophilus meningitis. If he does or you suspect he has, contact your doctor and postpone the appointment; it could actually put him at risk for contracting the bacterial infection.

"Hemophilus bacteria from an infected playmate or family member can take up residence in your child's nose or throat," says Dan Granoff, M.D., professor of pediatrics at Washington University School of Medicine in St. Louis. "The Hib vaccine may create a window of vulnerability by tying up the child's antibodies for a few days. With the body's normal defenses down, the bacteria already present has a chance to take hold and develop into meningitis."

Your doctor will probably postpone the shot for 10 days or so and prescribe the antibiotic called rifampin to wipe out the infection.

The Best Protection against Disease

Getting your child vaccinated means protection against major diseases. Polio, measles, mumps, German measles, whooping cough, diphtheria, tetanus, and hemophilus (Hib) infections can safely be avoided simply by following the following immunization schedule recommended by the American Academy of Pediatrics.

It's a good idea to check with your pediatrician to make sure your children are up-to-date on their shots.

Age	DPT	Polio	TB test	Measles	Mumps	Rubella	Hib	TD (tetanus, diphtheria)
2 months	■	■						
4 months	■	■						
6 months	■							
1 year			■					
15 months				■	■	■		
18 months	■	■					■	
4 to 6 years	■	■						
14 to 16 years								■

797. Switch to Aspirin Substitutes

Play it safe and never give your children aspirin when they are feeling ill. Instead, give them acetaminophen or ibuprofen.

Aspirin has been linked to Reye's syndrome, a potentially fatal disease affecting the brain. Doctors have found Reye's in children who were given aspirin while suffering from the flu or chickenpox. As a result, doctors have issued warnings about not giving aspirin to children suffering with these illnesses.

But not anymore. They're now saying the safest thing is to stay away from giving children aspirin altogether. "Refrain from using aspirin to reduce fevers in children and adolescents," says the California Medical Association. "Generally when treatment of a fever and associated symptoms is necessary, an aspirin substitute (acetaminophen) may be used."

The association states this is a good practice to follow until the child reaches the age of 18.

By the way, apparently a lot of parents are heeding this warning. There has been a marked decline in the incidence of Reye's syndrome in recent years. Doctors from the Centers for Disease Control in Atlanta say that cases have fallen 60 percent, even though the number of cases of chickenpox and flu has remained the same.

798. Pay Attention to Sore Throats

Ask your mother and father about their fears of rheumatic fever. Up until the pre-antibiotic days of the late 1940s, many a parent stood by helplessly and watched a child's sore throat develop into a permanently disabling heart condition known as rheumatic fever. By the 1970s, thanks to antibiotics, rheumatic fever had all but disappeared.

But now it's back. No one seems to know why. One theory claims that a stronger strain of streptococcus—the bacteria that produces what is commonly known as strep throat—may have evolved, but it has yet to be proven.

This doesn't mean that antibiotics can't kill a strep infection. They can—which is why doctors recommend that you should never ignore a child with symptoms of a sore throat. A sore throat that lasts more than a day or two, especially if it is accompanied by fe-

FACT OF LIFE

A Punch in the Nose for Kids

Nose drops are not quite as innocuous as they seem, say Swedish doctors. At least 6 infants and small children who were taking nose drops experienced side effects that involved their central nervous system. The effects ranged all the way from deep sleep to excitability, insomnia, and even convulsions. Given the central nervous system immaturity of young children, such effects may be life-threatening.

ver—should be checked out by a physician. A simple throat culture to test if strep is present can prevent problems of heart valve damage, due to rheumatic fever, from developing later in life.

It takes about 10 days of continual medication to get rid of the strep bug, so make sure your child keeps taking his medicine even if all the symptoms appear to be gone.

799. Don't Smoke in Front of Your Kids

You know smoking is harmful to *your* health, but did you know that your smoking can be harmful to your children's health as well? It's a fact.

The next time you light up and take a drag, watch where that smoke ring goes. You'll see it break up and drift away—right into the path and the lungs of those around you.

It's called passive smoking, and it's what happens when other people breathe in the smoke you exhale or the smoke that curls from your cigarette. The formaldehyde, ammonia, and hydrogen cyanide you're exhaling or emitting from a lit cigarette put your children (like yourself) at a much greater risk for a variety of symptoms and illnesses like asthma, upper and lower respiratory tract infections, bronchitis, pneumonia, and lung cancer.

In other words, it could damage their lungs for life. "The more attacks of bronchitis or pneumonia on the lung system, the greater the possibility of years of lung function impairment," says Frank Pedreira, M.D., clinical associate professor of pediatrics at George Washington Medical School in Washington, D.C.

"If you have a child at home, particularly an infant in the first year of life, don't smoke!"

800. Passive Smoking: Double Trouble for Boys

Boys going through puberty in smoking households have a greater chance of developing risk factors that lead to heart disease than boys living with nonsmoking families, one study shows.

"Chronic exposure to even low amounts of cigarette smoke affects the heart and blood fats of 12-year-old boys and may put them at higher risk of accelerated heart disease in the following decades of their lives," says William Moskowitz, M.D., assistant professor of pediatric cardiology at the Medical College of Virginia.

FACT OF LIFE

Everybody Gets Sick at Once

A six-year study of 2,591 children showed that the same children—representing 20 percent of the total group—got sick time after time. The reason? Heredity as well as social and environmental stresses all act together to produce illness-prone children. Moreover, these same youngsters, concluded the researchers, are likely to be tomorrow's illness-prone adults.

During puberty, varying levels of testosterone and other sex hormones in boys cause changes in the particles that carry fats and cholesterol in the blood. Those changes, explains Dr. Moskowitz, "promote atherosclerosis or hardening of the arteries."

In a study of a group of 11- and 12-year-old boys from families that smoke, Dr. Moskowitz found that the children had stiffer aortas, thicker heart walls, and lower levels of HDL2 (a protein that reduces the risk of atherosclerosis) than did boys from nonsmoking families.

The boys from smoking families had "significantly greater" coronary heart disease risk factors than boys from nonsmoking families. "This gives smokers another reason to quit, because they are damaging the long-term health of their children who involuntarily inhale the smoke."

801. Teens Should Run from Breast Cancer

Want to put your daughter on the right track to avoid cancer? Have her start running, swimming, or dancing.

A study conducted at the University of Southern California School of Medicine found that moderate exercises like running for as little as 2 hours a week can prevent teenage girls from ovulating.

Previous studies have shown that breast cancer rates are significantly lower among women who have fewer lifetime ovulatory cycles.

During ovulation, women produce estrogen in large quantities. Estrogen may be linked to breast cancer. The researchers believe that the less a women ovulates, the less estrogen she produces, which may result in less of a cancer risk. They also say the teenage years are the only time in a woman's life when it is easy to alter the menstrual cycle through physical activity.

802. Help the Overweight Lose Weight

If your child is overweight, exercise and a healthy diet can actually save his life. A study published in the medical journal *Pediatrics* reports that "obese adolescents are at a high risk for the development of coronary heart disease, and exercise, in addition to moderate diet restriction, can result in the reduction of multiple coronary heart disease risk."

For tips on losing weight, turn to chapter 3.

803. Think Twice about Incense and Drugs

You just wanted to have your house smell nice, but have you put your child at risk to develop leukemia because you burn incense?

Researchers at the University of Southern California recently found that children of parents who burn incense at home had a risk of leukemia almost three times greater than children whose parents didn't burn incense.

The same researchers questioned whether the incense was responsible for the increased risk or if it was due to something else that the researchers believe often goes hand in hand with incense burning: "marijuana or other drug use."

FACT OF LIFE

Making Fat Kids

It only takes an extra 50 calories a day to turn a small child with a tendency toward obesity into a small child who's fat, doctors say. Other causes of childhood obesity? Television (which turns children into inactive toadstools faster than the wicked witch), heredity, poor eating habits, and stringent dieting.

804. Get a Foothold on Emergencies

Where your children go, so too should go their medical history. It could prove an invaluable lifesaver during a medical emergency.

CRITIKID is a microfilm chip that attaches to your child's shoelace; during a life-threatening emergency, it could give him the foot up he needs to survive.

The chip contains your child's personal vital medical information, which emergency or hospital personnel can read by using a microscope or microfilm viewer.

You can call your local hospital to see if they distribute the CRITIKID tags, or you can buy them direct for about $11 by writing to CRITICARD Inc., 4M Plaza, 4 South 100, Rte. 59, Naperville, IL 60563.

Safety: First and Foremost

805. Introduce Your Kids to Fire Safety

We all know that smoke detectors installed near all the sleeping areas in your home will alert the family to a fire. But a smoke alarm alone isn't always enough to save the lives of your children. You need to plan what to do in case of a fire *before* you have a fire.

Fire officials state that children under 5 are at greatest risk of dying in fires because they panic and hide under beds or in closets where they can't be found in time.

Plan a fire escape route out of your house and show your children how to crawl through it. Always plan two ways to get out of every room and figure out how you would escape from the second or third floor if your house has more than one story.

Decide on a meeting place outside your house and plan who'll take charge of getting each child there. If you live in an apartment building, warn your children not to use the elevator and make sure they know where the fire escape is.

And maybe most important of all, check your smoke detector monthly to make sure it is operating properly. Don't just push the little red test button. Check it by using the real smoke of a candle held near the unit.

806. Baby Walkers: Unsafe at Any Speed

Had God wanted 5-month-old babies to walk, he might have equipped them with wheels at the end of their little legs. But he didn't. And for good reason. Infants don't understand danger.

Baby walkers are infant training wheels that unfortunately can propel a baby down a path to danger. "Babies and walkers tend to be top-heavy, and frequently the walker can flip over, causing severe injury to a child's head," says George Stern, M.D., chairman of the American Academy of Pediatrics.

That's why babies in walkers have plunged into pools, tumbled down stairs, scooted over to the stove and pulled pots of boiling water onto themselves, or even yanked on tablecloths, sending glasses and knives their way.

There are also developmental concerns surrounding walkers, says Dr. Stern. Studies have shown that children who use walkers are more likely to walk with their legs turned out in a tiptoe fashion, and there is even some suggestion that the child's heel cords tighten.

Your child will spend almost all his life getting around in an upright position. So let him enjoy a brief time of crawling before he enters a lifetime of walking.

807. Avoid Window Pains

Believe it or not, a young child can fall out a window that's open only 5 inches. To prevent that from happening, install window guards. Window screens are made to keep bugs out, not children in, so don't rely on them for protection.

If you don't have window guards, open your windows from the top if that's possible. And when your windows aren't open, keep them locked so they can't be opened without your knowing about it.

808. Block the Stairway to Heaven

For children aged 1 to 4, falls in the home are the leading cause of accidental death. Most of these deaths are caused by children tumbling down stairs.

To really see the danger, get down on your hands and knees at the bottom of your stairs and look up. That's how the staircase looks to your child—a Mount Everest of deep pile.

Put safety gates at the top and bottom of the stairs and attach the top gate to a wall. When you get gates, avoid the old accordion type that have large openings, because a child's head could become stuck in them.

If possible, carpet your stairs. It could cushion a fall. And never let your children play on or near the staircase.

809. Play It Cool with Your Tap Water

Kids are always getting into hot water. That's expected. But if they get into boiling water, it can cause the unexpected.

Think of your hot water tank as a big white teakettle. All you want to do with the water inside is to keep it simmering, not boiling, and you'll still be able to take a nice hot shower.

Turn the temperature setting outside the tank to no higher than 120°F. Even if a child turns on only the hot faucet, at that setting the child won't get scalded.

If you live in an apartment, you or your landlord can install a regulating valve that won't let the water go beyond a certain temperature.

810. Take the Back Burner to Safety

A watched pot never boils, but a boiling pot needs watching, especially if there are young children around. Turn the handles of pots and pans toward the back of the stove so a child can't reach up and pull them over. Better yet, to keep pots out of a kid's reach altogether, use the rear burners of your stove whenever possible.

811. Old Toy Chests Belong in the Attic

Remember that old wooden toy chest you had with Hopalong Cassidy painted on the side? Well, it could ambush your child if you've passed it on down to him, warns the U.S. Consumer Product Safety Commission.

Old toy chests have very heavy lids that can slam down on a child's head or neck when they reach in for a toy. If your child has a toy chest that has a free-falling lid, it's okay to still use it for storing toys only if you *remove the lid.*

If you're in the market for a new toy chest, the commission recommends you look for one with supports that will hold the lid open in any position. Toy chests with sliding panels or lightweight removable lids are just as safe.

812. Dispose of Disposable Lighters

You've told your child to never play with matches, and the matches you have around your house are kept well out of reach. But what about those cheap disposable butane lighters? You might not realize it, but they have become the "matches" of the present day.

According to the Shriners Burn Institute in Cincinnati, of the 70 reports they received concerning kids and fire, 1 out of 5 involved a disposable lighter. And we're not talking strictly big kids here—three of the children were less than 22 months old.

If you're wondering how a child that young could have the finger strength and dexterity needed to operate the lighter, you need to realize that he's not using it to light a cigarette but as a toy.

To a child, a wheel is a wheel, whether it's on a toy car or a butane lighter. Wheels are made to roll, and that's when the accident happens. The child uses the lighter as if it were a toy car, rolling it along on its wheel. A few good rolls can develop a spark, and if it's held in the right angle, the butane release valve will open, adding fuel to the fire. So, suddenly the "toy car"' the child thought he was rolling across the rug catches the child's clothes on fire.

Best advice: Keep your disposable lighter in the same spot you keep your disposable matches, out of your child's reach.

813. Leave Air Guns for the Air Force

Air guns do not shoot blanks; they shoot BB's, pellets, or even darts, all of which kill children every year.

Some of today's "toy" air guns have a muzzle velocity of 900 feet per second, which is dangerously close to that of a .22-caliber pistol. The U.S. Consumer Product Safety Commission warns that "parents don't realize the projectiles from high velocity air guns can penetrate the skull. They can kill."

If your child really must have an air rifle, look for one with a low velocity, less than 350 feet per second. Be warned, though, that even that speed is fast enough to put an eye out.

Whether your child owns a gun or not, it's important to teach him or her that these things are not toys but weapons, and they are very dangerous.

Your best bet: Buy your young Daniel Boone a water gun instead of an air gun. Tell him it's much better to give an unsuspecting squirrel a bath than it is to shower it with BB's.

814. Put Recliners Off Limits

If Dad's favorite chair is the recliner, then make it his private domain. The American Furniture Manufacturers Association wants parents to know that reclining chairs can be a hazard to young children. At least three children from the ages of 12 to 36 months have been killed playing in recliner chairs.

The children were apparently playing on the unoccupied chair while it was left in the reclined position. When they stuck their heads in the opening between the chair seat and the leg rest, they became trapped because the weight of their own body forced the leg rest down.

If you have a recliner in your house, always leave it in the upright, closed position when it is not in use. When shopping for a new recliner, look for a model that has a device installed on it that reduces the opening between the leg rest and seat cushion when the chair is in the reclined position.

815. Keep Outlets out of Reach

Anyone with young children around the house should cover *all* unused electrical outlets with safety caps. Anything with holes in it is a toddler's greatest temptation.

816. Kiddy Pools Need Lifeguards, Too

Never leave children unsupervised around water, whether it's a swimming pool, a kiddy pool, or even a bathtub. Children have drowned in as little as 2 inches of water.

If you have a pool, make sure you put a fence around it, not just for the safety of your kids but for the safety of all the children in the neighborhood. Even if the only pool you have is a little kiddie pool, never leave it standing with water in it. Drain it after every use.

817. This Three-Wheeler's Not for Kids

All-terrain vehicles (ATVs) are taking kids off the road and straight into the hospital. When the Centers for Disease Control conducted a statewide study of ATV accidents in a two-year period in Alaska, they found that 20 people had died while using the three-wheel ATVs.

Doctors at the University of Alabama at Birmingham Spinal Cord Injury Care System are well aware of the dangers of ATVs. "There is an inherent lack of stability of the vehicle due to the triangular wheelbase design. In addition, the ATVs generally lack a rear suspension system capable of absorbing shocks from bumps."

Even the four-wheel version, which will eventually phase out the three-wheeler, is considered a safety hazard because of the potential speed of the vehicle—up to 70 miles per hour.

If your children have access to an ATV, make sure they really know how to operate it, and that they do so under adult supervision. Also make sure they stay off public roads and away from hazardous or unknown terrain, and that they always wear protective clothing while riding it.

818. Toddlers Can Tumble

If you ride your bicycle with a toddler in a rear-mounted child seat, make sure you buy baby a helmet, too.

In a California study of 52 accidents involving parents riding with a child, 65 percent of the children suffered head or face injuries.

"Parents should be made aware of the risks involved with these carriers, especially the possibility of severe head injury," report the researchers. They say that the risk of serious injury could be reduced "if children using these seats wore appropriate helmets."

819. Practice Safe Driveway Tips

A Washington State five-year study found that in all its fatal pedestrian accidents involving children, more than half of those under age 4 died as a result of an accident in a driveway. And sadly, most times, it was the child's own driveway.

In 64 percent of the cases, the accidents occurred while a vehicle was backing up, with trucks and vans driven by friends or family being most often involved.

Start looking out for toddlers as soon as you start your car. Make sure the mirrors are adjusted for you, and that they give you a good view. If your children want to wave goodbye, have them do it from the lawn, and not the driveway. That way they'll also be able to wave hello when you come back.

820. Helmets Offer Top-Notch Protection

Head injuries cause three-quarters of all bicycle-accident fatalities, even at very low speeds. A fall from a bike also can permanently damage your child's brain.

When a child falls from a bike while wearing a helmet, the helmet and not his head takes the force of the blow. The liner inside the helmet crushes on impact, reducing the dangerous force to the head. Most helmets also give added protection by having a hard-shell covering which prevents any sharp object from penetrating.

Buying a helmet may be easier than getting your child to wear it. If you can, start him wearing the helmet while he is still young: That way, it will become a normal piece of bicycle equipment.

If your older kids tell you they feel like wimps wearing one, point out that nonwimp race car drivers and motorcyclists always wear helmets.

To show them how serious you are about it, the next time you go riding with your child, make sure you wear *your* helmet.

FACT OF LIFE

"Wheelies"—A Cause of Injuries

Two British emergency room teams report an "epidemic" of injuries to children riding BMX bikes. The Southampton General Hospital's emergency room treated 23 in 35 days—including a ruptured spleen—while the Sheffield emergency room saw 100 in 40 days.

At both hospitals, doctors found that most of the accidents had occurred while the riders were doing "wheelies" and other stunts; 23 of the Sheffield kids had been thrown over the handlebars in sudden stops. The Southampton doctors noted that only one of their patients had been wearing a helmet and elbow pads. Even he was injured.

821. Teach Your Child Street Smarts

Unless you live on Sesame Street, the street outside your house is a dangerous place to play. Young children think that since they can see the cars, the drivers of the cars can also see them. They think that cars can stop instantly, and they can't judge how fast traffic is moving.

They need to be taught about how to cross the street. The best way to do that is by taking them for a walk and showing them how.

Teach them to stop at the curb or edge of the street and never, never run out into traffic. Have them look to their right, and left, and right and left again. If they don't know their left from their right, tell them to "look this way, that way, this way, and back again."

Tell them to look and make sure the street is perfectly clear before stepping off the curb and to always keep looking until they're safely across.

822. Pickups Are for Cargo, Not Kids

If you don't know where children are supposed to ride in pickup trucks, just look for where the manufacturer put the seats. Chances are they put the seats *inside* the cab, not in the cargo area. That's the only place to put your children.

How much sense does it make to spoil all the fun kids can have in the back? In just one year, 80 children died in pickup accidents while riding in the open bed of the truck, reports the National Highway Traffic Safety Administration.

823. Car Seats Should Fit the Child

The use of child seats for those under age 4 is now law in all 50 states. But the seat you have will not give your child the best protection if it's not the right size. That means you will probably need more than one as your child grows.

When getting a car seat for your child, make sure you get one that makes a perfect fit. Babies under 18 to 20 pounds need rear-facing seats; after 20 pounds you can go for a front-facing seat. Older children weighing 30 to 60 pounds can use a booster seat with a front shield, and once they get around age 4 or 5 they can use the regular seat belts that are standard equipment now in all cars.

Here are some other tips on what to look for when buying a car seat.

- Look for car seats made after January 1, 1981. You can do that by checking the date tag or sticker on the back of the seat.
- Baby seats are not car seats, even though they look like they might be. You'll be able to tell the difference by looking for the word "safety" in the product description on the box.
- Avoid buying secondhand seats, if possible. If you must, avoid those with cracks in the plastic, dents in the framework, frayed and worn harness straps, or missing buckles or fasteners. Any of these defects could compromise the safety and structural integrity of the seat.

How important are car seats? According to the National Highway Traffic Safety Administration, in one year, 200 children's lives were saved in car accidents because they were in a car seat.

824. Give Your Kid a Belt

And make sure he uses it *all the time.*

Seat belts save lives. In one study conducted by the Centers for Disease Control in North Carolina, 1,100 lives were saved in one year as a result of seat belts. And the National Highway Traffic Safety Administration reports that seat belts are 45 percent effective in preventing fatalities.

If you've ever wanted to belt your kid, here's your chance.

FACT OF LIFE

Cars, the Number One Threat

Car accidents are the number one killer of children aged 2 to 6. Every year, 11,000 children are killed by cars. You don't need any better excuse than this to make sure your children use seat belts or car seats.

825. Carry On a Car Seat

Most parents know that the safest way for an infant or young child to travel in an automobile is strapped into a safety seat. But did you know that it's also the safest way for a child to fly?

A child held on your lap while on an airplane is not secure during a crash or even a bumpy ride. "During turbulence, a tightly held child can literally fly out of a parent's lap," says Richard Snyder, Ph.D., who directed crash-impact research for the University of Michigan's Highway Safety Research Institute.

A Harvard study concluded that use of infant restraints on commercial airplanes would save three babies' lives over five years. Yet, babies are the only airplane passengers who are not required to be strapped in during takeoff and landing. And in fact, many airlines permit children to fly free only if parents hold them in their lap.

If you want your child to travel in a safety seat, you'll have to take your own (since the airlines don't provide them), and you will probably have to pay the extra fare. You might be able to use the infant seat for free, however, if there are any empty seats on the flight.

826. Use DEET Prudently

Insect repellents are supposed to be toxic to bugs, but some may also be toxic to kids.

Diethyltoluamide (DEET), an ingredient found in most insect repellents, has been found to produce toxic reactions in some children after repeated applications, warns Lee A. Kaplan, M.D., of the University of California School of Medicine in La Jolla.

The chemical, which can irritate the skin, can also be absorbed into the bloodstream. Infants and chidren are particularly at risk because, proportionately, they have a greater skin surface area than adults. Once absorbed, DEET is carried to internal organs and can even affect the child's nervous system, resulting in slurred speech, headaches, and convulsions.

If your insect repellent contains DEET, use it sparingly on your child and don't use it for more than two consecutive days, advises Dr. Kaplan. It's best to apply a very small amount to his skin and use the remainder on his clothing or carrier.

Other kinds of insect repellents are available that contain the ingredient N, N-diethyl-methyl-toluamide. The label should list the

Life-Extension Tool

Pool Alarms

It's a splash no one hears. Screams and sirens are the only sounds that alert the neighborhood to the tragedy.

"Every year about 100 to 500 children drown in pools nationwide, and an additional 4,000 or so almost drown and need hospitalization," says Merle Stoner, president of Poolguard Industries, an Indiana distributor of one type of pool alarm.

"In children aged 1 to 5, drowning in pools is the second leading cause of accidental death in the home. In some states like Florida, California, and Arizona, where there are lots of pools, it's the number one cause. Most often it happens in the child's own backyard in an in-ground pool."

But it doesn't have to happen at all. If you have young children and a pool, you should also have a pool alarm. "Pool alarms are the last line of defense," says Stoner. "After fences and self-latching gates, when all the other barriers you've put up have been crossed, then a pool alarm is all that's standing between you and a drowning."

Like children, pool alarms come in a wide variety of sizes and shapes.

Wave motion detection devices. These products could probably be called the first generation of pool alarms. They're buoys with brains. "The alarm floats on the water, and when it detects a wave, it sounds an alarm both at the pool and inside the house," says Joanne Booth of Remington Products, one of the many distributors of floating pool alarms.

Some of these devices may give an alarm when triggered by wind-caused waves. Most, however, can be adjusted to eliminate these false alarms. Installation is easy: Just insert a battery and place the alarm in the pool. If your pool is more than 20 feet by 40 feet, it's a good idea to have two alarms. Prices for these devices range from $70 to $150.

Pressure-sensitive alarm. This L-shaped device detects changes in water pressure. "One end rests on the deck, and the other end goes into the water. When a child or pet falls into the pool, water is sent up the tube, which sounds an alarm at the pool and in your house," says Stoner. The suggested retail price for this product is around $250.

Aqualert Monitoring System. This system serves as an alarm for both your pool and your child. The Aqualert Monitoring System has

(continued)

Life-Extension Tool—*Continued*

three components: a sensor installed in the pool, a battery-operated alarm, and an electro-medallion that the child wears.

You attach the medallion to your child's clothing, or have the child wear it around his neck. Should the child fall into the water, contact is established between the medallion and the sensor, and a piercing alarm is sounded.

The suggested retail price of this system is about $300.

All of these pool alarm systems, along with other brands and varieties, can be found at your local swimming pool supply store or in many mail-order catalogs.

---

additive, followed by a percentage. The lower the percentage, the better. While it may not be as good as DEET in getting rid of the bugs, it won't be as potentially harmful to your child.

For infants, avoid repellents altogether and cover them up instead. If the temperature allows, dress your baby in long sleeves and cotton trousers and cover his crib or carrier with mosquito netting to keep the insects from reaching him in the first place.

827. Follow the Axiom "Out of Sight, Out of Reach"

Everything looks like food to a toddler, especially tiny little pills and medicines. Anything he can get his hands on, he can put in his mouth and usually will.

In a one-year period, over 60,000 cases of children under age 5 accidentally swallowing oral prescription drugs were reported to the American Association of Poison Control Centers. In a follow-up study of 306 child-resistant medicine containers, 65 percent were found not to be working properly. The study's authors warn, "Parents cannot rely upon packaging alone to prevent access by young children."

For that reason, keep all the medicine in your house in places that are out of a toddler's reach. Don't be lulled into a false sense of security because many of them may be in "childproof" containers. Given enough time and determination, children can open anything.

828. Put Medicines under Combination Lock

If you keep your medicines under lock, chances are your child knows where you keep the key. Inventive and determined children have been known to go after the "hidden" key when their parents are out of sight and then use it to open the medicine container.

To thwart this, use a container that has, or will allow you to use, a combination lock. Never let your child watch you when you dial in the numbers.

829. Flush Your Medicines Away

You may take great precautions locking up your medicines, but you just might toss all that safety out when you discard outdated medicines in the garbage.

A good way to make sure you won't trash your child's safety is to flush old medicines down the toilet when you know you no longer need them.

830. Childproof Grandma's House, Too

Your house may be childproof when it comes to medicines, but what about Grandma's house? Nearly 1 out of every 6 preschoolers poisoned by medications took their grandparents' medicine.

Many elderly people, because of arthritis, request that their prescriptions be put in containers that are not childproof, so they are easier to open. Let Grandma and Grandpa know of your concern and have them put their medicine out of reach when the grandkids come for a visit.

831. Put Purses out of Reach

Guests can bring danger to your house without even knowing it. Purses often contain such things as cosmetics, scissors, nail files, and medicines. A curious child doing what he shouldn't could be setting himself up for trouble.

Don't leave purses belonging to guests lying around on the floor or on a bed under a pile of jackets. Put the visitor's purse where you should be putting your own purse—out of a child's reach.

Children Are in Tune with Their Health

When children are allowed to make their own decisions regarding personal health, they generally perform exceptionally well. A University of California School of Medicine program shows that kids aged 5 to 12 are capable both of determining when they need medical help and at complying with medical advice on their own. They are also better than their parents at identifying particular stressors in their lives and figuring out how to deal with them.

All of this doesn't mean that parents shouldn't monitor their children's health, doctors say. It simply shows that kids are more in tune with themselves and their surroundings than adults generally give them credit for.

832. Keep Cleansers over the Counter

Putting cleansers and cleaners under the sink may be convenient for you, but it's also putting your child eye-to-eye with poison.

Move your cleaning supplies to the top shelf of a cabinet or closet. If it's inconvenient for you, you'll know it's probably impossible for your child.

833. Give Empty Jars the Boot

Mayonnaise jars are made to hold one thing, mayonnaise. The same goes for peanut butter jars, salad dressing bottles, and milk containers.

You may know that the old container that once contained lemonade now holds turpentine, but does your child know? To a child, turpentine, gasoline, or bleach are salad dressing when they're in the dressing jar.

834. Go Organic

To unsuspecting toddlers, the slug bait you use in your garden can look like a hidden cache of candy. The desire to take a handful and pop them into their mouths is irresistible. It's better to put up with pests in the garden then risk an unfortunate accident.

Also, research is showing that spraying new shrubs and plants with insecticides may increase the risk of leukemia in children.

Children have four times the risk of developing leukemia when pesticides are used in the home, and six times the risk when garden sprays are used on the lawn, according to the study.

If you do use insecticides, don't let your children play and roll around on your lawn.

835. Learn to Identify Pretty Poison

Plant poisonings account for about 75,000 calls to poison centers every year.

Philodendron, lily of the valley, English ivy, hyacinth, iris, daffodil, deadly nightshade (why else would they call it that?), rhododendron, azalea, dumb cane, and oleander are just a few of the plants toxic to children. So, too, are the common Christmas ornamentals holly, mistletoe, and poinsettia.

If your child should happen to eat all or part of these plants, call your local poison control center immediately. Luckily, most of the time kids rarely eat enough of the plant to cause them more than an upset stomach or mouth irritation.

836. Put Small Toys to the Test

Any caring parent knows not to give small toys to small children. They know the danger of getting the toy or part of the toy lodged in a child's throat. But how can you tell when a toy is too small?

You can buy a device called a No-Choke Testing Tube that will let you measure the toy in a matter of seconds. The tube has been used for years in federal toy testing labs and is available through Toys to Grow On, P.O. Box 17, Long Beach, CA 90801. The test is simple: Take a toy and see if it fits in the small cylinder device. If it does, it's a hazard and shouldn't be given to small kids.

837. Only Buy Pacifiers That Measure Up to This Test

If you've ever tried to pry a pacifier from a baby's mouth, you know the baby can develop quite a lot of suction. If the pacifier isn't big enough, the child could suck it back into the throat.

The U.S. Consumer Product Safety Commission warns that some commercial pacifiers are actually too small and pose a health risk to the baby using one of them.

To be safe, look for a pacifier that has a circumference of not less than 2¼ inches.

838. Leave the Nipples in the Bottles

The use of old baby-bottle nipples as a sort of homemade pacifier has killed 10 children in the last few years.

The New York State Department of Health says that many parents and hospital nurseries make pacifiers by sticking cardboard shields or other padding onto the back of baby-bottle nipples. The problem is that the backing can come off, and the child could then inhale or swallow the nipple. The report went on to say that all 10 deaths could have been prevented had a regular pacifier been used instead.

The Nutritional Edge

839. Let Fat Babies Be Fat

Don't worry about the rolls of fat on your baby's leg—babies need baby fat.

Experts will tell you that babies are constantly growing, and because of that they need and use calories much faster than an adult.

Researchers at New York's North Shore University Hospital found that when some parents put their babies on a low-fat, low-calorie regimen intending to prevent future obesity or heart disease, the children developed instead a condition called "nonorganic failure to thrive."

The infants, 7 in all, had poor weight gains and showed a decreased growth rate. The babies were only consuming 60 to 94 percent of the calories recommended for their age. Once back on a higher-calorie diet, the babies gained weight and started growing normally again.

It's best to wait until your child is age 2 or older, or showing doctor-diagnosed signs of obesity, before you start worrying about calories, say the researchers.

840. Breastfed Is Best

Research indicates that mother's milk may offer protection against some types of cancers.

According to work done at the National Institute of Child Health and Human Development, children who are breastfed for at least six months developed significantly fewer cases of lymphoma, brain tumors, and leukemia than did children fed only formula.

841. Try the Working Mother's Formula

Working mothers who want to breastfeed can help keep their baby on mother's milk around the clock by expressing milk into bottles and dropping it off with the baby at the day-care center.

842. Make the First Test a Cholesterol Test

What's in your blood could also be in your child's blood. The American Academy of Pediatrics is recommending that all children over the age of 2 with a family history of elevated blood-fat levels or early coronary heart disease get regular cholesterol testing.

The pediatricians say that "children with levels persistently exceeding 176 for cholesterol should be considered for dietary counseling."

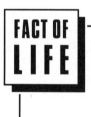

FACT OF LIFE

Breastfeeding Protects the Ears

Not only does breastfeeding protect children against middle ear infections during infancy, report researchers at the University of Helsinki, but the effect apparently lasts well into childhood. In one study, for example, only 6 percent of those who had been breastfed developed ear infections by the age of 3, while 26 percent of a formula-fed group had developed at least one. The delay is important, doctors say, because early ear infections seem to predispose children to recurrent bouts of infection that sabotage a healthy childhood.

843. Choose Foods from the Best-Fed List

It's not that you don't want to feed your children right; the problem is your children refuse to eat the foods you want to give them.
How do you deal with a finicky eater?

Below is a partial list of healthful foods that nutritionists say are
pleasing to kids and at the same time nutritionally good for them.
Feed these to your children to your heart's (and theirs) content.

- Low-fat milk
- Low-fat yogurt
- Cheese
- White potatoes
- Sweet potatoes
- Whole-grain bread
- Poultry without the skin
- Lean cuts of beef and pork
- Fish sticks (baked)
- Beans
- Carrots
- Strawberries
- Bananas
- Melon
- Figs
- Oranges
- Pineapple
- Broccoli
- Green beans
- Green peppers
- Whole-grain pasta
- Brown rice
- Whole-grain cereals
- Ready-to-eat cereals with low sugar

844. Make Baby's Bite-Sized

Hot dogs are one of kids' favorite foods. But in the past, hot dogs
have accounted for 17 percent of child deaths due to choking.

This doesn't mean you should deny your child his feast. Slice
the hot dog vertically first, then slice it horizontally into bite-sized
chunks.

845. Toe the Line on These Treats

Some foods should be used with caution when it comes to your child's eating habits. It's okay to give these foods to your child as long as you put a limit on them.

- Soft drinks
- Presweetened cereals with more than 6 grams of sugar
- Candy
- Cake and cookies
- Gelatin desserts
- Hot dogs
- Juice
- Sausage
- Bacon
- Pastries
- Potato chips, tortilla chips, and other fried snack foods

846. Go Slow in the Fast Food Lane

For a lot of kids, a three-course meal means a burger, Coke, and fries. And guess what—it's okay, as long as it's done occasionally.

The American Academy of Pediatrics says parents should attempt to follow the same guidelines for children that the American Heart Association has established for adults—that is, no more than 30 percent of calories should come from fat.

847. Exercise Is Important

If you can't get your child to exercise restraint over his diet, at least try to get him to exercise. In addition to keeping him in good shape, it will also help him fight high cholesterol.

In a study at the University of Virginia, a group of 16 boys aged 6 to 11 exercised for 30 minutes three times a week for 14 weeks. They exercised on weight machines, stationary bikes, and by doing sit-ups, in addition to their normal participation in sports.

At the end of the 14-week period, researchers discovered the boys' average cholesterol dropped by almost 16 percent. That's significant, since studies show that a 25-percent reduction in cholesterol levels can reduce the risk of coronary heart disease by 50 percent. So, keeping cholesterol levels down while you're young can have a big payoff later on in life.

Fast Action Ideas

848. Make Ipecac a Household Staple

The easiest way to get your child to vomit is to give him some Ipecac syrup. Having a bottle on hand in your first aid kit could save your child's life in an emergency.

If your child has ingested poison, call your poison control center right away. Many times the first treatment they will recommend will be to give Ipecac, so it's best to have it close by.

A bit of caution: Don't give Ipecac to children under 6 months, and be sure to describe to the person at the poison control center just what poison your child took. Some poisons such as lye or drain cleaners can cause additional harm if vomited.

849. Don't Treat Head Bumps Lightly

Any time your child gets a bump on the head and loses consciousness—even momentarily—he should be seen by a doctor right away.

Even if the child doesn't lose consciousness, watch for other symptoms like nausea or vomiting, changes in vision, a persistent headache, a large lump on the head that keeps getting larger, or any inappropriate behavior, such as loss of memory. All of these symptoms could be signs of a brain injury, so your child should be evaluated by a doctor.

850. The Right Move Is Don't Move

It may be tough not to run over and swoop an injured child up in your arms, but don't do it; you could cause even more injury. The only time you should think of moving a child hurt in an accident is if he is lying in a spot where he is in danger of being further injured. Then do it very carefully.

Try to remember all the details of what you saw when you arrived on the scene. Remember how he was lying when you found him. Was he bleeding? Was he breathing? Were his eyes open? Was he talking? Was he moving, or was he limp? All of this information will be valuable to the emergency medical personnel and physicians when they start to care for him.

Be Prepared and Save a Life

If a child swallows something poisonous, what you do in the next few minutes could mean the difference between life and death.

Stay calm and call your local poison control center and give the trained emergency medical personnel there the following information:

- Your name and telephone number
- The age of your child
- The weight of your child
- The name of the product and ingredients (keep the container handy and take it to the hospital with you, should your child be taken there)
- The time the poisoning occurred
- How much your child ingested
- What symptoms he may be experiencing
- What type of first aid was given to your child

The American Association of Poison Control Centers offers parents a free "Emergency Action for Poisoning" card that you can place in an easy-to-see place in your home. You can get this information card by sending a postcard to Emergency Action for Poisonings, Communications Department, McNeil Consumer Products Company, Camp Hill Road, Fort Washington, PA 19034.

851. Remember Your First Aid

If you must move a child who has suffered a head injury, remember to protect his neck as well as his head. Conscious or unconscious, the child could have a broken neck, and if moved, the spinal cord could be injured, resulting in permanent damage to his nervous system.

Parents should keep an updated first aid book on hand and familiarize themselves with it.

A
TAKE-CHARGE
GUIDE TO
MEDICAL
CARE

There's no place as lonely as a doctor's examining room when you're sick or hurt. Alone among the cottonball-stuffed glass jars and mysterious, tightly closed cabinet drawers, you can think only of yourself as you wait for the doctor to appear.

Questions race through your mind: Am I going to be all right? Why did this happen to me?

Every breath pounds in your chest, every stomach gurgle echoes off the spotless walls. And there you sit, crinkling the paper sheet on the examining table, listening for footsteps outside the door.

Now imagine a completely different experience. Imagine that you're sitting on the table, happily swinging your legs, listening to muffled laughter as your doctor shares a joke with someone in the examining room next door.

Laughter? In a doctor's office? Where people are sick?

Well, imagine people going to the doctor when they're well. Imagine that just as they take their children for well-baby checks, they take themselves for well-adult checks. Imagine people going to the doctor to prevent illness—not just to treat it.

This shouldn't be too hard to imagine at all—because that's the way it should be.

Preventive Care the Best Medical Care

When it comes to protecting your health, going to a doctor when you're well may be just as important as going when you're sick. According to a national task force, the best way to beat the 60 leading causes of death is to prevent the illnesses and conditions that trigger them in the first place. Magic bullets from the treatment arsenal of American medicine just cannot do the job as effectively as prevention. As your mother (probably) used to say, "An ounce of prevention is worth a pound of cure."

The U.S. Preventive Services Task Force—the task force that figured out that your mother was right—is a 20-member, blue-ribbon panel charged by the Assistant Secretary for Health with evaluating the scientific evidence in support of preventive health care services. It took the task force three years to pore over more than 2,400 scientific articles reviewing 169 different practices for the prevention of the 60 leading causes of death.

Their conclusion: Preventing disease is the single most important strategy in sidestepping premature death, and your family doctor—the medical system's point man, so to speak—is the key to helping you implement these changes.

"Your doctor can do more good for you by spending time looking at personal health behaviors that raise your risk for disease than by coming at you with a large battery of medical tests," says Steven Woolf, M.D., the scientific adviser to the task force. "Just talking to you about smoking, exercise, eating a good diet, sexual practices, injury prevention, alcohol abuse, things of this sort are very likely to improve your life and help you prevent disease . . . long after the office visit is over."

FACT OF LIFE

The High Cost of Health

Over a 20-year period, health-care costs have risen from 6 percent of the Gross National Product (GNP) to almost 11 percent. What does this mean in real dollars? Health-care expenditures in the United States total $458 billion, an average of about $1,837 for every man, woman, and child in America.

Defensive Action

But even when you and your doctor work hand in hand to prevent the diseases that can cause premature death, there comes a time in everyone's life when he needs medical care that involves diagnosis, treatment, and hospitalization.

Now, lying around in a hospital bed while men and women in white coats stab, poke, and otherwise abuse you is nobody's idea of fun. Nor are all the heavy-duty infections you can pick up from the experience. At least 20,000 people die each year from hospital-caused infections—20,000 people who might still be alive if they could have either avoided the experience or better defended themselves against it.

That's why this chapter not only includes tips on how to find the doctor who's best for you but also on how to intelligently participate in *all* facets of your medical care—even when it involves space-age diagnostic tests, hospitalization, and surgery. Your personal participation is your best defensive action in getting the medical care that will help you live a longer life.

Developing a Healthy Doctor/Patient Relationship

852. Form a Partnership

To make sure you get the best from your doctor, it's important that you develop a good doctor/patient relationship, says Daniel Johnson, M.D., a spokesman for the American Medical Association.

"The physician/patient relationship is a special kind of communication between two people," says Dr. Johnson. "Sometimes the language the physician uses gets in the way of your relationship, and you have to break through that. But good physicians judge what the patient can and cannot understand—and then they communicate in terms that the patient can relate to."

How you feel around your doctor is also important. "If your intuition says that this doctor isn't right for you, you need to respond to that," says Dr. Johnson. "Your relationship has to be built on confidence. And if you don't have that confidence, it's probably best that you keep searching for a physician you can trust."

Dreading illness is understandable. Dreading a visit to your doctor's office is a whole other story.

FACT OF LIFE

People Keep in Touch with Their Doctor

Most Americans keep in pretty close contact with their doctor. One survey indicates that every man, woman, and child gets in touch with their doctor an average of 5.4 times a year. In the survey, more than half the conversations were held in the doctor's office, 14 percent were in a hospital's outpatient department, and 13 percent were over the phone. Only 2 percent took place in the patient's home.

853. Choose a Physician Who Listens

"There's an old saying that if you listen to the patient long enough, the patient will give you the diagnosis," says Dr. Johnson. And it's true. But that means that your doctor needs to spend some time with you, not just run in and out of the examining room. So if your doctor looks at his watch more than he looks at you, suggests Dr. Johnson, it's time that you—rather than the doctor—move on.

854. Look into His Past

Don't just read the old magazines scattered around the waiting room when you're in a doctor's office—read the framed certificates that are hanging on the wall as well. Look to see where he went to medical school and if it's not a name you recognize, ask him where it is and what it's known for.

"The average physician in this country has had an extraordinary amount of education," says Dr. Johnson. "The quality of that education is excellent. The criteria set up for medical school and post-graduate study are extremely demanding and thorough. The chances are very high that your doctor is well qualified."

You can feel especially comfortable about a doctor's qualifications if you spot a document on the wall that indicates he's "board certified." Certification by a special medical board indicates that a doctor has trained for a number of years in his specialty and has passed a rigorous exam given by a jury of his peers.

And remember: Good physicians with good credentials will welcome your questions about their background. They're proud of all the hard work that went into earning those diplomas.

855. Look for a "Privileged" Character

Your doctor's hospital affiliation is another way you can get a feel for his competence. Good doctors are affiliated with good hospitals. Since doctors have to continually prove themselves to keep their affiliation, the annual appointment of privileges to a good hospital is a pretty good indicator of good performance.

856. Check Availability

You need to see your doctor as soon as possible when you're sick—not a week from Tuesday. It's important that you're able to get an appointment in a fairly reasonable time so that little problems don't become major ones.

857. And Convenience

It's also important to have a doctor who is located near where you live or work. Traveling long distances for medical help could turn a serious problem into a life-threatening one.

858. Examine Your Doctor Before He Examines You

Take a good look at your doctor. If it looks as though he ignores his own nutrition, fitness, and overall well-being, think about whether or not he'll help you achieve a healthy lifestyle. A doctor who tells you through his cigar smoke that you need to stop smoking might not be the best doctor to help you quit.

FACT OF LIFE

East Coast Boasts the Most Doctors

New England and the Middle Atlantic states (New York, New Jersey, and Pennsylvania) have the most doctors: about 26 private physicians for every 10,000 patients. On the other hand, the East South-Central states (Kentucky, Tennessee, Alabama, and Mississippi) have the fewest: 15 doctors per 10,000 patients.

Preventive Practices

859. Get a Complete Physical Every Three Years

"The complete physical is still a good idea," says Dr. Woolf. "Older people and young children need to be evaluated on a frequent basis, but the average healthy adult who has no history of medical problems doesn't need to be seen every year. Once every three years should do it.

"The exam should include a thorough medical history, along with a physical examination where the doctor searches your body for any signs of abnormalities."

860. Get a Second Opinion

If a tree fell on your house during a storm, you wouldn't let the first roofer who came to estimate the damage fix it, would you? Of course not. You'd get at least one more opinion. So why get only one opinion when it comes to taking care of your body?

If you've got a medical problem that needs some serious fixing—surgery or chemotherapy, for example—always get a second opinion before you decide on a course of treatment. And don't worry about offending your doctor. "A good physician," says Dr. Johnson, "is never going to mind having his judgment submitted to the judgment of another physician. If your physician balks at your getting a second opinion, then it may be time to change physicians."

861. Ask Lots of Questions

If you have a medical problem, chances are someone's developed a test to find it, define it, or elaborate on it. But how can you tell which tests are best? How can you tell if you need any of them?

Even the experts admit it's hard to know. "It's confusing," says the U.S. Preventive Services' Dr. Woolf. "Part of the problem is that a lot of these tests are promoted by people who have a very focused interest in that particular test, be it because that's what they specialize in or perhaps because they have some financial interest in it."

Of course, that's precisely why the federal government appointed the unbiased Preventive Services Task Force. It was the task force's job to sort things out.

"We went back to the scientific evidence for each of these tests and carried out a very systematic review of the evidence to determine which tests are effective," says Dr. Woolf. "We looked very

---

Making the Most of Home Medical Tests

With the advance of do-it-yourself medical testing, you now have the chance to self-detect some potentially life-threatening health problems, such as colon cancer, diabetes, or high blood pressure.

But to be able to do that, you need to make sure you do the test right. Here are some tips from the federal Food and Drug Administration to help you get the maximum benefits out of your home testing kit.

- Check the expiration date on the package. Chemicals used in some kits have a limited shelf life, after which they can cause inaccurate results.
- Store temperature-sensitive kits carefully. If a test is affected by heat, be careful not to leave it in an overheated car.
- Read the package insert thoroughly. Read the directions once to get an idea of what's supposed to happen, then go back and follow the instructions step by step.
- Don't guess at a step if the instructions aren't clear. Check to see if an 800 information number is listed on the package so you can call the manufacturer, or ask a pharmacist or other health professional to clarify the instructions.
- Some tests require you to detect a change in color. If you're color-blind, have a friend present to help you read the results.
- Look for special precautions to be taken before you perform the test, such as refraining from physical activity, food, or drink.
- Each step in a test must be performed in sequence and cannot be skipped. If the test calls for verification of a step, go back and do it again.
- If you need to collect a urine specimen, wash the container and rinse it thoroughly, preferably with distilled water.
- Be precise when timing the test. Use a stopwatch or kitchen timer if necessary.
- Accurately record the results.
- Keep any chemicals used out of the reach of children and dispose of them carefully and promptly when the test is done.

carefully at many different tests and found that, although there are some of definite value, there are many others of unproven value."

How can *you* know which is which? By grilling your doctor. If you need to have special tests, ask as many questions as it takes to get a clear picture of what's going to be done, why it's going to be done, and what the associated risks are. Ask if it's going to be painful, how much time it will take, and if it can be done in the office or must be done in the hospital. Ask if the potential advantages of the test outweigh its risk. And find out if the test itself is dangerous.

Also take the time to ask your doctor what would happen if you didn't have the procedure done. If your doctor says, "You'll die," then you'll want to go ahead with it. If, on the other hand, the reply runs along the lines of, "Nothing will happen—we'll just watch you for a few months and then reevaluate the situation," you might want to pass on the procedure for now.

862. Make Sure Your Tests Are Custom-Designed

"You need to make sure your doctor knows all the details of your medical history and then designs a package of tests that are appropriate for you," says Dr. Woolf. "A routine battery of tests performed on someone without regard to personal risk factors is not considered an effective strategy anymore. It's best to target the tests to the person."

863. Tests for Women Only

Basic tests for women should include a Pap smear, mammogram, and clinical breast examination.

"Pap smears should begin at age 18, or once the woman is sexually active and be repeated every one to three years at the discretion of your doctor," says Dr. Woolf. "We also recommend that Pap smears be performed beyond age 65 if you have not had consistently normal smears.

"At age 40 women should also have an annual breast exam performed by their doctor. Women with risk factors for breast cancer—like a relative who has had breast cancer—should begin younger than that.

"We don't recommend that mammography be performed routinely until age 50. This is different from other groups who say the testing should start at age 40. We feel that women after age 50 should have mammography done every one to two years."

Women with high risk factors for sexually transmitted diseases—individuals who have multiple sex partners or who have partners at risk for AIDS—would also benefit from routine screening tests for these types of diseases.

864. Basic Tests for Fifty-Plus

"Testing for colorectal cancer is important for men and women over 50," says Dr. Woolf, "but we only recommend it for people who have special risk factors for this type of cancer.

"There is insufficient evidence to advise blood stool testing or sigmoidoscopy as effective screening tests for colorectal cancer in people without symptoms or risk factors. It has been recommended by some that people have a sigmoidoscopy exam every three to five years once they are over age 50. We found that it really hasn't proven to reduce deaths from colorectal cancer, so we feel that it's premature to advise this test for everyone over age 50. It is important, though, that people with risk factors like polyps or family history have the exam done regularly."

865. Overweight People Need These Tests

"If you are obese, more than 20 percent above your desirable weight, you're at increased risk for heart disease," says Dr. Woolf. "You need routine checkups to screen for high blood pressure, cholesterol, diabetes, and other disorders."

866. Get Your Cholesterol Checked Once Every Five Years

The National Cholesterol Education Program's coordinating committee suggests that all adults over the age of 20 get their cholesterol checked at least once every five years.

Any test that shows a cholesterol level over 200 should be repeated to verify the results, the committee recommends. It should then be retested in a year. You should also repeat the test and get a more detailed analysis of your cholesterol if it's over 240.

What are you looking for? The amount of high-density lipoprotein (HDL) and low-density lipoprotein (LDL) in your blood, and the ratio between the two. These three numbers will tell your doctor what's going on inside your arteries and what your chances are for a heart attack or stroke. (For more on HDL and LDL and what the numbers mean, see chapter 2.)

High-Tech Tests That Could Save Your Life

867. Nuclear Scans Can Locate the Problem

When your doctor suspects a serious problem and needs help in locating it within your body, he's likely to turn to one of the new space-age imaging devices that can see into the deepest recesses of your body.

One such device is a nuclear scan, which basically comes in two forms: a bone scan and something called ventilation-perfusion scintigraphy—otherwise known as V-P scanning—which is used to examine your lungs.

Both scans work by using radioactive compounds, also called radioisotopes or radionuclides, which attach to body tissues. After a radioisotope is introduced into your body, you're positioned under a large instrument called a gamma camera. This device maps the distribution of the radioisotope in your body by translating it into spots of light on film.

Radiologists use bone scans to check your skeleton for tumors, infections, injury, or a source of unexplained pain. The scan will point out hot spots—areas of increased activity that indicate abnormalities in bony structures—weeks to months before they can be detected by standard x-rays.

V-P scanning can provide physicians with valuable information about your lungs. Ventilation refers to breathing; perfusion refers to blood flow. And both can be measured using radioisotopes and a gamma camera. In fact, by comparing two measurements and looking for a "V-P mismatch," radiologists can detect a pulmonary embolism, a potentially fatal condition involving blood clots in the lungs, and stop it before it hurts you.

868. This Computer Detects Heart Disease

When coronary artery disease is suspected, testing with the help of single photon emission computed tomography (SPECT) can be particularly useful in evaluating the condition of the heart muscle.

SPECT features three innovations over the conventional nuclear scan: Its gamma camera rotates to shoot from a variety of angles, it produces images of thin sections of your body, and the computer produces a three-dimensional picture.

To prepare for this test, you first exercise to get your heart in gear. Then a radioactive tracer such as thallium–201 is injected into your body.

"The heart is a big muscle surrounded by a lot of air," says Philip Alderson, M.D., professor and acting chairman of the Department of Radiology and director of the Division of Nuclear Medicine at Columbia-Presbyterian Medical Center in New York City. "When you inject thallium, it's pretty easy to see the heart muscle."

SPECT photographs the image after the thallium injection and then again several hours later. Together, the two sets of images indicate any heart blockages that may be causing angina or other troublesome symptoms.

FACT OF LIFE

Doctors Really Rate

A *Prevention* magazine survey found that 83 percent of the people polled rated their doctor's competence as very good to excellent, and 75 percent felt that their doctor expresses personal concern for them.

869. The Best Test to Spot a Stroke

Angiography has been used for years to help doctors diagnose clogged arteries and prevent strokes. After injecting contrast dye into a suspicious artery through a catheter, radiologists can pinpoint any trouble spots both present and future.

Digital subtraction angiography (DSA) is a recent advance in imaging that has become an important complement to angiography. Through this technique, unwanted x-ray detail is subtracted from the angiographic image, thus offering a clearer outline of veins and arteries.

In addition, DSA requires less contrast material to produce an image than angiography alone. This means that narrower, more comfortable catheters can be used, and best of all, it also means less radiation exposure for you.

870. CAT Scanners Find Tumors

Take an x-ray tube, a fixed ring of very sensitive detectors, add a computer, and you have the granddaddy of modern imaging: the computerized axial tomography (CAT) scanner.

Called the biggest imaging advance since the discovery of x-rays, the CAT scanner looks more like a gigantic washing machine. What it does is create detailed two-dimensional pictures of the entire body so that the computer can put it together to form three-dimensional images. The whole technological jigsaw puzzle comes together in just 40 seconds.

The CAT scanner can distinguish tumors from normal tissues and determine their size and volume in the process. And scanning the skull, chest, and abdomen of an accident victim can provide the physician with a prompt diagnosis that speeds the treatment of internal injuries.

871. MRI: Detection without Radiation

The magnetic resonance imaging (MRI) machine is a powerful magnetic coil with up to 30,000 times the strength of the earth's magnetic field. Unlike a standard x-ray or CAT scan, it uses no radiation. And, as far as the experts know, it involves no risks or side effects.

MRI performs its magic by an ingenious combination of magnetic field, radio waves, and computer. The device is useful in the study of musculoskeletal diseases and has the potential to detect changes in joint tissue early on so that people with rheumatoid arthritis or osteoarthritis can get a jump on their treatment.

A tumor or large cystic spaces within the spinal cord can also be detected. MRI can also be used to study biochemical activity in tissue at the very early stages of disease.

872. Ultrasound: A Picture of Health Problems

Ultrasound, or sonography, is another alternative to using radiation to see inside your body. Here high-frequency sound waves are emitted from a transducer that is passed over various areas of your body.

As the transducer is held over a particular part of your body, sound waves bounce off structures within and echo back into the transducer. This information is then electronically transformed into a picture.

Ultrasound's value lies in its ability to examine soft-tissue densities and discriminate among them. "It's an indicator as to what needs to be studied further," says George Leopold, M.D., professor and chairman of radiology at the University of California, San Diego.

Ultrasound can also be used to study not only the structure of blood vessels but also the flow within them. And a new technique allows urologists and radiologists to detect early cancer of the prostate.

873. This Test Measures Blood Flow

If you've ever listened to the declining pitch of a train's whistle as the train disappears down the track, you've observed the Doppler flow imaging effect: The pitch of a sound rises as the source approaches, decreases as it moves away.

Recently, the same principle has been applied to the study of blood flow, resulting in the creation of a Doppler flow imaging ultrasound beam.

"If the beam hits a moving target, the signal we get back is altered," says Dr. Leopold. And linked with ultrasound images, the signal can be used to evaluate blood flow, even in vessels deep within your body. The result is a clear profile of any partially blocked blood vessels that might one day contribute to a heart attack or stroke.

Color Doppler flow imaging, the latest development in Doppler testing, samples all areas of flow within the vessels simultaneously. Then by assigning a different color to each flow speed, the radiologist can quickly spot areas of slowdown or blockage.

874. PET Targets Heart and Brain

Beyond the imaging of anatomy, soft tissues, and blood flow, there enters a technique that uses radioactive tracers to take a look at the metabolic activity going on inside an organ.

The brain and heart have been the prime targets for the new experimental test known as positron emission tomography (PET). Radiologists can use PET to study brain-related disorders such as epilepsy, Alzheimer's disease, schizophrenia, and Parkinson's disease. PET can also evaluate the vitality of your heart muscle before you undergo surgery.

Life-Extension Tool

MediScope

Here's a piece of jewelry that could save your life. MediScope is a 1-inch-long gold pendant with a powerful lens on one end and a microfilm capsule on the other.

Your entire medical history can be transcribed on the microfilm so that, in a crisis, all emergency room personnel need do is tilt the pendant up to the light to know all about your health problems, medications, and allergies. There's even room for your personal doctor's telephone number.

The pendant can dangle on a key chain or be worn on a chain around your neck or wrist. And the medical information inside can be easily updated by notifying the manufacturer.

This device, which costs about $20, can be purchased at many retail stores or directly from Med-Tech Marketing, 2230 S.W. 70th Avenue, Davie, FL, 33317.

A Preventive Health-Care Plan

After three years of intensive scientific scrutiny of preventive medical care, the U.S. Preventive Services Task Force has come up with a checklist of age-specific medical exams, tests, and immunizations that they think can help prevent premature death. The recom-

Age and Schedule	Physical Exam

19–39: Every 1–3 years unless otherwise indicated

EVERYONE ▶	Blood pressure Height and weight
THOSE AT RISK FOR SPECIFIC DISEASES ▶	Breast (women 35 and older with family history of breast cancer) Oral cavity (includes smokers, alcoholics) Skin (persons with personal or family history of skin cancer: persons with increased exposure to sunlight, such as outdoor workers; persons with suspicious skin lesions) Testicles (men with history of testicular disorders)

Leading Causes of Death: Ages 19–39

Motor vehicle crashes

Homicide

Suicide

Injuries (non-motor-vehicle)

Heart disease

mended schedule applies only to the periodic visit itself. The frequency of preventive care should be left to the discretion of you and your doctor. Here's a list of the basic preventive procedures the task force recommends for healthy adults.

Tests and Procedures	Immunizations
Cholesterol, nonfasting Pap smear (women)	Tetanus-diphtheria booster (every 10 years)
Blood sugar, fasting (persons who are obese, persons with family history of diabetes, or women who developed diabetes during pregnancy) Colonoscopy (persons with family history of intestinal polyps and/or intestinal cancer) Hearing (persons regularly exposed to excessive noise) HIV (AIDS) (includes homosexual or bisexual men, IV drug users, persons with multiple sex partners, persons whose sex partners have had multiple sexual contacts, persons with history of blood transfusions between 1978–1985) Mammogram (women 35 years or older with family history of breast cancer) Rubella immunity (women who have no record of previous immunization) Sexually transmitted diseases—syphilis, chlamydia, gonorrhea (includes persons with multiple sex partners, persons whose sex partners have had multiple sexual contacts) Urine (diabetics)	Hepatitis B vaccine (includes homosexuals, IV drug users) Influenza vaccine (annually; includes residents of chronic care facilities, persons with chronic cardiopulmonary disorder, immune system or kidney disorders) Measles-mumps-rubella vaccine (persons born after 1956 who have no record of previous immunization) Pneumococcal (pneumonia) vaccine (includes persons with chronic cardiac or pulmonary disorders, diabetes, alcoholism, kidney disease)

(continued)

A Preventive Health-Care Plan—*Continued*

Age and Schedule	Physical Exam

40–64: Every 3 years unless otherwise indicated

EVERYONE ▶ Blood pressure
Breast (annually for women)
Height and weight

THOSE AT RISK FOR SPECIFIC DISEASES ▶ Arteries, exam with stethoscope
(includes persons with risk factors
for stroke and cardiovascular
disease)
Oral cavity
(includes smokers, alcoholics)
Skin
(persons with personal or family
history of skin cancer; persons
with increased exposure to
sunlight, such as outdoor workers;
persons with suspicious skin
lesions)

**Leading Causes
of Death:
Ages 40–64**

Heart disease

Lung cancer

Stroke

Breast cancer

Colorectal cancer

Obstructive lung disease
(chronic bronchitis,
emphysema, asthma, etc.)

Tests and Procedures	Immunizations
Cholesterol, nonfasting Mammogram (1–2 years, women aged 50 and older) Pap smear (women)	Tetanus-diphtheria booster (every 10 years)
Blood sugar, fasting (persons who are obese, persons with family history of diabetes, or women who developed diabetes during pregnancy) Bone mineral content (includes women at increased risk for osteoporosis) Colonoscopy/blood stool (persons with family history of intestinal polyps and/or intestinal cancer) Electrocardiogram (men with two or more cardiac risk factors, such as high blood cholesterol, high blood pressure, diabetes, smoking) Hearing (persons regularly exposed to excessive noise) HIV (AIDS) (includes homosexual or bisexual men, IV drug users, persons with multiple sex partners, persons whose sex partners have had multiple sexual contacts, persons with history of blood transfusions between 1978–1985) Sexually transmitted diseases—syphilis, chlamydia, gonorrhea (persons with multiple sex partners, persons whose sex partners have had multiple sexual contacts) Sigmoidoscopy/blood stool (includes persons aged 50 and older with family history of colon or rectal cancer; women with history of breast, ovarian, or uterine cancer	Hepatitis B vaccine (includes homosexuals, IV drug users) Influenza vaccine (annually; includes residents of chronic care facilities, persons with chronic cardiopulmonary disorders, immune system or kidney disorders) Pneumococcal (pneumonia) vaccine (includes persons with chronic cardiac or pulmonary disorders, diabetes, alcoholism, kidney disease)

(continued)

A Preventive Health-Care Plan—*Continued*

Age and Schedule	Physical Exam
65 and over: **Every year**	

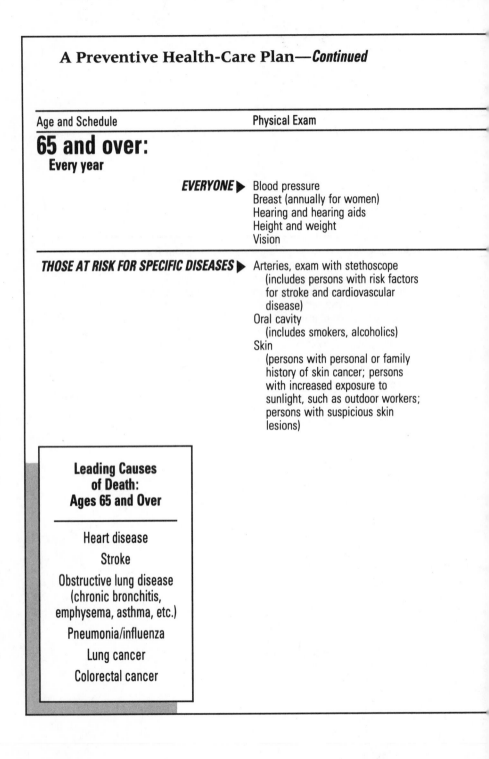

EVERYONE ▶
Blood pressure
Breast (annually for women)
Hearing and hearing aids
Height and weight
Vision

THOSE AT RISK FOR SPECIFIC DISEASES ▶
Arteries, exam with stethoscope
(includes persons with risk factors
for stroke and cardiovascular
disease)
Oral cavity
(includes smokers, alcoholics)
Skin
(persons with personal or family
history of skin cancer; persons
with increased exposure to
sunlight, such as outdoor workers;
persons with suspicious skin
lesions)

**Leading Causes
of Death:
Ages 65 and Over**

Heart disease

Stroke

Obstructive lung disease
(chronic bronchitis,
emphysema, asthma, etc.)

Pneumonia/influenza

Lung cancer

Colorectal cancer

Tests and Procedures	Immunizations
Cholesterol, nonfasting Mammogram (1–2 years for women until age 70, unless abnormality is detected) Thyroid (women) Urine, dipstick	Influenza vaccine (annually) Pneumococcal (pneumonia) vaccine Tetanus-diphtheria booster (every 10 years)
Blood sugar, fasting (includes persons who are obese, persons with family history of diabetes or women who developed diabetes during pregnancy) Colonoscopy/blood stool (persons with family history of intestinal polyps and/or intestinal cancer) Electrocardiogram (men with two or more cardiac risk factors such as high blood cholesterol, high blood pressure, diabetes, smoking) Pap smear (women who have not had previous consistently negative tests) Sigmoidoscopy/blood stool (includes persons with family history of colon or rectal cancer; women with history of breast, ovarian, or uterine cancer)	Hepatitis B vaccine (includes homosexuals, IV drug users)

Seeking "Hospital-ity"

875. Don't Be Afraid to Speak Up

Face it, no one feels that they have any control over what goes on when they're wearing a hospital gown that's slit all the way down the back. But even in the hospital, you do have a say in how your medical care is conducted.

"Hospitals are becoming more and more consumer-oriented," says Alexandra Gekas, spokesman for the American Hospital Association and director of the National Society for Patient Representation and Consumer Affairs. They're less defensive when asked for information than they used to be and more aware that patients have the right to ask for more information so they can say yes or no or question their other options.

876. Pick the Hospital That Suits Your Needs

Are you a generalist or a specialist? Do you buy shoes in a shoe store or a department store? How you answer those questions may help you decide whether you would rather be in a general or specialty hospital.

What's the difference? Well, general hospitals handle all sorts of problems from fevers to fractures, infections to injuries. Specialty hospitals handle only one thing, be it cancer, children, orthopedic problems, or eyes, ears, noses, and throats. They concentrate on one

FACT OF LIFE

Competitive Hospitals Are More Hospitable

Hospitals in communities that have several hospitals keep their patients longer than those in areas having a single hospital, reports a study in the *Journal of the American Medical Association*. Researchers found that hospital stays averaged almost 17 percent longer in competitive markets than in areas where there is only one hospital. The competition, it appears, makes hospitals more inclined to oblige doctors and patients who request longer stays.

problem day in and day out. As a result, the people who work there become experts dealing with it. That's good if your problem matches their mission. But specialty hospitals have one drawback: They have limited emergency facilities. Say you choose an orthopedic hospital to have hip surgery, and while being operated on, you go into cardiac arrest. The surgical team isn't going to let you die because all they happen to care about are knees and hips, of course. But all they might be able to do is stabilize the emergency and send you off to another hospital. The specialty hospital might not have the facilities, technology, or expertise needed to do much more.

General hospitals aren't necessarily better than specialty hospitals, but they're equipped to handle a larger variety of medical eventualities. They are, literally, a bunch of little specialty hospitals under one roof.

877. Get Insider Information

Want to know if a specific hospital is really any good? If you do, a good way to find out is to ask someone in a position to really know. Ask your doctor, for example, "If you were sick, what hospital would you go to?" Or if you know any nurses or paramedics, ask them the same question. Medical personnel who deal with hospitals all the time know which hospitals are best.

878. Go See for Yourself

Most hospitals have already established tours, and they'd be happy to show you around. Call the hospital's community relations or administration department and tell them that you may be having surgery soon and you'd like to see their facility. Most tours are done on a monthly basis, so ask if you can tag along on the next one.

While on the tour, ask questions. Ask to see specific departments that will deal with your ailment. And make sure you see enough to get a feel for the place. Is it clean? Does it feel orderly or chaotic? Do the people who work there seem friendly or harried? Do you feel comfortable there? All of these impressions will help you get a sense of the hospital's efficiency—and the level of competent care.

879. Avoid Hospitals on Wednesdays in July

Wednesday is the worst day to be treated in a hospital—doubly so if it happens to be a Wednesday in July.

Why? Scientists suspect it's because Wednesday happens to be when most doctors take a day off, and July happens to be the month in which new interns and residents replace more experienced staff.

Significantly, researchers at California's Kaiser Permanente Hospital have found that more high-risk surgery patients die on Wednesday than any other day of the week, while researchers at the Denver Veterans Administration hospital have found that more things go wrong in a hospital during the month of July than at any other time during the year.

When's a good time to be in the hospital? The Denver researchers discovered that May and June, near the end of the more experienced staff's term, were the least risky months.

880. Don't Be Afraid to Complain

If medical personnel who care for you are not responding to reasonable requests, complain. "The Joint Commission on Accreditation of Health Care Organizations has implemented a standard requiring every hospital to have a patient complaint mechanism," says Alexandra Gekas. And hospitals are required to tell you what it is.

Most hospitals, for example, have an ombudsman or patient representative who will act as a liaison between you and the hospital. Ask to meet with this individual if you feel your problem isn't being handled properly. Ten-to-one the ombudsman will get people moving to your satisfaction.

If he doesn't, you still have another option: Contact the state department of hospital licensing with your complaint. Your hospital will have the phone number, and they must give it to you whether they want to or not.

If your complaint involves problems with specific doctors, nurses, or medical technicians, however, contact the regulatory agency that monitors their profession. For doctors, it's the Board of Medical Examiners; and for nurses, it's the Board of Nurse Examiners. For other medical personnel, contact the Office of Occupational or Professional Licensing. Again, the hospital will have these phone numbers.

What to Do Once You're Inside

881. Ask for Library Privileges

Use your time in the hospital to learn about your condition. Ask if you can use the medical library. If it's strictly for physicians, ask if there is a library set aside for patients. Or contact the Nursing Education Department in the hospital and ask if there is a nursing library and if you can use it. Nursing libraries have many technical and nontechnical health information sources that the nurses use to continually update their education. An educated patient is a patient who can more wisely evaluate his medical options.

882. Block Hospital-Caused Infections

Where are you more likely to pick up an infection than at a place where people go to get rid of them? Infectious agents abound in hospitals, which is why hospitals go to such great lengths to keep the place clean. Hospitals don't smell like disinfectant because that's their fragrance of choice.

Despite the precautions, however, infections can be spread through the hospital in a variety of ways. They can be transmitted in food or water, in transfused blood, on towels and sheets, even by a nurse who forgot to wash her hands after treating someone else.

So be on the lookout for ways that infections could be passed to you. And work to block their route.

When you're out and about in the hospital, for example, wash your hands as soon as you get back to your room. If you're given a gown to wear, make sure it's just back from the laundry. And if you visit other patients, don't enter a room without first finding out if there's a chance you could catch what they've got.

883. Say Goodbye to Infected Roommates

If your roommate has an infection, find out exactly how infectious it is. If it's a serious infection, ask if you can be moved to another room. But make sure you emphasize that *you're* willing to be the body that's moved. You'll have a much better chance of getting away from an infected person if you don't ask them to move someone who may be seriously ill.

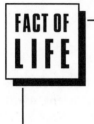

Ten Percent of the Sick Get Sicker

Sometimes you get more than you bargained for when you enter a hospital. Infections caught in the hospital, or nosocomial infections, strike 5 to 10 percent of all patients (about 2 million people) and add an extra four days to their hospital stay. They cause death in 3 percent of the cases.

884. Slow the Flow of Blood

Harvard Medical School researchers studied the rate at which blood is taken for testing in hospitals and found that the average patient has blood taken slightly more often than once a day. In fact, reported the researchers, the average patient loses about ¾ cup of blood to tests during the average stay.

In many of these patients, this bloodletting caused anemia and contributed to the need for later transfusions. And in this day of widespread infections, transfusions are not without risk.

Moreover, taking all that blood simply isn't needed, argued the researchers. Current laboratory instruments require so little blood for testing that the small specimen tubes normally used for children would be sufficient even for an adult. Switching to these smaller tubes would cut blood loss by 40 to 50 percent.

The doctors also observed that many tests can be done on a single tube of blood. The inefficient practice of drawing a new tube for each test is unnecessary.

What can you do to slow the flow of blood? Keep a daily tally of how much blood is taken from you and show it to your doctor. Tell him it's getting to be a pain in the, uh, arm and ask if there's anything he can do about it. Once you show him proof on paper, he may reduce the blood flow to a trickle.

885. Remind Your Doctor How Much You Weigh

In a study at Harvard Medical School, researchers found that older, underweight people frequently take prescription drugs in too high a dose because their doctors fail to take into account their age or weight when prescribing medication. People weighing 110 pounds or less are at greatest risk, the researchers found, and receive dosages 31 to 46 percent higher than they need.

"If you are very thin," suggests the study's organizer, Edward Campion, M.D., "it's worthwhile to remind your doctor how much you weigh." Overmedication can cause kidney damage, confusion, or deadly drug interactions.

886. Put the Hospital Dietitian on Your Team

Try to meet with the hospital dietitian for a nutritional counseling session. Let him know why you are in the hospital and whether or not you have any food sensitivities or allergies. Explain your nutritional goals and ask how he can help you meet them while you're in the hospital. Try to foster an atmosphere in which the dietitian will be an important member of your medical team.

887. Think about Vitamin Supplements

A study conducted by the home economics research center of Washington State University concludes, "It may be advisable to consider vitamin supplementation for hospital patients, especially those on restricted diets or with limited appetites, whose needs may not be met with institutional foods."

If you take vitamin and mineral supplements at home, ask your doctor if it's okay for you to continue taking them while you're in the hospital. If he says it's fine with him, make sure he marks it on your chart so that other hospital personnel don't get nervous when they see you popping some extra pills.

888. Bring Your Own Food

If you suspect the hospital will not be able to meet your own particular dietary needs, check with your doctor first and then supplement the hospital diet by bringing in a few of your own foods. Prepare the food at home and place it in clearly labeled containers with your name on the outside. Don't bring in things that will take up lots of storage room, such as a watermelon. But if it's watermelon you crave, simply cut it into chunks, place it in a small container, and tote it along.

Low-Risk Surgery

889. Know Your Surgeon's Batting Average

The time to meet your surgeon is not while you're lying on the operating table. Meet him well ahead of time to discuss the surgical procedure. Ask him how many times he's done the kind of surgery that he's going to perform on you—you don't want someone who's done it once or twice, do you?—and how many times his patients have developed complications such as infection or delayed healing.

Postsurgical infections can be life-threatening, so it's only fair that you know your surgeon's batting average.

890. Talk to the Anesthesiologist

Usually an anesthesiologist will pop his head into your room a couple of hours or the night before your surgery, ask a few questions, and leave. The only other conversation you'll have with him is when he tells you to start counting backward from 100. That conversation won't last long, either.

Yet the two of you need to exchange some pertinent information if your surgery is to go as smoothly as it should. So instead of waiting for your anesthesiologist to find you, you should find him. Make an appointment to sit down and talk. Ask what kind of anesthesia will be used on you and why. Ask how long you will be in recovery, and whether he will be there with you.

And while you have your anesthesiologist's ear, tell him if anyone in your family has died or had a serious reaction to anesthesia. Doctors used to call it an "act of God" when a young, healthy person died during surgery. Now they're more likely to suspect a rare genetic condition called malignant hyperthermia.

People who have this condition react to general anesthesia with a skyrocketing fever and rigid muscles. And if the person is to survive, the reaction must be quickly reversed with ice packs and injections of the drug dantrolene—which some hospitals don't stock. That's why your anesthesiologist needs to be forewarned that malignant hyperthermia may run in your family.

Once your anesthesiologist knows of this potential problem, switching anesthetics—to a local anesthetic or nitrous oxide, perhaps—may be all that's needed to avert a tragedy.

891. BYOB

That's "bring your own blood." And in this day of global germs that cause life-threatening infections—AIDS, for example—storing your own blood in the hospital blood bank in case it is needed is not a bad idea. Contact your hospital's blood bank administrator to make the necessary arrangements.

892. Find Out Who Your Roommate Is

If you're checking into a hospital for surgery, having a roommate who's just had surgery and is well on the road to recovery may help *your* recovery.

A study of 27 patients found that those rooming with someone whose surgery was a success were less anxious before surgery, walked more afterward, and left the hospital a day and a half sooner than did people who had nothing in common with their roommates.

"We think patients were reassured that they would be okay after watching their roommates make it through a difficult surgery," says researcher James Kulik, Ph.D., who conducted the study at the University of California, San Diego. Moreover, roommates tend to share little tips—that walking speeds recovery, for example—that may make recovery easier.

893. Stop Smoking

If you're a smoker who's about to go under the knife, quit smoking, even if it's only 12 to 24 hours beforehand.

Smoking puts a strain on your body's ability to recover from trauma, experts say, and even a temporary halt to your habit can lessen that strain.

894. Build Your Infection-Fighting Power with Food

Surgery puts a tremendous amount of stress on your body, which can, unfortunately, suppress your immune system right when you need it the most. That's why a good diet, high in immune-boosting vitamins and minerals, should be one of your top priorities as you prepare for surgery.

The most important nutrients in terms of wound healing and infection fighting are vitamins A and C and the mineral zinc. Yellow and orange vegetables and fruits and leafy green vegetables are good sources of vitamin A. Citrus fruits, green peppers, broccoli, brussels sprouts, and cantaloupe are good sources of vitamin C. And low-fat beef, lamb, chicken, pumpkin, and sunflower seeds provide a nice supply of zinc.

895. Avoid a Close Shave with Infection

If you need to be shaved for surgery, don't let the hospital staff use a razor. One study found that people who were shaved had an infection rate of 5.6 percent, while people who had their unwanted hair removed with a chemical depilatory had an infection rate of only 0.06 percent.

896. Don't Be Cool When It Comes to Surgery

The anesthetic inhalants, spinal blocks, and muscle relaxants usually administered just prior to surgery can prevent your body from generating enough heat to keep you warm, just when the combination of surgery and anesthesia is lowering your normal body temperature. Unfortunately, the combined effects could cause a surgically induced hypothermia—especially in older people. It's a serious situation that can lead to heart failure, circulatory problems, severely low blood pressure, and respiratory complications.

It is possible, however, to prevent hypothermia from happening. Here's what the experts suggest you do to ensure a warm reception in surgery.

- Ask that several warm blankets be on hand to cover you when you arrive in the operating room.
- Ask that the room temperature of the operating room be raised above 69.8°F prior to surgery so that your body temperature has a better chance of remaining within normal limits during surgery.
- Ask that a portable radiant heat lamp be available for additional heat should your body temperature drop. Lengthy surgical procedures involving large incisions can cool even the warmest body.

897. Pack Some Paderewski with Your Pajamas

When music is played for patients before, during, or after surgery, it reduces anxiety, lessens pain, speeds recovery, and reduces the need for preoperative and postoperative medication.

One study found that when relaxing music was piped into the operating room throughout surgery, the amount of sedative required by patients was cut in half. In another study, the investigators estimated that music had an effect comparable to that of an intravenous dose of 2.5 milligrams of Valium, which may explain a third study, which revealed that patients who listened to music before and during surgery had less stress hormones in their blood.

898. Get Clearance from Your Doctor Before You Take Off

If you're thinking of visiting a brother in Buffalo or a sister in Sausalito after your surgery, check with your doctor before you make any airline reservations. Traveling in an aircraft too soon after surgery can cause problems, because air and gases in the body expand. Don't fly until at least three weeks after heart, lung, or gastrointestinal surgery, and wait at least two weeks after eye surgery.

899. Listen to Positive Messages

You may have a quicker recovery if you listen to positive suggestions while under anesthesia. At least that's what a group of English doctors found when they studied 39 women who were undergoing hysterectomies.

Half the women listened to blank tapes during the operation, while the other half heard tapes with positive messages that suggested, "You will not feel sick. You will not feel pain. The operation seems to be going well. How quickly you recover from your operation depends on you. The more you relax, the more comfortable you will be."

The results? Women who heard the positive messages spent less time in the hospital, had fewer days of postoperative fever, and were less likely to have problems with gas, diarrhea, or constipation than women who heard the blank tape. Women who heard the positive messages were also rated as having a better-than-normal recovery by nurses who didn't know which tape the patients had heard.

The researchers speculated that the tape may have reduced anxiety by obscuring operating room conversation and noise. Or, they say, the odd state of awareness sometimes experienced during anesthesia may make people more open to suggestion, just as they'd be while under hypnosis.

900. Walk through Recovery

"Most of the time, recovery from surgery is a four- to eight-week process," says D. W. Edington, Ph.D., director of the University of Michigan Fitness Research Center.

But walking will put you on the right track. It's the perfect choice for recovering patients, says Dr. Edington. "They get a general improvement in body tone, in aerobic health, and in overall body function, without stressing the body too much."

Get moving as soon as your doctor liberates you from all the IVs and catheters. And keep moving after you get home. Strive toward gentle walking for 20 minute stretches, three to four times a week, suggests Robert Goldszer, M.D., an assistant professor of medicine at Harvard Medical School. Easy bicycling and swimming will also put your body on the road to recovery.

INDEX

Boldface references indicate tables.

Rodale Press, Inc., publishes PREVENTION, America's leading health magazine.
For information on how to order your subscription,
write to PREVENTION, Emmaus, PA 18098.